Medical Immunology
Text and Review

———◆———

Medical Immunology
Text and Review

◆

James T. Barrett, Ph.D.
Professor
Department of Molecular Microbiology and Immunology
University of Missouri-Columbia
Columbia, Missouri

F. A. DAVIS COMPANY • Philadelphia

Printed in the United States of America

Last digit indicates print number: 10 9 8 7 6 5 4 3 2 1

NOTE: As new scientific information becomes available through basic and clinical research, recommended treatments and drug therapies undergo changes. The author and publisher have done everything possible to make this book accurate, up-to-date, and in accord with accepted standards at the time of publication. The author, editors, and publisher are not responsible for errors or omissions or for consequences from application of the book, and make no warranty, expressed or implied, in regard to the contents of the book. Any practice described in this book should be applied by the reader in accordance with professional standards of care used in regard to the unique circumstances that may apply in each situation. The reader is advised always to check product information (package inserts) for changes and new information regarding dose and contraindications before administering any drug. Caution is especially urged when using new or infrequently ordered drugs.

Library of Congress Cataloging-in-Publication Data

Barrett, James T., 1927–
  Medical immunology : text and review / James T. Barrett.
    p.   cm.
  Includes bibliographical references and index.
  ISBN 0-8036-0664-8 (alk. paper)
  1. Clinical immunology.   2. Immunology.   I. Title.
  [DNLM: 1. Allergy and Immunology.   2. Immunity.   QW 504 B274m]
RC582.B377   1991
616.07′9--dc20
DNLM/DLC
for Library of Congress   91-16140

Preface

◆

A recent survey of a national organization of physicians indicated they agreed quite closely on what aspects of infectious disease should be presented to students. Topics such as venereal disease, bacterial meningitis, tuberculosis, antibiotic resistance, and others were all considered essential in biomedical curricula, but a similar inquiry about key subjects in immunology resulted in a mixed response. Some practitioners thought a full discussion of blood grouping was very important; others thought it of marginal value. Mixed opinions were also seen in responses seeking the value of tumor immunology, lymphocyte populations, phagocytosis, asthma, and so forth, in the curriculum.

One explanation for this dichotomy is that physicians in all areas of infectious disease are presented with very similar problems regardless of their specialty. The micro-organisms involved, their epidemiology, their virulence, their potential for antibiotic resistance, do not change radically from one area of medicine to another.

This consistency is not seen in immunology. Although transplant and tumor immunologists may confront similar problems, their problems are quite different from those encountered by allergists, pediatricians, gynecologists, and others. Thus immunology is, in this sense, a broader subject than microbiology. Its emphasis varies markedly from one specialty area to another.

All this goes to say that this is a book in basic immunology, a text that cannot include every immunologic detail for the wide audience of immunologists. What this text does offer is a general, basic background in the major areas of immunology, current in its factual content, and presented in an organized and readable style with many figures and tables throughout.

But, more than that, it contains a section of sixteen color plates and virtually every chapter has a case study in which an immunomedical situation is presented, queried, and discussed. Each chapter has a glossary and a set of review questions, with a final examination at the end of Chapter 14. Annotated answers are included for every question including those in the final examination section. These self-review aids will be useful in evaluating each reader's information base for his or her own interest or in preparation for national exams.

Authors probably receive undue credit for their work; in fact, many hours of labor from Karen Ehlert, Nyla Snyder, Jeanne Toma, Brad Cowan, and others at the Manning Company, and from Elaine Ewing and others at F. A. Davis Company were necessary to make the text what it is. I thank them all.

James T. Barrett

Contents

◆

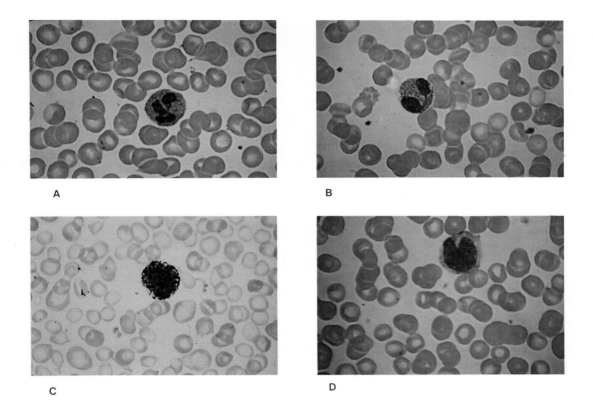

A

B

C

D

Figure 2–2. The separate panels in this figure show the appearance of *(A)* a polymorphonuclear neutrophilic leukocyte, *(B)* an eosinophil, *(C)* a basophil, and *(D)* a monocyte in stained preparations of human blood.

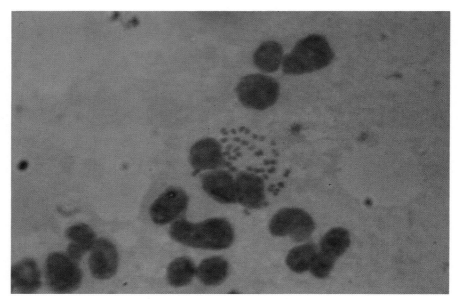

Figure 2-5

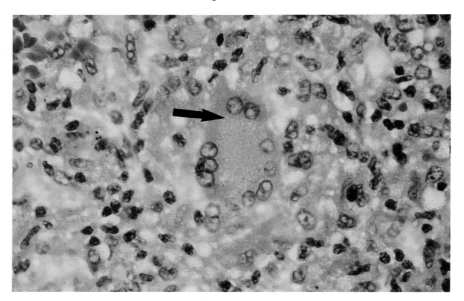

Figure 2-7

Figure 2-5. A neutrophil is shown phagocytizing bacteria. Because of the acid condition of the preparation, the phagocytes are stained atypically.

Figure 2-7. The large structure in the center is a multinucleated giant cell.

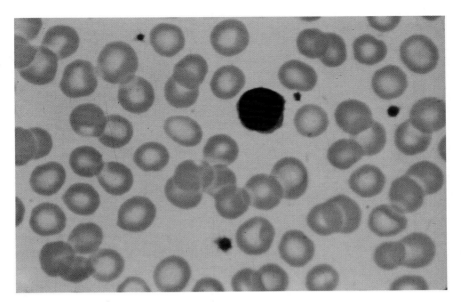

Figure 3-1

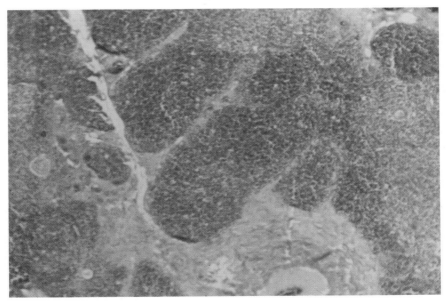

Figure 3-2

Figure 3-1. The central dark staining cell is a typical lymphocyte displaying its scant cytoplasm and large nucleus.

Figure 3-2. Notice the many lobes that house the lymphocytes in the thymus.

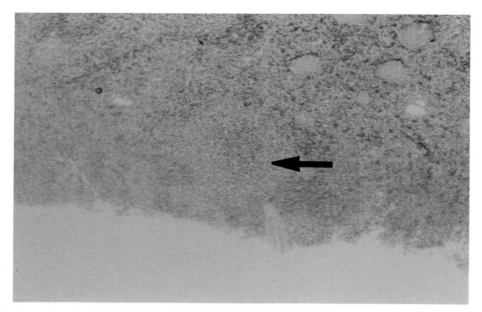

Figure 3–3

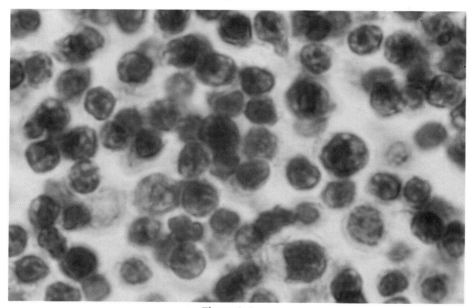

Figure 4–1

Figure 3–3. This preparation from a human spleen reveals a cluster of lymphocytes in a spherical structure known as a germinal center.

Figure 4–1. In the thymus, a dense population of lymphocytes—largely T cells—is detectable in tissue specimens.

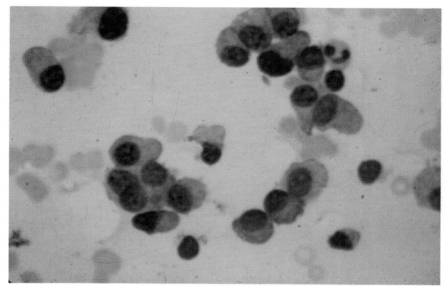

Figure 5-7

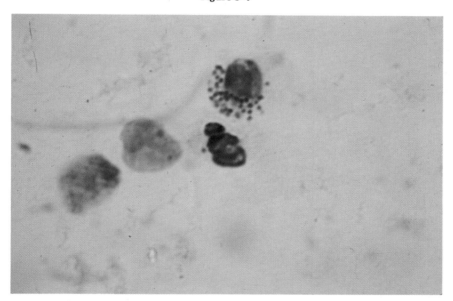

Figure 7-2

Figure 5-7. This cluster of malignant plasma cells is typical of those seen in malignant myeloma.

Figure 7-2. This phagocyte (upper center) has engulfed numerous bacteria.

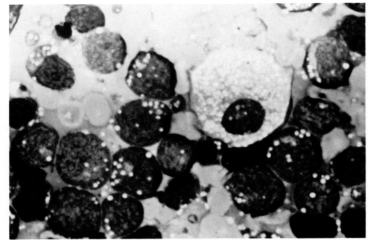

Figure 10-1

Figure 10-1. The smaller, dark-staining cells are typical of Burkitt's lymphoma and are of B-cell lineage.

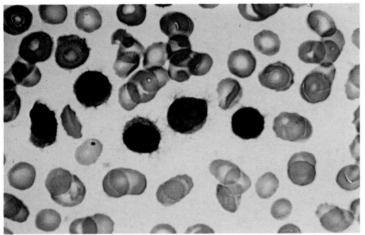

Figure 10-4

Figure 10-4. Hairy-cell leukemia was so named because the malignant B cells had fine hairlike protrusions, which are barely visible in this photograph.

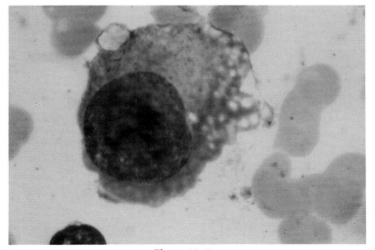

Figure 10-5

Figure 10-5. This abnormal B cell (plasma cell) was seen in a blood smear of a patient with malignant myeloma.

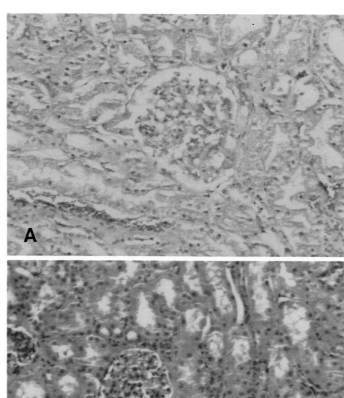

Figure 11-4 A and B. A normal kidney is seen in *(A)*, and the congested kidney of a patient with poststreptococcal glomerulonephritis in *(B)*.

A

B

Figure 11-4 A and B

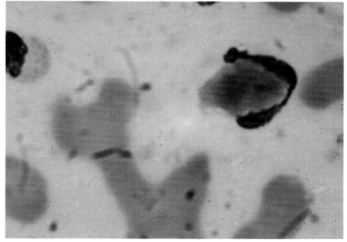

Figure 11-5. This photograph shows an LE cell, a phagocytic cell that has ingested the damaged nucleus of another cell.

Figure 11-5

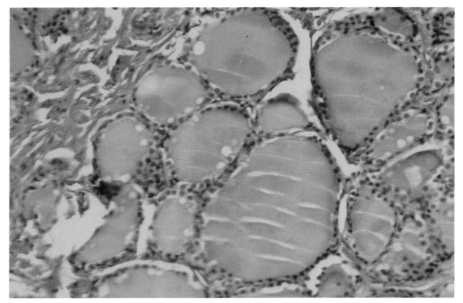

Figure 11-6

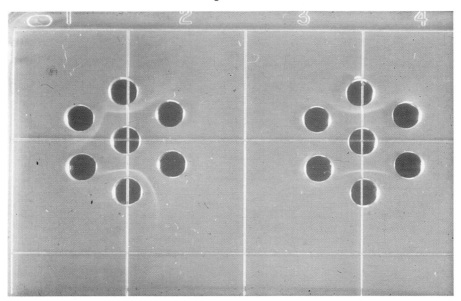

Figure 14-9

Figure 11-6. Normal thyroid as shown here has stored protein (colloid) in the acellular space. In thyroiditis the quantity of colloid is decreased and mononuclear cells infiltrate the area.

Figure 14-9. These immunodiffusion plates contain antibody to hepatitis B virus in the center well and patient sera in the outer wells. The presence of a precipitate is evidence of a hepatitis virus in the patient's specimen.

Introduction: Synopsis of Immunology

In the past century, immunology has broadened its original base in the areas of immunity and infectious disease to include those of chemistry, genetics, molecular biology, medicine, and surgery. The expanding interest and knowledge about immunology has been so great that a special jargon has emerged. Old terms are being used in new ways, and new terms are being originated. Unfortunately this has resulted in duplicate definitions and vague or imprecise descriptions. Normally the vocabulary for a science develops gradually as knowledge of the science itself grows, but whenever uncertainty exists, reference to a dictionary or glossary becomes inevitable. Such a glossary is found at the end of each chapter in this book. Although it might be possible to memorize a brief glossary, a better appreciation of the manner in which immunologic terms are used may be conceived from a condensed introductory sketch of immunology.

Immunology is so interlaced with itself that it is often difficult to decide where to begin. For example, to explain how vaccines (antigens) stimulate the antibody response, it is necessary to describe the cells that act on the vaccine. However, these cells use antibody to capture the vaccine. Should one begin by describing the antigens, the cells, or the antibodies? It is just

this problem that has dictated the need for this synopsis. Here, part of the vocabulary of immunology is introduced with a quick appraisal of how the parts of the immune response interact with each other. In the early chapters that follow, the details of the system are described. In later chapters, the application of this information to several facets of medicine, allergy, immunity, immunodeficiency, and the like, are presented.

The Immune Pathway

Immunology is dynamic in the sense that it analyzes the body's response to foreign substances. The first foreign substances that come to mind are bacteria, viruses, or other infectious agents that the immunologist calls **antigens**. These cells are composed of many antigenic molecules, but individual proteins and polysaccharides may be antigenic too. The body can also respond to many nonantigenic substances called **haptens** but only when these are linked to antigens in hapten-antigen conjugates. Haptens are customarily of lower molecular weight and are simpler structures than antigens. Thus, the animal body has evolved a method of reacting to simple molecules as well as to those that are complex. This response can be magnified if the antigen is presented to the animal with an **adjuvant.**

Adjuvants improve the immune response ("immune response" is the term used, even though the antigen or hapten may have no connection with an infectious agent). Tissue **macrophages,** a type of **phagocyte,** engulf and partially degrade the antigen, passing on **antigenic determinants** (epitopes) to **B** and **T lymphocytes.** The macrophage can capture antigen by random phagocytosis or via the assistance of antibody on its surface that reacts with a specific antigen.

The epitope is held on the macrophage surface by a **DP, DQ,** or **DR** protein that will react only with that epitope. These proteins are products of **immune response (Ir) genes** that are a part of the **major histocompatibility complex (MHC).** It will be necessary to discuss the MHC in detail later in this chapter.

B lymphocytes receive antigen from the macrophage via an immunoglobulin (antibody) on its surface. This antibody is limited to reaction with this single epitope that the macrophage is offering. B lymphocytes are so named because in birds they pass through and are altered by a cloacal gland called the **bursa of Fabricius.** Humans do not have a bursa but possess cells with the same properties as B cells. After leaving the bursa, the B cell is patterned to respond to antigen and to stimuli from **T lymphocytes** by a reproductive burst that terminates in the **plasma cell.** Although the B cell has antibody on its surface, it does not secrete antibody until it becomes a plasma cell. The antibodies are found in the gamma globulin fraction of the blood. Several structural variations of these antibodies are synthesized, each by a different line of B cells. *The five major classes (isotypes) of antibody are IgG, IgM, IgA, IgD, and IgE,* "Ig" being the abbreviation for immunoglobulin. Various subclasses of these antibodies are also produced.

Some antigens do not stimulate an immune response unless they also activate T lymphocytes. These are the **T-dependent antigens.** T cells are influenced by the thymus; hence the designation "T." Like B cells, they receive antigenic determinants from the macrophage's DP, DQ, or DR protein. The T-cell protein that accepts the antigen is called the **T-cell receptor (TCR).** Simultaneous with antigen presentation the macrophage secretes a hormonelike protein called a **monokine.** This monokine, **interleukin 1 (IL-1),** stimulates the T cell to respond to the antigen. This first reacting T cell is called a **helper T (T_H) cell** because it helps the B cell to become a plasma cell. The T_H cell also assists other T cells in their response to antigen. The other T-cell subclasses include the **suppressor T cell (T_S),** the **delayed-type hypersensitivity T cell (T_{DTH}),** and the **cytotoxic T lymphocyte (CTL or T_C).** All of these cells receive the growth factor, **interleukin 2 (IL-2),** from the T_H cell. The T_H cell also secretes other interleukins that influence B and T cells.

A brief aside is needed to clarify some of these new terms. A **monokine** is a protein produced by monocytes that encourages a kinetic response in another cell. A **lymphokine** is similar except that its source is a lymphocyte. These fall under the broader title of **cytokines.** Moreover, because cytokines often act on other white blood cells (leukocytes), they are also known as interleukins.

As just mentioned, the T_H cell *helps the antibody response* via the B cell. *The T_S cell restrains this response so that the antibody response does not dominate the metabolism of the individual. The T_C cell is important in halting viral and other intracellular agents by killing the cells they invade. The T_{DTH} cell is responsible for aspects of allergy.* The participation of these T cells in the immune response is the basis for the term **cell-mediated immunity**, as opposed to **humoral (blood) or antibody–based immunity** controlled by B cells.

Another aspect of humoral immunity involves the **complement system**, a collection of blood proteins that react with antibody although there is also a nonantibody alternative method for activation of these proteins. *Complement proteins aid phagocytosis when they behave as opsonins. They cooperate with IgG and IgM to lyse some infectious agents.* Complement-derived peptides, *the anaphylatoxins, participate in the inflammatory response* by creating edema. Three of the complement proteins are determined by genes in the MHC, and now it is time to examine some of the details of the MHC since proteins controlled by the MHC regulate the immune response.

The Major Histocompatibility Complex

The genes of the human MHC are situated on chromosome 6. One set of these genes, **the HLA-A, HLA-B, and HLA-C** genes, regulates transplant rejection or acceptance through the *class I MHC proteins.* This is the basis for the designation of genes on this chromosome as part of the major histocompatibility complex. The early description of these histocompatibility proteins as human leukocyte antigens accounts for their designation as HLA proteins. ⟨H L A⟩

A second set of genes on this same chromosome regulates the immune response capability of an individual. These are the immune response (Ir) genes, which determine the structure of the *class II proteins, products of the human DP, DQ, and DR genes.*

The third set of genes regulates the structure of the *class III proteins,* three proteins of the complement system (Fig. I–1).

THE CLASS I GENES AND PROTEINS

Each of the class I genes is polymorphic. Currently 15 specificities have been assigned to the A locus and 21 to the B locus. In addition, 9 probable A and 30 probable B genes designated "A workshop" (Aw) or "B workshop" (Bw) are expected to have a definite assignment to the A and B genes in the future. Assignment of the C genes is insecure; 11 are designated "Cw" with no definite C genes yet assigned.

These HLA genes are codominant, allelic genes, inherited and expressed so

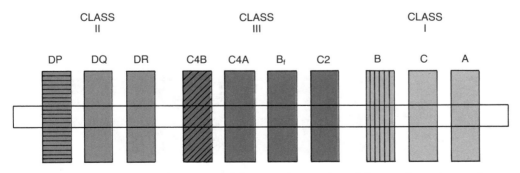

Figure I–1. The human major histocompatibility complex consists of three major regions on human chromosome 6. The class I genes dictate the structure of the transplantation (histocompatibility) antigens. The class II genes are immune response genes. The class III genes relate to complement molecules. The genes for tumor necrosis factors α and β are not included among the class III genes.

that each person has *two proteins from each of HLA-A, B, and C genes* on virtually all nucleated cells. Each of these proteins is *approximately 45,000 Mr* relative mass and can be described in terms of its five domains. The extracytoplasmic portion of the protein consists of approximately 270 amino acids and is divisible into the $\alpha 1$, $\alpha 2$, and $\alpha 3$ domains. These three domains house about 90 amino acids each. Disulfide bonding and the β pleated sheet alignment in two of these domains resemble those seen in immunoglobulins and several other proteins described as the **immunoglobulin supergene family.** These three extracellular domains are followed by a transmembrane section of about 40 amino acids and a cytoplasmic region of about 30 amino acids. Of these approximately 345 amino acids, the amino acid sequence of the $\alpha 1$ and $\alpha 2$ domains is the most varied when different HLA proteins are compared. It is this region that behaves as a foreign antigen that prompts an immune response in T_H and T_C cells when tissue is grafted into a nonidentical recipient. The class I proteins are the major proteins that regulate graft rejection.

The **$\beta 2$ microglobulin** (12,500 Mr) is always noncovalently associated with the class I protein. All samples of this protein are sequence invariant, thereby eliminating any influence of this protein on transplant success or failure. Both the $\beta 2$ microglobulin and the HLA proteins have internal disulfide bonds and a mixed α helix–β plate structure first emphasized as a constant part of the *immunoglobulin supergene family.* These proteins are not genetically related, however.

THE CLASS II GENES AND PROTEINS

The human DP, DQ, and DR class II immune response genes are separated from the class I genes by the interposition of the class III genes. Each member of this D-gene triad encodes a two-peptide protein. *Each D protein has an α and a β peptide of essentially the same size.* The DP gene contains two α peptide and two β peptide subgenes. This is also true of the DQ gene, except the first α-β gene set is now being segregated and may be accepted as a separate DX gene. The DR gene has four subgenes for the β peptide and one for the α peptide. Considerable variation in the DR gene product is possible because the α peptide can be matched with any of four β peptides. The total number of DP, DQ, and DR specificities is not entirely known. Currently 6 DPw, 9 DQw, and 13 DRw have been agreed upon but, as the "w" indicates, these assignments are not yet final (Fig. I–2).

The α and β chains of the D proteins

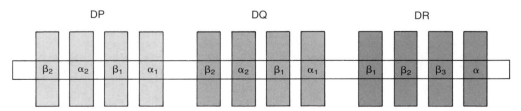

Figure I–2. This fine detail of the immune response reveals that the DR locus differs from the DP and DQ loci by having only a single α sublocus to be used with one of the three β subloci chosen.

are similar in size at approximately 30,000 Mr. The α and β chains have two extracellular domains of about 90 amino acids, an intramembrane sequence of about 30 amino acids, and a cell anchor of 10 to 15 amino acids. In the β chain both of the extracellular domains are disulfide bonded and are similar in structure to β chain fellow members in the immunoglobulin supergene family. The outermost domain of the β chain is the sector with the greatest amino acid sequence variability and that which provides epitope specificity. The α chain has little direct influence on antigen recognition. Only the innermost of the two extracellular domains of the α chain is disulfide bonded, but it, like the β chain, is an immunoglobulin supergene protein.

Although class I proteins are present on most nucleated cells, *the class II protein distribution is largely limited to antigen-presenting cells* (ie, macrophages, **dendritic cells, Langerhans' cells,** B cells). Both the class I and class II proteins are important in cell-to-cell interactions. For example, T_H cells react with MHC class II proteins on self-antigen–presenting cells, T_C cells interact with class I proteins on altered or foreign cells, and T_{DTH} cells react with class II and T_S cells with class I proteins.

THE CLASS III GENES AND PROTEINS

The complement-determining genes for the C2, C4, and factor B proteins, though important to the interaction of the complement proteins with one another, do not participate as directly in immune functions as do the C3 and C5 proteins. More details of the complement system are presented in Chapter 6. Tumor necrosis factors α and β are also class III molecules.

IMMUNOLOGIC REACTIONS

The union of an antigen with its antibody with or without the participation of complement is the subject of serology. When the antigen is soluble, the reaction is a **precipitation reaction.** Serologic precipitates can also form when the reagents diffuse through gels and combine with each other. There are many variations to such **immunodiffusion tests**—radial immunodiffusion, double diffusion of the Ouchterlony type, immunoelectrophoresis, crossed immunoelectrophoresis, counterimmunoelectrophoresis, and so forth.

When the antigen is cellular or particulate, the serologic reaction is **agglutination** or, in the case of erythrocyte antigens, hemagglutination. Fluid antigens can be adsorbed to cells to convert precipitation tests to **passive agglutination tests.** When complement proteins are present, they become bound into the serologic reaction (**complement fixation**), and this may be measured as a cytolytic reaction (bacteriolysis or hemolysis). When phagocytic cells are present, the serologic reaction may favor **phagocytosis** of the antigen because antibody and complement are both opsonins. Occasionally no outward sign of an antigen- or hapten-antibody reaction may be noted. This situation may demand the use of **fluorescent antibody procedures, radioimmunoassay (RIA), enzyme-linked immunosorbent assay (ELISA), or antiglobulin (double antibody) techniques.**

The result of in vivo immunologic reactions that destroy or resist foreign cells or their products is immunity. This explains the origin of the terms *transplantation immunity,* and *tumor immunity,* because tumors usually have a new set of antigens that makes them foreign. Foreign cells present many new antigens to the graft recipient. When the immune response is directed against self-antigens, an autoimmune disease may result. This may take the form of an antibody-mediated disease such as myasthenia gravis or may be associated with misdirected T-cell activities as in postinfectious encephalomyelitis.

Diseases that result from immune responses to external antigens are usually labeled **allergies,** or **hypersensitivities.** One class of allergy relies on the attachment of IgE to the surface of mast cells. Combination of this IgE with antigen initiates **mast cell degranulation** with the liberation of vasoactive amines such as **histamine.** Other pharmacologically active substances are released that contract smooth muscle (**leukotrienes**) or that influence the activity of platelets (**platelet-activating factor**) and eosinophils (**eosinophil chemotactic factors**). Antihistamines and β-adrenergic drugs such as adrenalin modify these toxic reactions. In their milder forms, these reactions are associated with the **atopic illnesses, hay fever** (or other **respiratory allergies**), and **food allergies.** In their more severe form, these are seen as life-threatening **anaphylactic reactions.**

T-cell activities may also be expressed as allergies. **Contact dermatitis** including reactions to cosmetics, dyes, animal products, and poison ivy, share T-cell activities that are seen in the **tuberculin reaction,** a form of delayed-type hypersensitivity.

From this compact overview of immunology it is apparent that the expanse of immunology is enormous. The antigens that activate immunocytes are covered in Chapter 1. This is followed by a consideration of the macrophages and lymphocytes in Chapters 2, 3, and 4. Products of these cells are discussed in all these chapters, with Chapter 5 being devoted to the immunoglobulins. Complement is described in Chapter 6. Thereafter, separate chapters will fill in the details of B and T-cell–mediated immunity (Chapter 7), immunodeficiency (Chapter 8), transplant and tumor immunity (Chapters 9 and 10), and autoimmunity (Chapter 11). The allergies and diagnostic serology are described in the final three chapters.

CHAPTER 1

◆

Antigens and Haptens

Immunology is one of the fastest-growing biologic sciences. A century ago immunology was no more than the study of immunity. This early focus on immunity included the nature of vaccines, the use of immune sera in therapy, and some aspects of the serologic diagnosis of disease. By midcentury, several events began to reshape immunology: The ABO and Rh blood groups were discovered, allergy was recognized as a new subdivision, and the chemical nature of vaccines (antigens) fell under intensive study. Soon the chemical nature of antibodies (immunoglobulins), the discovery of autoimmune and immunodeficiency diseases, new adventures in transplantation, and studies of the cellular basis of the immune response expanded both the immunochemical and immunocellular aspects of immunology. Within the past few decades, immunology has moved into many new areas—embryology, biochemistry, molecular biology, genetics, cell physiology, cancer, and radioisotopic and enzyme immunochemistry. Because of the borderless nature of modern science, a knowledge of immunology is useful in the study of many biologic sciences.

In these early chapters, the nature and progress of antigens through the antigen-processing cells to their contact with the B and T lymphocytes is described as it ultimately leads to the

7

secretion of the immunoglobulins. In this chapter, only the first stage of this process is considered, that of antigens and haptens. Here the chemical and physical nature of these substances is presented against the host background —the immune response genes and T-cell response—that permits the immune response to occur. Thus, the size, chemical complexity, foreign nature, and ability to catalyze only B cells or both T and B cells precede a glimpse of haptens as a useful sequence in describing antigens, class 1 and class 2 T-cell–independent antigens, and epitopes and agretopes.

Antigens

The resistance we develop from contracting an infectious disease or from an injection of a vaccine depends upon what immunologists call the immune response. This is an immune response specific to molecules in the vaccines known as antigens. Antigens as the stimuli of immunity are the major subject discussed in this chapter.

FUNCTIONAL DEFINITION OF ANTIGENS

Antigens are substances that catalyze lymphocytes to proliferate and to secrete their unique metabolic end-products. As will be described in Chapters 3 and 4, there are two major classes of lymphocytes. *The B lymphocytes produce antibodies and the T lymphocytes secrete interleukins, also called lymphokines.* Collectively, these B- and T-cell activities dominate the antigen-specific phase of the immune response.

The term **antigen** is often used as a synonym for **immunogen,** yet it has a broader meaning than the latter. Liter-

ally, "antigen" means antigenerator, which we know to be principally antibody. "Immunogen" means immune generator. Immunogens generate immunity, but because antibodies are an important component of our immunity, antigens are also immunogens. By far the largest number of antigens have nothing to do with immunity, and "immunogen" should not be substituted for "antigen" in these cases. In the following chapters, antigen will be used almost exclusively.

CHEMICAL DEFINITION OF ANTIGENS

The separation of the active and inactive components of complex vaccines such as bacterial cells, viral particles, or complex mixtures of molecules eventually permitted description of antigens in chemical terms. The three major chemical attributes of antigens are their large size, internal complexity, and degradability by enzymes contained in phagocytes (Table 1–1).

Large Size

The size threshold that separates antigens from nonantigens is inexact because several other characteristics also regulate antigenicity. *Most antigens are molecules of 10,000 Mr or greater.* In general, the larger a molecule, the easier it is to demonstrate its antigenicity. Nevertheless, several molecules less than 10,000 Mr are proven antigens. Insulin (5700 Mr), histones (6000 Mr), and several low molecular weight polymers of amino acids are antigenic, though much weaker than serum albumin (45,000 Mr), tetanus toxoid (55,000 Mr), and thyroglobulin (669,000 Mr).

Table 1-1
IMPORTANT FEATURES OF ANTIGENS

Feature	Comments
Size	Usually larger than 10,000 Mr, with exceptions
Complexity	Must contain amino acid or monosaccharide sequence variation
Stability in vivo	Must be degradable by phagocytic cells
Relationship to host	Must come from nonidentical genetic source; ie, must be foreign
Responding cells	Usually both B and T lymphocytes
Genetics of response	Controlled by DP, DQ, and DR immune response (Ir) genes

Internal Complexity

Certain large molecules are not antigens. One cause of this is that the molecule, in spite of its size, has no structural complexity. Chemists can synthesize long linear polymers containing only lysine or styrene, for example. Neither polylysine nor polystyrene is an antigen. Each of these polymers consists of a simple unit structure repeated indefinitely, which confers little complexity on these molecules.

In contrast, most antigenic proteins are composed of 20 different amino acids. These are assorted in irregular sequences characteristic for that protein. Likewise, oligosaccharides are constructed from a selection of several monosaccharides, and many complex sugars are antigenic. Because of cross-linking in proteins and polysaccharides, an additional level of molecular complexity is added in the form of their three-dimensional structure. Assembly of these macromolecules into quaternary structures adds further to their structural complexity.

Degradability

Cellular or insoluble antigens must be degraded in order to release their antigenic constituents in a soluble form. Antigen digestion is also necessary for all large antigens. This function is the duty of phagocytic cells. Through a process labeled "antigen processing," *phagocytic cells preserve critical smaller fragments of macromolecular antigens.* If a molecule resists attack by the digestive enzymes in these phagocytic cells, the molecule cannot function as an antigen. For this reason, polypeptides made of D amino acids or complex plastic materials fail to meet this criterion of antigenicity despite their suitable size and internal complexity.

MEMORY CHECK 1-1

Antigens
1. Stimulate new, adaptive responses in B and T lymphocytes
2. Are usually large molecules
3. Must have chemical complexity in addition to a large size
4. Must be digestible by phagocytes

Host Control of Antigenicity

It could be argued that the degradability requirement of antigens is as much an aspect of host control as it is a chemical attribute of the antigen. However, it is antigen chemistry that permits or denies its degradability. Other features are more clearly host restrictions.

FOREIGN NATURE OF ANTIGENS

Although each person has molecules that clearly fulfill the requirements of antigenicity listed earlier, these proteins, oligosaccharides, and other molecules lack the fourth criterion of foreignness. It is not absolutely true that we treat these self-proteins as nonantigens, but it is rare that we respond to them as we do to true antigens. When blood transfusion is done we do not respond to the proteins in blood as we would were the blood from a lower animal. Human serum albumin is a nonantigen for humans, but bovine serum albumin is a potent antigen. *If a protein comes from a distinctly different genetic source than the immunized recipient, it will usually be treated as an antigen.*

IMMUNOLOGIC TOLERANCE

It is said that *the failure of an individual to respond to self-antigens is due to immunologic tolerance. This is an antigenic specific state.* Immature individuals become tolerant to self-antigens because their immune system encounters these antigens when still undeveloped. It can be shown that the injection of antigen A into a fetal animal will render it tolerant to a second exposure of antigen A in adult life, at a time when the animal will respond to other antigens (Fig. 1–1). *Both B and T lymphocytes can be tolerized*, the T lymphocytes maintaining their tolerance for a longer time and being more sensitive to low doses of antigen.

Adult tolerance can also be demonstrated. *The intravenous injection of large quantities of soluble antigens favors immune tolerance*, compared with other injection routes or antigen formulations. Tolerance is not permanent; the animals will eventually recover from the tolerant state as new nontolerized lymphocytes mature. However, administration of repeated doses of the **tolerogen** (antigen used to induce tolerance) will maintain the individual in the tolerant state. Polysaccharides are often more tolerogenic than proteins.

IMMUNE RESPONSE GENES

Even if all conditions are perfectly poised for an immune response, there invariably will be an individual who will not respond. It has been deter-

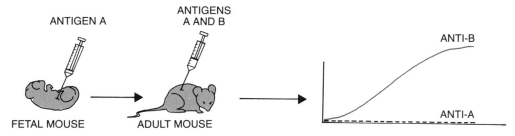

Figure 1–1. Immune tolerance is easily created by fetal exposure of an animal to an antigen. As an adult, that animal will respond to other antigens but not the one encountered in fetal life.

mined both in humans and in experimental animals that an *individual's genetic make-up also controls the immune response*. Breeding experiments in mice have shown that some strains respond to some antigens, and other strains to different antigens. This quality is inherited by ordinary mendelian transmission as a dominant trait.

These **immune response (Ir) genes** are most easily analyzed when simple antigens are used. When large, complex antigens are evaluated nearly everyone is a responder. One individual may respond to portion A of the antigen and a second individual may respond to portion B, but both are responders. As will be expanded later in this chapter, this implies that an antigenic molecule may have several distinct parts that are responsible for its antigenicity. These parts are called antigenic determinant sites, or epitopes. It is possible to identify proteins on the surface of lymphocytes that are controlled by the Ir genes. *In the human, these are the DP, DQ, and DR proteins*, the class II MHC proteins. These class II MHC proteins enable phagocytes and B lymphocytes to be recognized by T lymphocytes. Not all antigens require cooperation between two classes of lymphocytes to generate an immune response. Some antigens are T-cell dependent and others are T-cell independent.

MEMORY CHECK 1–2

Antigens

1. Must come from a genetically different source than the animal being immunized
2. May also be tolerogens
3. Cannot stimulate an immune response if the host lacks the proper immune response genes

---

T-CELL DEPENDENCY OF ANTIGENS

T lymphocytes are not required for the antibody response to all antigens. This enables a classification of antigens as either T-cell dependent (TD) or T-cell independent (TI) (Table 1–2). TD or TI refers only to T helper cells. Other T-cell subsets influence responses to both TD and TI antigens.

Table 1–2
RELATIONSHIP OF T-CELL–DEPENDENT AND
T-CELL–INDEPENDENT ANTIGENS

	T-Cell–Dependent Antigens	T-Cell–Independent Antigens
T_H cell need	Require T cells for antibody response	Do not require T_H cells
Macrophage processing	Small peptides processed from entire antigen are functional	May not require antigen processing
Chemistry	Chemically complex	Chemically simpler
Primary response	Induce full array of antibody classes	Dominated by IgM response
Secondary response	Good booster response	Feeble booster response
As tolerogen	Poor	Good
Other T cell	Influenced by all T-cell subsets	Do not require T_H cells, influenced by other T-cell subsets

T-Cell–Dependent Antigens

TD antigens are structurally more complex than TI antigens. Most proteins are TD antigens. Conjugates of proteins—nucleoproteins, glycoproteins, and lipoproteins—are also TD antigens. These antigens usually stimulate the *full array of the antibody response,* resulting in the production of IgG, IgM, IgA, and the two lesser immunoglobulins. When an animal is reexposed to a TD antigen, *very high levels of IgG are quickly achieved.* This heightened response to a second exposure to antigen is called the **anamnestic, booster, or memory response.** This memory response is important in immunity because most viruses, bacteria, and other pathogens are TD antigens.

T-Cell–Independent Antigens

Most T-cell–independent antigens are structurally simple, even if macromolecular. Among the intensely studied TI antigens are pneumococcal polysac-charide, dextran, polyvinyl pyrroli-done, and bacterial lipopolysaccharide. *IgM dominates the response to TI antigens,* and IgM does not display a memory response. Although some evidence indicates TI antigens can use T-cell help, it is of a different nature or magnitude than the T-cell contribution to the TD antigen response.

TI-1 and TI-2 Antigens

A subclassification of TI antigens developed from a study of *xid* mice. These sex-linked immunodeficient mice respond to certain TI antigens as do neonatal mice. (Normally, newborn mice are poor responders to antigens.) These have been designated TI-1 antigens. TI-2 antigens do not stimulate *xid* mice or normal mice until they are about 2 weeks old. The *xid* and immature mouse B-cell population does not have protein Lyb-3 or Lyb-5 on its surface (Lyb meaning lymphocyte). Lyb-3^-5^- mice respond to TI-1 antigens, and only when normal mice begin to develop Lyb-3^+5^+ lymphocytes are they enabled to respond to TI-2 antigens. The TI-1 response is high in IgM with some IgG subclass 2 and 3 antibodies. TI-2 antigens elicit primarily IgM and IgG subclass 3 antibodies. Pneumococcal polysaccharide and polyvinyl pyrrolidone are examples of TI-2 antigens. Bacterial lipopolysaccharide is a TI-1 antigen. Some of the TI-1 antigens are nonspecific B-cell mitogens; they stimulate mitosis in all B cells regardless of the antigen specificity of these cells.

Absolute proof of a separate human response to TI-1 and TI-2 antigens may not exist. Nevertheless, the poor response of the human infant to pneumococcal polysaccharides and to the polysaccharides in the meningococcal group B and *Haemophilus influenzae B*

MEMORY CHECK 1–3
◆

Antigens

1. Cause B cells to make antibodies

2. That require B cell–T cell interaction are called T-dependent antigens

3. Are more often T-dependent than T-independent

4. Of the TI type are simpler than TD antigens

5. Of the TI type do not stimulate a good booster response

6. Of the TI type stimulate IgM synthesis, but little of the other antibodies are formed

Table 1–3
COMPARISON OF TI-1 AND TI-2 ANTIGENS

	TI-1	TI-2
B-cell stimulation	Polyclonal, most B cells respond	Fewer B cells respond
Reactive B cell in mice	Lyb 3⁻,5⁻	Lyt 3⁺,5⁺
Response in *xid* mice	Yes	No
Antibody response	IgM, some IgG2 and IgG3	IgM, little IgG2, IgG3
Examples	Lipopolysaccharide, trinitrophenylated *Brucella* bacteria	Pneumococcal capsule, polyvinyl pyrrolidone

vaccines indicates they are behaving as type 2 TI antigens, parallel to their behavior in mice. In contrast, the human infant does respond adequately to the meningococcal group A and C vaccines, indicating that these are type 1 TI antigens (Table 1–3).

SUPERANTIGENS

A novel class of TD antigens has supported our earlier ideas of how T lymphocytes help B lymphocytes. For several years the dogma has been that a receptor protein for antigen on T cells (T-cell receptor, or TCR) held a part of the antigen while the B cell held a different part. The antigen receptor on the B cell is immunoglobulin. When antigen links the two cells through these receptors, the T cell releases hormones called either lymphokines or interleukins. These cause the B cell to differentiate and to synthesize and release antibody into the blood stream.

Superantigens do this but in a completely different way. First of all, they are not processed by phagocytes. Second, instead of fitting into internal grooves of the TCR and immune-associated protein, *superantigens bind simultaneously to the periphery of the TCR and the DP, DQ, or DR protein on the antigen-presenting cell.* This stimulates the T cell to help the B cell (Table 1–4).

A third remarkable feature of this is the manner in which superantigens fit with the TCR (Fig. 1–2). Normally the TCR is specific for and reacts with a single antigen. However, superantigens react with a large number of TCR molecules *because they combine with a*

Table 1–4
PROPERTIES OF SUPERANTIGENS

Property	Remarks
Type of lymphocyte stimulated	T_H and T_s cells, probably others
Cell population activated	Large number of T cells
Basis of T-cell activation	Combines with β chain of TCR
Needs antigen-presenting cell	Yes
Binding site on presenting cell	MHC class II protein
Examples	Staphylococcal enterotoxin, streptococcal toxins

14

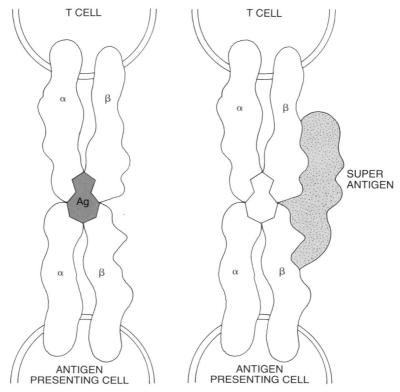

Figure 1–2. A superantigen does not link the TCR and class II proteins by fitting into the cleft between these proteins as is the situation with epitopes. Instead, superantigens link the exterior of the two proteins, usually to the β chain of the class II protein on the antigen presenting cell.

part of the TCR molecule that is identical or similar in many TCR proteins. Several superantigens are toxins; toxins of staphylococci and streptococci are examples. It is considered for-tunate that these toxins are superantigens because they engage a massive number of T cells and B cells in a protective antibody response.

Antigenic Determinant Sites

EPITOPES

Molecules that behave as antigens have discrete structures within them that are responsible for this function. This arrangement mimics that seen in enzymes that have a distinct catalytic site, except that *antigens typically have several such sites, their antigenic determinant sites or epitopes.* For low molecular weight antigens there is

Table 1-5
CHARACTERISTICS OF EPITOPES

Characteristic	Comment
Number per antigen molecule	Usually several, always two or more
Size	5 to 10 amino acids or monosaccharides
Position	May be sequential or conformational
Cell receptor	Antibody on B cells, TCR on T cells
Other functions	May behave as a tolerogen
Relationship to hapten	Hapten is a single epitope

roughly one epitope for each 10,000 Mr, a figure that does not apply to larger molecules (Table 1–5).

In proteins, *an epitope consists of about six amino acids and a similar number of monosaccharide units in antigenic oligosaccharides.* The epitope is the central participant in the reaction of an antigen with its specific antibody, although the entire combining site may encompass another 10 to 12 residues.

An epitope may consist of a **sequential or linear array** of amino acids, or a **conformational or topographic arrangement.** In nonsequential epitopes the active site is created by a folding or cross-linking of the peptide chain (Fig. 1–3).

It is difficult to predict exactly which parts of a molecule will function as its epitopes. One theory is based on the supposition that any given sequence could function as an epitope in some species, or some individual under the correct circumstance. The opposite opinion suggests that certain amino acids tend to appear more frequently in epitopes. Examples can be cited that support both views. It is well known that different species of laboratory animals respond to different epitopic regions in myelin basic protein. A recent analysis of a small peptide whose

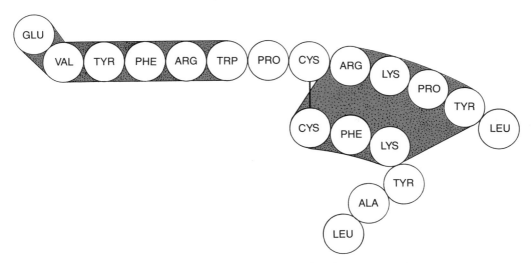

Figure 1–3. Sequential and conformational epitopes in the above peptide fragment of a protein encompass the shaded amino acid residues.

amino acid composition was varied identified phenylalanine, tyrosine, and tryptophan more frequently in epitopes than valine, leucine, or several other amino acids. The *most potent epitopes for T lymphocytes were amphipathic helices*—that is, they were highly polar on one side of the helix and apolar on the other side. Epitopes can overlap one another, and a section of amino acids can be antigenic in one strain of mice but be tolerogenic in another.

Some epitopes provoke the formation of more antibody than others and are rightly termed the immunodominant epitope or determinant of an antigen.

AGRETOPES

The epitopic zone of an antigen reacts with antibody and the TCR. *That part of the antigen that binds to the class II MHC protein is its agretope.* Superantigens bind to different sites of the TCR and DP, DQ, or DR proteins than do the epitopic and agretopic residues in regular antigens. This will undoubtedly spawn another set of descriptors.

MEMORY CHECK 1–5

◆

Facts related to epitopes and agretopes include:

1. Epitopes are the size of about six amino acids or six mono-saccharides.
2. Epitopes bind to the interior of the T-cell receptor.
3. Epitopes may be sequential or conformational.
4. Agretopes bind to the class II MHC protein of the antigen-presenting cell.

HAPTENS

Definition

Haptens are low molecular weight, nonantigenic substances by definition, but they modify existing antigens to create a new antigenic determinant site that includes the attached hapten. These antigen-hapten complexes are described as **conjugated antigens or neoantigens** and are prepared by coupling a simple chemical grouping such as the dinitrophenyl radical to an antigen (Fig. 1–4). This can be done by

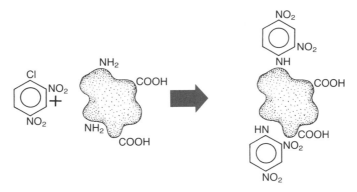

Figure 1–4. When a hapten couples to an existing antigen, it creates a new epitope.

mixing dinitrochlorobenzene with a protein. A condensation reaction occurs in which chlorine is lost from the hapten and hydrogen from the antigen as the dinitrophenyl antigen is formed. Injection of this conjugate into an animal will stimulate antibody formation against the new as well as the old determinant sites. Antibody against the haptenic portion of the conjugated antigen is demonstrable in several ways. In one scheme, a radioisotopically labeled dinitrophenol can be shown to combine with the antiserum. In the other, dinitrophenyl groupings attached to an unrelated protein can be shown to react with the antiserum. These reactions demonstrate that haptens can react with antibodies directed against them but do not themselves provoke antibody formation.

Autocoupling Haptens

It would be futile to inject dinitrobenzene into an animal with the intention of producing antibodies. However, the injection of dinitrochlorobenzene would not be futile because this compound can combine with tissue proteins and create new, partially foreign epitopes to which the animal will respond. *Haptens that spontaneously couple* with existing tissue proteins or polysaccharides are sometimes referred to as **autocoupling haptens.** Allergies to poison ivy, poison oak, and poison sumac; contact dermatitis to leather products, dyes, and cosmetics; and allergies to penicillin and other drugs develop as the result of neoantigen formation with such autocoupling haptens. It is not essential for a hapten to establish a covalent bonding with its carrier antigen; firm ionic bonding may be enough to maintain the hapten so closely associated with the antigen that it appears as a new antigenic determinant to antigen-handling cells.

MEMORY CHECK 1–6

Haptens
1. Are not antigenic
2. Create new antigenic determinants in an existing antigen
3. React with antibodies to hapten-antigen conjugates
4. May have highly reactive groups that favor self-coupling to antigens

---

Antigen Nomenclature

Many prefixes or modifiers are used to illustrate the source, use, or other properties of antigens. Antigens are often named according to their cellular or tissue origin: tumor antigen, blood group antigen, transplantation antigen, nuclear antigen, flagellar antigen, and cell surface antigen will all be encountered in later chapters of this book.

A conjugated antigen has two or more parts, one of which must be antigenic. For example, a lipoprotein in which the lipid is not antigenic but the protein is. A related term is neo-antigen—a new antigen, modified from its earlier form. If a nonantigen such as a lipid is added to an antigenic protein, the product could be labeled a neoantigen or conjugated antigen.

SPECIES ORIGIN OF ANTIGENS

A frequently used series of prefixes refers to the species origin of an antigen or antibody in relation to the species receiving the antigen or making the antibody. These prefixes also apply to the term "immunization." *An* **autoantigen** *or* **autologous antigen** *is a self-antigen;* an isologous antigen is one from the same species. **Alloantigen** *is* *also from the same species, but from a genetically different individual.* A xenoantigen is from a different species. (Because most antigens, especially those in vaccines, are from different species than the animal being immunized, xenoantigen is an unnecessary redundancy.) If an antigen is widely distributed through unrelated species, it can be described as a **heterophil or heterogeneic antigen.**

USES IN SEROLOGY

Special terms are given to antigens when they engage in serologic reactions with their antibodies. Precipitating antigen, agglutinating antigen, and so on, refer to the physical form of the serologic test. The antigen first used in immunization and then later in a reaction with antibody is the **homologous antigen.** If a different antigen is used in the serologic reaction, it is a **heterologous antigen.** Heterologous antigens are used to validate the specificity of the antibody. If the heterologous antigen reacts with the antibody it is a **cross-reactive antigen** (and the antibody is also cross-reactive). If this cross-reactive antigen is widely distributed in nature, it could be called a heterophil antigen. Antigens become cross-reactive when they share identical or similar epitopes (Fig. 1–5).

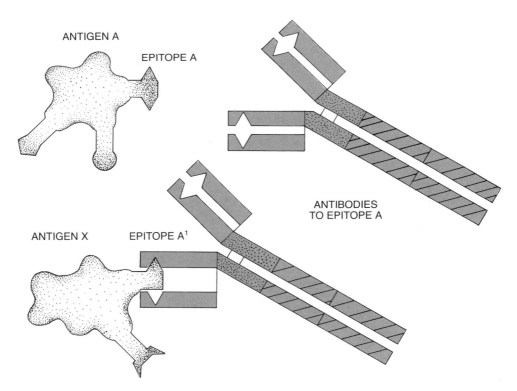

Figure 1–5. Cross-reactive antigens are structurally and/or physically similar, so that each can combine with a single antibody or single TCR molecule. Here it can be seen that an epitope on the lower antigen molecule is sufficiently similar to an epitope on the upper antigen that it will cross-react with the antibody to antigen A.

References

Atassi, MZ, (ed): Immunobiology of Proteins and Peptides. Vols 1–5. Plenum Press, New York, 1982–1989.

Berzofsky, JA: Intrinsic and extrinsic factors in antigenic structure. Science 229:932, 1985.

Coffman, RL: T-helper heterogeneity and immune response patterns. Hosp Pract 24(8):101, 1989.

Cresswell, P: Antigen recognition by T-lymphocytes. Immunology Today 8:67, 1987.

Sercarz, EE and Berzofsky, J (eds): Immunogenicity of Protein Antigens: Repertoire and Regulation. CRC Press, Boca Raton. FL, 1988.

Sercarz, EE (ed): Antigenic Determinants and Immune Regulation. Karger, Basel, 1989.

QUESTIONS AND ANSWERS

1. Epitope is synonymous with
   A. Hapten
   B. Agretope
   C. Neoantigen
   D. Antigenic determinant site
   E. Superantigen

Answer D

A hapten may be part of an epitope but is not usually the full epitope or antigenic determinant site. The agretope is that portion of an antigen that combines with the MHC class II protein. A neoantigen is a hapten-antigen pair. Superantigens combine with the TCR and DP, DQ, or DR protein but not by the usual epitope and agretope interaction with their receptors.

2. TI antigens
   A. Are usually proteins
   B. Stimulate a strong IgG response
   C. Fail to muster a memory or booster response
   D. Are not influenced by any type of T cell
   E. Bind and deactivate the TCR

Answer C

TI antigens are usually structurally simple antigens such as polysaccharides rather than proteins, and they stimulate a feeble IgG response but a good IgM response. Thus, answers A and B are both wrong and answer C is correct. TI antigens are subject to control by some T-cell subsets but are poorly regulated by T helper cells. TI antigens neither bind nor deactivate the T-cell receptor.

3. Which of the following is *not* required of antigens?
   A. Must contain a haptenic epitope
   B. Must be from a species source foreign to the animal being immunized
   C. Must be large
   D. Must be degradable by antigen-processing cells
   E. Must have structural complexity

Answer A

All the qualifications listed are required of antigens, except A. Antigens must contain epitopes, but these need not be haptenic in character; they must, however, be foreign, large, complex, and degradable.

4. An antigen
   A. Is sometimes a tolerogen
   B. Is constructed of epitopic and nonepitopic regions
   C. May contain only linear epitopes
   D. May be chemically identical or semi-identical from different species sources
   E. All of the above

Answer E

Under different circumstances a molecule may be either an antigen or a tolerogen. The number of epitopes in an antigen varies with its size, but the largest part of most antigens consists of nonepitopic sites. The epitopes may be either linear or conformational. Heterophil antigens are defined by answer D. The answer to the question is E.

5. Which of the following is an example of host control over antigenicity?
   A. The greater antigenic potency of proteins compared to polysaccharides
   B. The failure of an animal to make antibodies to its own blood proteins
   C. The ability of haptens to add new epitopes to an antigen
   D. The existence of linear and conformational epitopes in some antigens
   E. All of the above

Answer B

Proteins are normally more complex structures than polysaccharides, which is a feature of antigen chemistry, as is the ability of haptens to contribute to new epitopes. The sequential or topographic configuration of epitopes is again a matter of antigen chemistry. Only answer B exhibits host control over substances that are fully antigenic.

Case Study: Heterophil Antigen

Sara, a 20-year-old college student, consulted her physician because of a sore throat that had persisted for 4 days. She had felt feverish and had had a headache for a few days prior to the development of her sore throat. Physical examination revealed a modest bilateral enlargement of cervical lymph nodes, pharyngeal inflammation and edema, and a temperature of 38.4°C (101.2°F). Infectious mononucleosis was considered a strong possibility in the differential diagnosis when throat cultures showed normal flora, and white blood cell counts revealed a prominent lymphocytosis (68% lymphocytes). A serologic test for heterophil antibody was requested. The results were Paul-Bunnell titer 1:3584, and differential absorption by guinea pig kidney 1:1792. The serologic findings were confirmatory, and a diagnosis of infectious mononucleosis was established.

Questions

1. How is a heterophil antigen associated with infectious mononucleosis?

2. What is the Paul-Bunnell test and its interpretation?

3. Describe differential antibody absorption in infectious mononucleosis.

Discussion

Heterophil antibodies are those that react with apparently unrelated antigens of diverse sources. People receiving injections of horse serum, for example, develop antibodies that clump (agglutinate) sheep and beef red blood cells, and a small percentage of apparently healthy individuals have antibodies that will agglutinate sheep red blood cells. Forssman's antigen was originally described as an antigen on guinea pig cells, except erythrocytes, that would induce the formation of antibodies that would agglutinate sheep red blood cells. Persons with infectious mononucleosis have similar antibodies. In human medicine the term "heterophil antibody" usually refers to one that will agglutinate sheep red blood cells. Because there are several of these, they must be distinguished before they can be used to diagnose disease.

Forssman's antigen has been partially characterized. It is truly heterogeneic, being present in corn, in *Streptococcus pneumoniae*, in sheep red blood cells, and in chicken, carp, toad, tiger, whale, and horse tissues. Resistance of the antigen to heat indicates it is a polysaccharide. Because extensive purification results in a loss of antigenicity, the probability exists that Forssman's antigen is actually a hapten. Chemically, it is similar to human blood group A antigen. The heterophil antigen in horse serum and that associated with infectious mononucleosis are largely uncharacterized.

Most of the attention given to heterophil antigens has focused on their antibodies. In 1932 Paul and Bunnell discovered that the serum of patients with infectious mononucleosis would clump sheep red blood cells, and they suggested this as a diagnostic aid for the disease. The sheep cell agglutinin in normal human sera can rarely be diluted more than 1:28 and still retain activity, so elevated titers were of some aid but did not distinguish true Forssman or serum sickness agglutinins from those of mononucleosis. This came about by the use of differential absorption of these antibodies by guinea pig kidney and beef cells, known as the differential or Davidsohn differential absorption test. This test is applied to sera that have a presumptive titer (unabsorbed serum plus sheep erythrocytes) greater than 1 : 28. Guinea pig kidney removes the "serum sickness" antibody but removes none (or only very little) of that associated with mononucleosis. Bovine erythrocytes remove the serum sickness antibody and most of the infectious mononucleosis and Forssman antibody.

Heterophil titers in infectious mononucleosis have reached 1 : 14,336, but figures between 1 : 28 and 1 : 3584 are more typical. After the third week of the disease, 100% of all patients have a titer of at least 1 : 14 after guinea pig kidney absorption. This is an increase from 76% in the first week. Forssman antibody titers range up to 1 : 112 and are deleted by kidney absorption. Serum sickness titers range between 1 : 56 and 1 : 224 and are largely eliminated by absorption.

GLOSSARY

---

agretope   That part of an antigen that binds to class II MHC proteins on the antigen-presenting cell.

alloantigen   An antigen present in another member of one's own species.

antigen   A macromolecule that will induce the formation of immunoglobulins or sensitized cells that react specifically with the antigen.

antigen determinant sites   Unique portions of the structure of the antigen that are responsible for its activity.

autoantigen   A molecule that behaves as a self-antigen.

autocoupling hapten   One that can combine spontaneously with a carrier.

conjugated antigen   An antigen covalently joined to a hapten.

cross-reactive antigen   An antigen so structurally similar to a second antigen that it will react with antibody to the second antigen.

epitope   An antigenic determinant.

hapten   A nonantigenic material that, when combined with an antigen, conveys a new antigenic specificity to the antigen.

heterophil antigen   An antigen that is broadly distributed in nature.

immunodominant region   The most potent epitope in an antigen.

immunogen   Antigen.

immunologic tolerance   A failure of or depression in the immune response on proper exposure to antigen.

isoantigen   An antigen present in another member of one's own species.

neoantigen   An antigen with a specificity altered by addition of a hapten.

superantigen   An antigen that binds to the MHC class II protein and receptor protein on many T cells.

T-cell–dependent antigen   An antigen that requires T and B cell cooperation to induce specific antibody formation.

T-cell–independent antigen   An antigen that does not require that T cells assist B cells in the production of its specific antibody.

tolerance   Failure to respond to an antigen.

tolerogen   An immunogen used under circumstances that produce tolerance rather than immunity.

CHAPTER 2

◆

Macrophages and Their Response to Antigen

In this chapter, two major subgroups of phagocytic cells are considered: the macrophages ("big eaters") and the granulocytes (granulated cells). Even though the phagocytic destruction of pathogenic microbes justifies an extensive discussion of these cells, the macrophages share with a few other cells several other important steps in the immune response. These include a phase of macrophage activity termed **antigen processing**, followed by **antigen presentation**. Macrophages contribute additionally to the immune response through the secretion of interleukin 1, interleukin 6, tumor necrosis factor, and a large number of other bioactive molecules. The multiple roles of macrophages in the early aspects of the immune response are the basis for their description in an early chapter of this book.

Also discussed in this chapter are the colony-stimulating factors—a series of hormones that is essential in the maturation of these phagocytes and other cells. The expression of specific cell surface markers on macrophages is useful in distinguishing them from other phagocytic and antigen-processing cells. Among the latter included in this chapter are dendritic cells, Langerhans' cells, and B cells. Considera-

25

tion of these cells is delayed until the destructive attack of phagocytes on their targets through their oxygen-independent and oxygen-dependent pathways is described.

The Hematopoietic System

In the strictest sense, hematopoiesis means the development or production of blood cells. Until about the second month of fetal development, the yolk sac is the chief hematopoietic organ, after which it is superseded by the liver and to a lesser extent by the spleen. The liver continues to contribute to the development of blood cells until birth. The bone marrow, which will be the only significant hematopoietic tissue after birth, begins to function by the fourth month of intrauterine development. It gradually replaces hematopoiesis by the liver over the succeeding months.

BONE MARROW

The average adult has about 3 kg (1.5 to 4 kg) of bone marrow, which is the largest organ of the body, surpassing the liver in both weight and volume. About half of the bone marrow is hematopoietically active. The marrow completely fills the shaft of the long bones and is divisible into two distinct halves—the white (or yellow) marrow and the red marrow. The white marrow consists chiefly of fat cells and tends to be more centrally placed. The red marrow, located more toward the perimeter, is the source of the blood cells. In the red marrow precursors to erythrocytes are blended together with stem cells of the lymphocytes, granulocytes, and monocytes.

COLONY-STIMULATING FACTORS

The leukocytes of the blood are derived from undifferentiated stem cells of the bone marrow. **Colony-stimulating factor (CSF)** products from macrophages, fibroblasts, T lymphocytes, and other cells are required for differentiation and maturation of these cells to form the major blood lines (Fig. 2–1). The activity of these products was first observed in cell cultures. A rather unusual method to demonstrate the activity of CSF was to detect the growth of cells in the spleen of lethally irradiated animals that were injected with stem cells from bone marrow. The CSF proteins induce the growth of different cell lines depending upon their specificity (Table 2–1). *The CSF for macrophages is M-CSF, for granulocytes G-CSF, and for both macrophages and granulocytes GM-CSF; one product is known as a multi-CSF, which is a synonym for interleukin 3.* Except for G-CSF, these growth factors originate from human chromosome 5.

M-CSF

M-CSF behaves as a dimer, and in some circumstances as a polymer, a fact that has confused molecular weight determinations. Calculation of the molecular weight of M-CSF from its DNA suggests a protein of 84,000 Mr, but its size appears to be nearer to 77,000 Mr. Fibroblasts, macrophages, and other cells elaborate M-CSF. *Aside from stimulating the maturation of monocytes, M-CSF stimulates macrophage secretion of numerous products and enhances macrophage killing.*

G-CSF

G-CSF is a 19,500-Mr glycoprotein secreted by activated fibroblasts, kera-

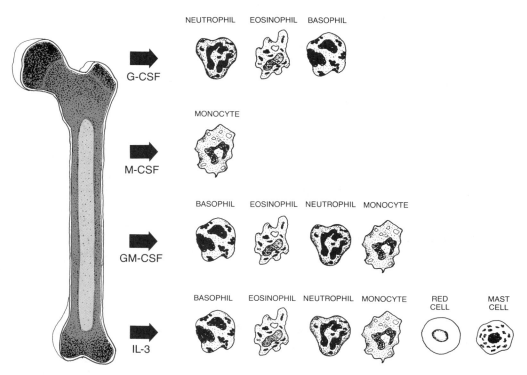

Figure 2–1. Specific colony-stimulating factors (CSF) accelerate the maturation of separate cell lines from stem cells in bone marrow. Granulocyte (G)– and monocyte (M)–stimulating activities are present in individual molecules and are combined in a second molecule. IL-3 is also known as multi-CSF because it stimulates maturation of the six cell lines indicated in the figure.

Table 2–1
HUMAN COLONY-STIMULATING FACTORS

Factor	Source	Target Cells	Chromosome Origin	Mr
M-CSF	Macrophages Fibroblasts Epithelial cells	Macrophages	5	76,000
G-CSF	Fibroblasts Ketatinocytes	Granulocytes	17	19,500
GM-CSF	T lymphocytes Macrophages Fibroblasts Endothelial cells	Granulocytes Macrophages T lymphocytes	5	22,000
IL-3 (Multi-CSF)	T lymphocytes	Progenitors to granulocytes, macrophages, erythrocytes, and mast cells	5	23,000

tinocytes, and endothelial cells. Its origin is chromosome 17. *G-CSF increases the number of all three types of circulating granulocytes.* The neutrophils and eosinophils are both cytocidal. The basophils have little phagocytic capacity.

GM-CSF

GM-CSF is produced by activated T cells, fibroblasts, endothelial cells, and even macrophages. This 22,000-Mr glycoprotein *stimulates both granulocyte and monocyte proliferation.* In contact with GM-CSF, these cells become aggressive phagocytes.

Interleukin 3

IL-3, or multi-CSF, is derived from stimulated T lymphocytes as a 23,000-Mr protein. This CSF is active on progenitors of monocytes, granulocytes, erythrocytes, and mast cells. IL-3 is associated with *an increase in 20-α steroid dehydrogenase* in exposed stem cells, but it is uncertain how this enzyme is integrated into the maturation of these cells.

Cells of the phagocytic system, referred to in the earlier literature as the reticuloendothelial system, are divisible into two distinct morphologic forms. The **mononuclear phagocytic system** is characterized by two types of cells: the monocytes and the macrophages. In general, these cells have a large nucleus that is circular in profile and possibly indented, and they contain numerous cytoplasmic granules, vacuoles, and inclusions. The other cell system includes the *three granulocytic phagocytes.* Three cell forms are present among the granulocytes, the most important in terms of phagocytic activity being the polymorphonuclear neutrophilic leukocytes. Eosinophils and basophils are important in the al-

lergic response to antigens but are feeble phagocytes.

Granulocytic Phagocytes

The cells of the granulocytic series of phagocytes are cytodestructive but do not function in the processing or presentation of antigen. Neither are they as important as the monocytes in secretory functions. Monocytes are known as the source of proteins in the complement system, in the blood clotting system, and the acute inflammatory response proteins.

POLYMORPHONUCLEAR NEUTROPHILS

The polymorphonuclear neutrophilic leukocytes represent about 60% to 70% of the 5,000 to 10,000 circulating white blood cells in each milliliter of blood. These cells are easily recognized in stained blood smears by their *multilobed nucleus, often connected by thin strands of nuclear material* (Fig. 2–2). Their cytoplasm is filled with *small granules that do not stain readily with either acidic or basic dyes; that is, they are neutrophilic.*

The granules in neutrophils are of two different types. **Primary granules,** also known as azurophilic granules, are the first to appear in the cell maturation sequence; these represent about a third of the granules in the mature neutrophil. The primary granules contain a number of enzymes, the most important of which may be **myeloperoxidase** and **lysozyme.** The **secondary or specific granules** become more numerous during later stages of maturation. These granules may also contain lysozyme, but they lack myeloperoxidase. *Myeloperoxidase is considered a*

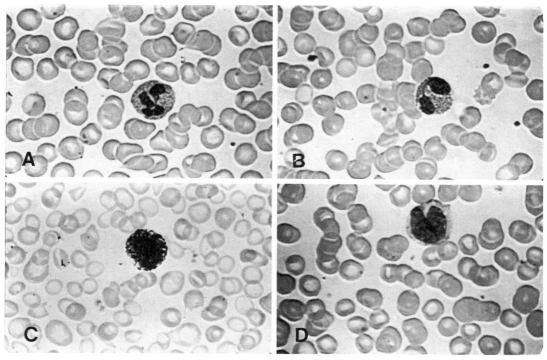

Figure 2-2. The separate panels in this figure show the appearance of (A) a polymorphonuclear neutrophilic leukocyte, (B) an eosinophil, (C) a basophil, and (D) a monocyte in stained preparations of human blood. (See color figure after Table of Contents.)

key cytotoxic agent used by phagocytes in the destruction of bacteria and other living parasites.

EOSINOPHILS

Eosinophils are white blood cells whose granules stain with acid dyes. These cells represent about 3% of the circulating white blood cells. *The granules in eosinophils* are unlike those seen in neutrophils because they *contain a large crystalloid core.* This unique structure is a concentrated source of the **major basic protein (MBP).** This 6000-Mr protein is the antimicrobial agent used by eosinophils in their destruction of bacteria and animal parasites. Although eosinophils contain numerous peroxidases, nu-

cleases, proteases, and other enzymes, they are considered to be less cytodestructive than neutrophils.

BASOPHILS

The basophils are the rarest of the circulating white blood cells, usually representing less than 1% of the total. These cells get their name from the basophilic character of the granules contained in their cytoplasm. The granules in basophils differ considerably from those in eosinophils and neutrophils. *These granules contain heparin, a powerful anticoagulant, and histamine, a powerful vasoactive amine.* These same products are also found in the granules of tissue mast cells. During certain forms of allergic reactions, the blood basophils and mast cells transport their granules to the cells' surface, from which they are discharged. The histamine and heparin released from these granules cause serious physiologic changes in a condition known as anaphylaxis (see Chapter 12).

MEMORY CHECK 2 – 1

◆

Phagocytes

1. Arise from stem progenitor cells of the bone marrow
2. Mature in response to colony-stimulating factors
3. In the granulocytic series include the neutrophils and eosinophils

---

The Mononuclear Phagocytes

The mononuclear phagocytes consist of the circulating monocytes and the free and fixed macrophages. The macrophages are derived from monocytes.

MONOCYTES

The monocytes, present in human blood at a level of 300 cells per milliliter, represent 1% to 3% of all circulating white blood cells. These cells are characterized by a large spherical, often indented, nucleus that occupies more than half the cell space (Fig. 2–2). The diameter of these cells ranges from 10 to 20 μm. *Monocytes have a short half-life in blood*, averaging about 10 hours. When they disappear from the blood, the monocytes are not removed as dead or damaged cells, but rather *enter the tissues and are converted to macrophages*.

TISSUE MACROPHAGES

Macrophages are found in virtually all soft tissues of the body, although spleen and liver are the most heavily populated. *Macrophages are named according to the tissue in which they reside*. Macrophages are called histocytes in connective tissues, Kupffer's cells in liver, dust cells in lungs, and so forth. These cells were named differently because, despite their common origin and properties, they do not have an identical morphology. Their metamorphosis from the monocytic to the macrophage stage is influenced by the tissue in which this transformation takes place, which results in morphologic variation. These mononuclear end cells are large, perhaps 50 μm in diameter, and have an ovoid to block-shaped nucleus. Their cytoplasm is filled with lysosomal granules and vacuoles. Macrophages are characterized by an ameboid mobility that enables them to move across surfaces of the body where they attack and phagocytose object particles. In many instances, phagocytic destruction is the primary result of this activity. In other circumstances, antigen is captured and partially degraded, and its essential parts salvaged. This is called **antigen processing**. The macrophages then present critical epitopes to B and T lymphocytes as antigen-presenting cells. Macrophages secrete more than 30 proteins, not including the enzymes shed from their granules.

Resident Macrophages

Because of the ease by which they can be captured from the peritoneal space and alveolar washings, macrophages from these sources have often received the most attention. *Macrophages can be thought of to exist in three separate stages of activation*. Those that are washed from the untreated peritoneal space or lung by normal buffers or saline are referred to as the **resident macrophages**. *These represent "normal" or resting macrophages.* These cells are capable of phagocytosis and are cytodestructive to any foreign cells or matter that they ingest. They adhere readily to surfaces and display ameboid motility.

Stimulated Macrophages

Irritation of the peritoneal cavity with nonantigenic irritants draws additional macrophages to the peritoneal space. These cells are more mobile, have a greater phagocytic activity, and are *more cytotoxic than resident macrophages.* These cells are **stimulated macrophages**.

Activated Macrophages

The third-level macrophage is the most ambitious, the most mobile, and most cytodestructive phagocyte. This macrophage can be harvested again from the peritoneal space, after treatment of the space with antigenic or mitogenic materials. These **activated macrophages**, also called "armed" or "professional" macrophages, rely on messages from T cells to reach the ultimate level of activity possible by these cells.

SURFACE PROTEINS ON MACROPHAGES

Although staining techniques have made it possible to recognize macrophages and to distinguish them from other cells, these cells are often identified by a combination of morphology and phagocytic ability. Recently, antibodies directed against surface proteins have been used to map the outer membrane of macrophages. Macro-

phages possess several surface proteins that are entirely specific for them (Fig. 2–3). In addition, they have surface markers that are shared by quite different cells. The most important of these proteins are those that relate to macrophage function. These include the Mac1-CR3 protein, the FcγR receptors, the class II MHC proteins, the lectinlike receptors, and the CR1 receptor (Table 2–2).

The Integrin: Mac1-CR3

The Mac1 protein has several synonyms. It is referred to as **the M1 or Mo protein**, but the most useful synonym is **CR3**. *The CR3 receptor binds various forms of the C3b molecule from the complement system.* The Mac1 protein is not found on other cells besides monocytes and macrophages but has a structural relationship to similar proteins found on other cells. These proteins are described as **integrins** *because of their role in cell-to-cell adhesion. Leukocyte functional antigen (LFA-1) and glycoprotein gp150/95 are two additional members of the integrin family.*

Each of the integrins consists of two noncovalently joined peptides. The β peptide is identical in each of the proteins and has a molecular size of 95,000 Mr. In each case, *the α chain provides molecular specificity.* The α chain of Mac1-CR3 has a molecular size of 170,000 Mr, that of the LFA-1 molecule 180,000 Mr, and that of gp150/95 obviously 150,000 Mr. Protein gp150/95 is probably complement receptor CR4. It is present on macrophages and several other cell types.

Fc Receptors

Macrophages may have immunoglobulins on their surface. These antibodies attach by noncovalent binding to the

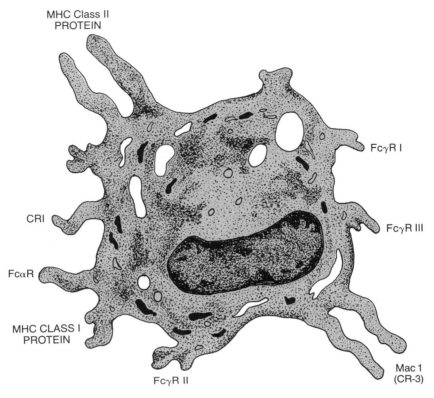

MHC Class II
PROTEIN

FcγR I

CRI

FcγR III

FcαR

MHC CLASS I
PROTEIN

Mac 1
(CR-3)

FcγR II

Figure 2–3. This macrophage has been drawn to demonstrate the numerous surface proteins needed for its function and also useful in its identification.

Fc receptors found on the macrophage. *There are three different receptors for IgG.* The first receptor, **FcγRI (CD64)**, a 72,000-Mr protein, binds IgG1, 3, and 4 but not IgG2. It is present on both macrophages and monocytes. **FcγRII (CD32)**, only 40,000 Mr, binds all four IgG isotypes. This receptor is also present on monocytes and macrophages but also has been detected on B

Table 2–2
SELECTED MACROPHAGE SURFACE PROTEINS

CD	Protein	Status	Function
CD11b/18	Mac1 (CR3)	One of the integrins, unique to macrophages	Binds C3b of the complement system
CD64	FcγRI	On monocytes and macrophages	Binds IgG1, 3, and 4 but not IgG2
CD32	FcγRII	On monocytes, macrophages, B cells, neutrophils	Binds all IgG isotypes
CD16	FcγRIII	On monocytes, macrophages, B and T cells, neutrophils	Binds IgG
	Class II MHC	DP, DQ, and DR proteins	Holds antigenic determinants
CD35	CR1	On macrophages, B and T cells, neutrophils	Binds C3b and C4b of the complement system

cells, neutrophils, and eosinophils. **FcγRIII (CD16)** is also present on several cell types—T cells, large granular lymphocytes, as well as the same cells that have FcRII. FcγRI is a member of the immunoglobulin supergene family (see Chapter 5) and RIII is relatively unique in that it uses a lipid tail for cell anchoring. These Fc receptors are highly specific for immunoglobulin G. Recently, receptors for IgA on monocytes have been reported.

The designation CD for proteins on white blood cells refers to cluster designation. CD is always followed by a number that identifies the protein.

Class II MHC Proteins

The class II MHC proteins are products of the immune response genes. In humans, three structural variations of these proteins are known as the **DP, DQ, and DR proteins**. The DP and DQ proteins are found on 50% or less of the macrophages but DR is found on the majority of these cells. Each of these is encoded by a gene on human chromosome 6. *Each protein consists of two peptides*—**the α and β peptides**. Both peptides are approximately 30,000 Mr and *have a sufficiently large number of structural variations to account for all existing agretopes.* Variation in the amino acid sequence of the β chain confers specificity for the agretope, holding the antigenic determinant so that the TCR on the T cell can contact the epitope.

Not all macrophages possess these surface proteins. DP-, DQ-, or DR-deficient macrophages may be cytodestructive, but they are not antigen-processing or -presenting cells. Other antigen-presenting cells—Langerhans' cells, dendritic cells, B lymphocytes, and a few others—also bear these proteins on their surface.

The Lectinlike Receptors

Monocytes and macrophages have at least five different receptors on their surface that combine with polysaccharides and glycoproteins. These receptors may be relatively scant on the resting cell but increase upon exposure to steroid hormones. *These lectinlike receptors for sugar residues are useful in the attachment phase of phagocytosis for bacteria and fungi.*

CR1

Another **complement receptor** found on the surface of macrophages has been called **CR1 (CD35)**. CR1 was first recognized as present on erythrocytes, but it has also been found on other cells, including monocytes, granulocytes, and both B and T lymphocytes. Because of the disparate nature of these cells, it is presumed that the CR1 molecule has different functions on each. CR1 binds to forms of C3b and C4b of complement. The CR molecules are discussed also in Chapter 6.

MACROPHAGE SECRETORY PRODUCTS

Nearly 75 export products have been identified as originating from monocytic cells. Many of the products are proteins and several are enzymes (Table 2–3). Oxygen intermediates and bioactive lipids form other groups. One group, the monokines, is composed of hormonelike reagents that activate other cells. The CSF proteins described earlier belong to this group of cell stimulants or cytokines. Other monokines are discussed subsequently.

Interleukin 1

An important pleiotropic protein secreted by macrophages is **interleukin 1**

Table 2–3
SELECTED SECRETORY PRODUCTS FROM MACROPHAGES

Protein	Symbol	Function
Interleukin 1	IL-1	Stimulates T-cell growth
Tumor necrosis factor α	TNFα	Hemorrhagic destruction of tumors, acts as cachectin
Endothelial leukocyte adhesion molecule	ELAM-1	Aids adhesion of leukocytes to blood vessels and cells
Interleukin 6	IL-6 Interferon $\beta2$	B-cell stimulatory factor
Complement molecules	C1, 2, 3, 4, 5; factors B, D, and P	
Miscellaneous		Blood clotting factors, interferons, transferrin

(IL-1), *a monokine best known for its ability to stimulate the growth of T lymphocytes* and formerly known as lymphocyte-activating factor. *IL-1 is the endogenous pyrogen,* the agent responsible for the fever that accompanies infections. Among the other functions of IL-1 are the stimulation of ELAM 1 synthesis and the production of CSF by endothelial cells. IL-1 is cytostatic for tumor cells, stimulates proliferation of B cells, is chemotactic for lymphocytes and neutrophils, and activates natural killer cells.

Two forms of IL-1 are encoded by separate genes on human chromosome 2. IL-1α, with an acidic isoelectric point, and IL-1β, the isoelectrically neutral molecule, are secreted as 17,500-Mr peptides. The initial transcript, proIL-1, is found in the cytoplasm as a 31,000-Mr precursor. The α and β forms of IL-1 have only a 25% amino acid homology but use the same receptor on the cells they activate. Short amino acid stretches of strong homology may allow the two proteins to bind the same receptor. The IL-1 receptor (IL-1R) is a 60,000-Mr protein that is heavily glycosylated and has a full size of 80,000 Mr. Very few molecules of IL-1R are present on resting T cells, but a 10-fold increase follows T-cell exposure to antigen. Binding of IL-1 to the receptor is presumed to activate the T cell via the G protein–cAMP pathway rather than the Ca^{2+} phosphatidylinositol-protein kinase C system. Cell proliferation of helper T cell is necessary for the full participation of B cells and the other T-cell subsets in the immune response.

Tumor Necrosis Factors

The *injection of bacterial lipopolysaccharide into tumor-bearing animals may result in a hemorrhagic dissolution of the tumor.* The **tumor necrosis factor (TNF)** responsible for this is a product of macrophages. TNF is secreted by these cells after exposure to many stimuli—the bacille Calmette-Guérin (BCG) vaccine for tuberculosis and lipopolysaccharide (LPS) being most commonly used.

TNF is a peptide of 17,500 Mr with a sharp structural resemblance to lymphotoxin (LT), a lymphokine produced by lymphocytes. TNF and LT both have their origin from human chromosome 6, are essentially the same size, have a 30% amino acid homology, attach to the same cell receptor, and are active against tumor cells. TNF is now referred to as TNFα and LT as TNFβ.

TNFα has numerous biologic activities in addition to its antitumor function. It has antibacterial and antimalarial activity; it induces interferon (IFN) and IL-1 production, stimulates phagocytosis, and causes a set of responses termed cachexia—weight loss, fever, chills, nausea, anorexia, lowered blood pressure, and so on. **Cachectin** *is a synonym for TNFα.* The nonspecific or adjuvant therapy of tumors (see Chapter 10) is based on a stimulation of TNFα. Pure recombinant TNFα is also effective but produces a number of toxic side effects that prevent the use of this product in human patients.

Endothelial Leukocyte Adhesion Molecule 1

TNFα and IL-1 are able to activate the endothelium so that monocytes and neutrophils adhere to the endothelial surface. This is the first step in diapedesis, the migration of phagocytes from the blood vessels into neighboring tissues. The *molecule responsible for adhesion—endothelial leukocyte adhesion molecule 1 (ELAM1)—is a member of a large group of molecules whose structure contains tandem repeats of 60 amino acids.* Most of these molecules regulate the complement system and are described more fully in Chapter 6 as the **RCA molecules, regulators of complement activation**. ELAM 1, by its lectinlike grasp of neutrophils, holds these phagocytic cells against the blood vessel wall, where phagocytosis is much easier accomplished than in the blood stream. Alternatively, the phagocytes transgress the blood vessel wall and enter areas of inflammation.

Interleukin 6

The **B cell stimulatory factor 2 (BSF-2) and interferon β2** have been identified as identical molecules with multiple activities and **have been renamed interleukin 6 (IL-6)**. As is true of most interleukins, IL-6 is produced by several cell types, including T lymphocytes and monocytes. It is discussed extensively in Chapter 4.

Complement Components

Eight different proteins of the complement system plus two regulators of that system are produced by macrophages. The eight proteins are C1, C2, C3, C4, C5, and factors B, D, and P (see Chapter 6).

Miscellaneous Products

Among the other products originating from macrophages are plasminogen activator, α2-macroglobulin, transferrin, prothrombin, factors IX and X of the blood clotting system, prostaglandin E_2, erythropoietin, transcobalamin, and many others. Interferon, also produced by macrophages, is described in Chapter 4.

MEMORY CHECK 2–2
◆

Important monokines include

1. The endogenous pyrogen and T-cell stimulant, IL-1
2. Tumor necrosis factor α
3. IL-6, a B-cell stimulatory factor

Phagocytosis and Antigen Processing

The ingestion and destruction of living cells or nonviable antigens by phagocytic cells is divisible into several stages: chemoattraction or opsonization, endocytosis, intracellular death, and digestion (Table 2–4). These are all necessary preliminary events to a

Table 2–4
CONTRIBUTORS TO PHAGOCYTOSIS

Phagocytic Stage	Contributors
Chemotaxis	C5a from complement
	Tuftsin
	Formyl peptides f Met Met Phe
	f Met Leu Phe
	Eosinophil chemotaxins (ECF-A)
	Arachidonic acid derivatives
Attachment	IgG
	C3b
	ELAM-1
Endocytosis	
Intracellular death	Singlet oxygen, $^1O_2$
	Hydrogen peroxide, H_2O_2
	Hypochlorite, ^-OCl
	Hydroxyl radical, $\cdot OH$
	Superoxide, $\cdot O^-_2$
	Defensins

critical early stage in the immune response, antigen presentation.

CHEMOATTRACTION

The first problem faced by the phagocyte is how to reach the victim cell or particle. In the blood stream this may be a chance encounter of the circulating phagocyte with the victim particle. Moreover, as the blood passes through the soft tissues, the dense population of macrophages at the surface of the blood vessels contact and engulf their prey. The earliest phases of leukocyte margination are the effects of platelet-activating factor (PAF) and complement protein C3b. (These agents are described in Chapters 12 and 6, respectively.) Later the appearance of ELAM-1, synthesized in response to IL-1, adds to macrophage accumulation at the blood vessel surface. Probably of equal importance is the ability of phagocytic cells to emigrate from the blood and to accumulate at inflammatory foci. This is aided by several events. **A chemoattractant**, released

from bacteria at the site of the infection or by injured tissue cells, **will draw phagocytes from the blood**. Antibody may activate the complement system to release a chemotaxin. More than 15 chemotaxins are known to act upon monocytic cells. Many of these also stimulate granulocytes. Only a few of these can be mentioned here (Table 2–5).

C5a from Complement

An important chemotaxin is generated from the complement system as the result of a combination of antigen with certain isotypes of IgG or with IgM. A nonantibody-dependent pathway of complement activation also releases this chemotaxin. The cleavage product C5a is derived from the fifth component of complement. This molecule is a low molecular weight protein of approximately 16,000 Mr that contains only 77 amino acids and considerable polysaccharide. *C5a is a chemoattractant for all types of phagocytic cells*—macrophages, neutrophils, eosinophils, and even basophils.

Table 2–5

CHEMOTACTIC AGENTS ACTIVE ON MONOCYTES AND MACROPHAGES

Factor	Mr	Origin
C5a	7,400	C5 of complement system
Tuftsin	400	Tetrapeptide from immunoglobulin
Formyl peptides	300	Bacteria
Thromboxane β_2 other lipids	3,500 varies	Arachidonic acid
TNFα	17,500	Macrophages
Macrophage chemotaxin	12,500	T lymphocytes

Tuftsin

A tetrapeptide consisting of the residues Thr Lys Pro Arg known as **tuftsin** *is chemotactic for both granulocytes and macrophages.* Tuftsin is released from a large protein, probably a gamma globulin, by hydrolysis of specific peptide bonds. Tuftsin deficiency is associated with an increase in bacterial infections.

Formyl Peptides

Peptides of low molecular weight in which the terminal amino group is a formylated methionine are chemotactic. Two of these are well known: **formyl Met Leu Phe** and **formyl Met Met Phe**. It is interesting that the formyl group is required for their chemotactic function—the unsubstituted peptides are inactive. The presence of the formyl Met residue at the amino terminal end indicates that these *are portions of bacterial peptides* whose synthesis was interrupted. The formyl Met group is the initiating group for extension of protein synthesis at the ribosomal level in bacteria but not human cells.

Eosinophil Chemotaxins

Mast cells that undergo degranulation during allergic reactions release two peptides that are specific in inducing the chemoattractant response in eosinophils. These peptides described as **eosinophilic chemotactic factors of ana-** phylaxis (ECF-A) have the sequence Val Gly Thr Glu and Ala Gly Thr Glu. These peptides exist preformed in mast cells and are released when the mast cells are stimulated to degranulate by a combination of IgE antibody and antigen on its surface.

Arachidonic Acid Metabolites

In addition to ECF-A, mast cells and cells damaged by trauma or infection may release fatty acids from their cell membrane. One of these lipids is the 20-carbon acid with the scientific name **icosatetraenoic acid** and the common name **arachidonic acid**. Arachidonic acid is degraded by two separate pathways known as the lipooxygenase pathway and the cyclooxygenase pathway. **Chemotactic derivatives** are formed in both of these pathways. In the lipooxygenase pathway two compounds called **12-hydroxy and 5-hydroxy icosatetraenoic acid** are powerful chemotaxins for granulocytes (Fig. 2–4). The leukotrienes are also chemotactic. In the cyclooxygenase pathway, the compounds **thromboxane B_2 and hydroxytetraenoic acid** are chemotactic for neutrophils and eosinophils.

Miscellaneous Chemotaxins

T lymphocytes can secret a macrophage-specific chemotaxin when stimulated by antigens or by mitogens. A

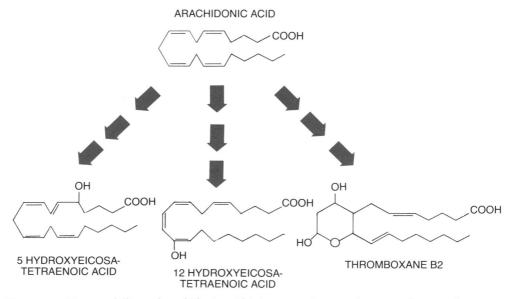

ARACHIDONIC ACID

5 HYDROXYEICOSA-
TETRAENOIC ACID

12 HYDROXYEICOSA-
TETRAENOIC ACID

THROMBOXANE B2

Figure 2–4. The metabolism of arachidonic acid is important in several aspects of immunology. Here the structure of three chemotaxins derived from arachidonic acid is illustrated. (See Chapter 12 for the role of arachidonic acid in IgE-mediated allergy.)

wide array of other compounds have chemotactic activity including bacterial endotoxins (LPS), lysosomal enzymes, collagen, fibrin, thrombin, and others.

CELL BINDING — OPSONIZATION

Once the phagocytic cell is drawn near its victim, phagocytic engulfment may or may not occur. Many bacteria produce capsules that maintain phagocytic cells at a distance. If the bacterium or other particle is on a surface, the ameboid motion of the phagocyte favors contact and engulfment. A number of molecular factors called **opsonins** *promote adhesion of the phagocyte with its object particle.*

*The most potent opsonins are immunoglobulins that bind to the Fc recep-*tors on macrophages and neutrophils. Immunoglobulins G1 and G3 are extremely potent opsonins. Immunoglobulin binding via the Fc region of the immunoglobulin leaves the antigen-binding sites of the molecule free. Thus, the phagocytic cell and its victim particle are only one molecule in length from each other. *Opsonic activity of the complement molecules is also* important in continuing the attack of phagocytic cells on bacteria. The complement molecule C3 is split after antigen-antibody combination and interaction with complement to form two peptides: the C3a low molecular weight molecule, and the larger C3b residue. The C3b residue remains attached to the antigen-antibody complex. Because of the presence of the Mac1 receptor for C3b on macrophages, the phagocytic cell is closely linked to the antigen-antibody aggregate.

CELL ENGULFMENT — ENDOCYTOSIS

Exactly how the phagocytic particle is taken into the cell without a loss of cytoplasm continues to be a mystery. Time-lapse cinematophotography has shown that the cytoplasm of the phagocytic cell flows around and completely surrounds the target cell. The cytoplasm apparently fuses with itself, capturing the particle in a vesicle known as the **phagosome**. By virtue of this fusion, the phagosome is surrounded by an inverted cell membrane. The phagosome is transported centrally and comes in contact with the lysosomal granules present in phagocytic cells. The lysosome disintegrates, releasing its hydrolytic enzymes into the structure now known as the **phagolysosome** (Fig. 2–5).

INTRACELLULAR DEATH

For years acceptance of the premise that hydrolytic enzymes of the lysosome were responsible for the cytocidal event blocked further study of the chemical nature of this process. More recently, it has become apparent that there are both oxygen-dependent and oxygen-independent avenues for this process.

Toxic Forms of Oxygen

The resting phagocyte generally uses anaerobic glycolysis as its major pathway of carbohydrate metabolism and energy source. During this process, lactic acid is formed and no oxygen is consumed. During the phagocytic act, however, the phagocytes shift to the higher energy-yielding hexosemonophosphate shunt. This causes a 100-fold increase in oxygen consumption above the resting state.

Superoxide anion. Associated with the hexosemonophosphate shunt is the enzyme nicotinamide adenine dinucleotide phosphate dehydrogenase. This enzyme is physically associated with chemoreceptors on the cell surface and is activated during chemoattraction and phagocytosis. This enzyme, also known as **NADPH oxidase**, *reduces normal oxygen to the superoxide anion.* The superoxide anion, since it has an unpaired electron, is highly reactive and carries a negative charge. At one time it was thought that these superoxide radicals were responsible for the lethal hit of white blood cells on internalized bacteria, but this belief is fading under the weight of other evidence (Fig. 2–6).

Singlet oxygen. *The enzyme* **superoxide dismutase** *scavenges superoxide and, by the addition of hydrogen pro-*

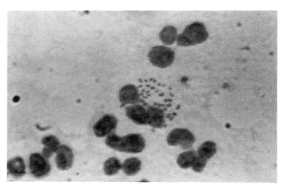

Figure 2–5. A neutrophil is shown phagocytizing bacteria. Because of the acid condition of the preparation, the phagocytes are stained atypically. (See color figure after Table of Contents.)

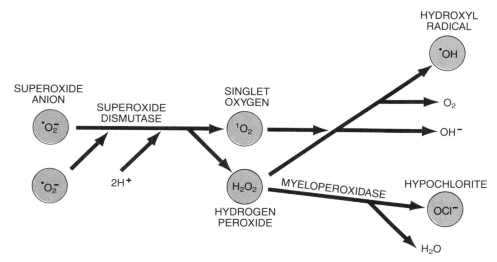

Figure 2-6. The interlaced relationship of the toxic forms of oxygen generated by phagocytic cells is presented here. Potentially, the hypochlorite ion and hydroxyl radical are the most toxic.

tons, *produces hydrogen peroxide and singlet oxygen.* When singlet oxygen, itself an unstable molecule, returns to the ground state of normal oxygen, light is emitted. This chemoluminescence is detectable by instrumentation. It is known that phagocytic cells engaged in phagocytosis emit light, and it is therefore felt that the return of singlet oxygen to normal oxygen is important in the phagocytic attack upon target cells. Certain dyes and pigments will absorb and quench the light formed by the shift of singlet oxygen to normal oxygen. Microorganisms that contain a high concentration of these pigments are more resistant to intraphagocytic death than are mutant cells that lack these pigments.

Hydrogen peroxide and hypochlorite. Hydrogen peroxide has long been considered a bactericidal agent by microbiologists, but the evidence for this has not always been convincing. Catalases and peroxidases quickly destroy peroxides. *Hydrogen peroxide may be bactericidal in living systems by virtue of its conversion to the hypochlorite ion by the enzyme myeloperoxidase.* The hypochlorite ion is known to be antimicrobial and is the form of chlorine in

water from water treatment plants. The potential for hypochlorite or hypoiodite formation by phagocytic cells is significant because the primary granules of phagocytic cells contain myeloperoxidase to the extent of about 5% of the entire cell weight. Deficiency of myeloperoxidase impairs cell killing by phagocytes and causes an increase in bacterial infections.

Hydroxyl radical. Another potentially cytotoxic form of oxygen is derived from hydrogen peroxide when it interacts with the superoxide radical. In this reaction, oxygen is reformed along with hydroxyl ions but neither of these is considered to be toxic. The third product, the **hydroxyl radical**, *has been described as the most powerful oxidizing form of oxygen in living systems* and is considered as the most toxic form of oxygen produced by phagocytes.

Oxygen-Independent Cell Killing

Several oxygen-independent factors also contribute to the elimination of bacteria from inflammatory sites. The intracellular accumulation of **lactic acid** within phagocytic cells creates a bacteriostatic environment. **Lysozyme** released into the phagolysosome is able to digest the cell wall of gram-positive bacteria, causing them to rupture. Cationic proteins, known as **defensins**, recently described in phagocytic cells, interfere with the cell transport functions and cause the death of both gram-positive and gram-negative bacteria. **Transferrin** and **lactoferrin** may bind iron and remove it from the nutrient supply necessary for microbial growth.

CELL ELIMINATION — DIGESTION

Nonviable antigens within phagocytic cells are quickly *digested by enzymes released into the phagolysosome.* Many living organisms are resistant to these enzymes but become sensitive upon their death. Among the enzymes that we find present in lysosomes are various proteases, phosphatases, ribonucleases, collagenases, esterases, glactosidases, glucosidases, lipases, and so on. This vast array of hydrolytic enzymes will ultimately digest all biomolecules to a soluble state. When this does not occur, the macrophages may fuse to form a multinucleate giant cell (Fig. 2–7).

MEMORY CHECK 2–3

In phagocytosis

1. ELAM-1 aids attachment of macrophages to blood vessels after its up-regulation by PAF and C3b.
2. C5a, tuftsin, formyl Met peptides, ECF-A, and arachidonic acid metabolites assist as chemotaxins
3. The two most important opsonins are antibody and C3b
4. Cell death occurs through oxygen-dependent and -independent pathways
5. Toxic forms of oxygen, especially OCl^- and $\cdot OH$, are key compounds

---

Antigen-Presenting Cells and How They Do It

The mononuclear phagocytes and granulocytes are nonspecific cells. They will ingest any particle regardless of its antigenic nature and they will even ingest inert plastic or glass beads. In contrast to phagocytes, each B cell

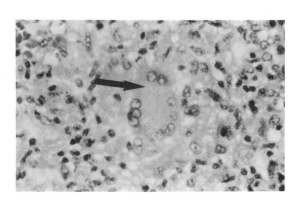

Figure 2–7. The large structure in the center is a multinucleated giant cell. (See color figure after Table of Contents.)

and T cell is patterned to respond to a specific antigen. The T cell responds not to the complete antigen but to the processed antigen. This processed epitope must be offered by a qualified antigen-presenting cell. *Antigen-presenting cells (APC) must have class II MHC proteins on their surface to activate the helper T cell.*

MACROPHAGES

The DP, DQ, and DR class II MHC proteins are present on macrophages, as described on page 33. *Macrophages are the most important antigen presenters.*

DENDRITIC CELLS

The **dendritic cell**, a recognized antigen presenter, is derived from a precursor in bone marrow. After exiting the marrow, this precursor matures in tissues. Only the brain remains free of these cells.

Dendritic cells have an eccentrically placed nucleus in a cell with an irregular outline. Morphologically they resemble macrophages even to the extent of possessing lysosomal granules and vacuoles, but they *are not phagocytic.* When interlaced with lymphocytes and macrophages, dendritic cells have been *described as interdigitating cells* because of their starlike projections thrust between their neighbors. It is this stage of cell interaction in which antigen presentation is most likely to occur.

The presence of DP, DQ, and DR proteins on dendritic cells is necessary to their function as antigen-presenting cells. Fc receptors may also serve in this function by presenting antigen that has already been bound into an immune complex. This may establish a larger role for dendritic cells in the memory than in the primary response.

Dendritic cells are Den1+, class II, MHC+, but Mac1−.

LANGERHANS' CELLS

Within the last several years, cells known as **Langerhans' cells** have garnered considerable attention as antigen-presenting cells. Langerhans' cells *represent 5% to 10% of all cells in the epidermis.* These cells are very irregular in profile, having an indented nucleus and a cell body somewhat larger than that of monocytes. Long, spider-like extensions spread from their cell core. These extensions often contain the rod-shaped Birbeck granules, considered a key identifying structure. Langerhans' cells can be found in lymphoid organs such as the tonsils and the lymph nodes, where they are seen as interdigitating cells. It has now been recognized that Langerhans' cells *sequester antigen through the agency of their FcγR and CR1 receptor.* Langerhans' cells also possess on their surface the MHC class II proteins needed for antigen presentation.

B CELLS

Evidence that neoplastic B cells could serve as antigen-presenting cells detracted from reports that normal B cells could effect this transfer equally well. It is now accepted that *B cells can function in two directions with T cells — delivery of antigen and receipt of interleukin assistance for antibody formation.* Immunoglobulin and MHC class II proteins on the B-cell surface enable antigen capture and presentation.

ANTIGEN TRANSFER

The dual peptide structure of both the DP, DQ, and DR proteins on antigen-presenting cells and the T-cell receptor

(TCR) protein on the antigen-receiving cell has simplified the concept of how antigenic determinants are offered to the T cell. The determinant is held by its agretope domain to a groove between the α and β peptides of the class II MHC protein. The α and β peptides of the TCR grasp the epitope. This is the first stage in activation of the T cell. Adsorption of IL-1 by receptors on the T-cell surface is the second stage. These events catalyze the T cells to produce several lymphokines that activate B cells and make other adjustments in their metabolism. These events are described in Chapter 4.

MEMORY CHECK 2−4

◆

Antigen presentation

1. Requires the DP, DQ, or DR protein on the presenting cell
2. Is a normal activity of macrophages, dendritic cells, Langerhans' cells, and B cells
3. Is accompanied by IL-1 stimulation of T cells
4. Requires the TCR protein on T cells
5. Can be considered as a sequence of DP, DQ, or DR protein−agretope-epitope-TCR

References

Beutler, B: The tumor necrosis factors: Cachectin and lymphotoxin. Hosp Pract 25:(1):45, 1990.

Dexter, TM, Garland JM, and Testa NG (eds): Colony-Stimulating Factors. Marcel Dekker, New York, 1990.

Dinarello, CA: Interleukin-1 and its biologically related cytokines. Adv Immunol 44:153, 1989.

Kishimoto, TK, et al: The leukocyte integrins. Adv Immunol 46:149, 1989.

Martin, M, and Resch, K: Interleukin 1: More than a mediator between leukocytes. Topics Pharmaceutical Science 9:171, 1988.

Mauri, C, Rizzo, SC, and Ricevuti, G (eds): The Biology of Phagocytes in Health and Disease. Pergamon Journals, Oxford, 1987.

Mizel, SB: The interleukins. FASEB Jour 3:2379, 1989.

Pernis, B, Silverstein, SC, and Vogel, HS (eds): Processing and Presentation of Antigens. Academic Press, San Diego, 1988.

Sbarra, AJ, and Strauss, RR (eds): The Respiratory Burst and its Physiological Significance. Plenum Press, New York, 1988.

Thomas, ML: The leukocyte common antigen family. Annu Rev Immunol 7:339, 1989.

Zembala M, and Asherson, GL (eds): Human Monocytes. Academic Press, San Diego, 1989.

QUESTIONS AND ANSWERS

1. Which of the following markers on the macrophage surface contributes to the attachment phase of phagocytosis?
   A. MHC class II protein
   B. MHC class I protein
   C. FcγR
   D. GM-CSF receptor
   E. Myeloperoxidase

Answer C

Class II proteins are recognition proteins for T cells in the cooperative events leading to T-cell activation and eventually to antibody formation by B cells. All macrophages and most other nucleated cells have surface MHC I proteins. The Fcγ receptor binds IgG, and any antigen bound to the Fab portion of IgG is directed in this way to the macrophage surface. FcγR is a key contributor to opsonization. The receptor for GM-CSF is important in binding that agent to immature granulocytes and macrophages. Myeloperoxidase is a lysosomal enzyme that is useful in the cytocidal phase of phagocytosis.

2. All of the following are chemotaxins *except*
   A. C5a
   B. Tuftsin
   C. Formyl Met Met Phe
   D. IgG
   E. Thromboxane B_2

Answer D

IgG is a powerful opsonin, but it is not a chemotaxin. Tuftsin, derived from immunoglobulins, is a chemotactic tetrapeptide. C5a is a powerful chemotaxin generated from the complement system. The formyl peptides are derived from bacteria, and thromboxane B_2 comes from host cell membranes.

3. Which of the following is a member of the integrin family of proteins?
   A. Mac1 protein
   B. FcγRI
   C. GM-CSF
   D. C5a
   E. IgG

Answer A

The integrin family of proteins all share a 95,000-Mr β peptide and have different α peptides. These proteins are involved in intercellular adhesion. The Mac1-CR3 protein is the integrin member on this list. FcγRI and IgG are both part of the immunoglobulin supergene family. The GM-CSF and C5a molecules are not structurally related to each other. C5a is related to other molecules in the complement system.

4. Myeloperoxidase
   A. Converts H_2O_2 to H_2O and $1/2\ O_2$
   B. Is found in primary granules of macrophages
   C. Is considered an important secretory product of macrophages
   D. Is the source of superoxide radicals in macrophages
   E. Participates in oxygen-independent killing by phagocytes

Answer B

Peroxidases decompose H_2O_2. Myeloperoxidase uses halides for this purpose and produces H_2O + OCl$^-$ if chloride ion is used. Found in the primary granules of macrophages, this enzyme is an important lethal enzyme. Superoxide radicals are produced by nicotinamide-adenine dinucleotide phosphate dehydrogenase. Answer E is erroneous.

5. Which of the following is *not* produced by macrophages?
   A. G-CSF
   B. IL-1
   C. Complement molecules
   D. Defensins
   E. ECF-A

Answer E

Of the colony-stimulating factors, G-CSF and GM-CSF can be produced by macrophages. IL-1 is a critical interleukin from macrophages required to stimulate T and other cells. Numerous complement proteins including C1, C2, C3, and C4 have macrophages as their source. Defensins are cationic defending proteins found in macrophages. ECF-A, of which there are two closely related forms, is produced by mast cells.

Case Study: Chernobyl and GM-CSF

Tanya is the 8-year-old daughter of Petra and Vassily Rostov, whose farm was in the path of radiation fallout from the Chernobyl accident in the USSR. When the accident occurred, Tanya had been on a walk through neighboring meadows to pick wildflowers. She remained in the meadow for an undetermined period of time unaware of the accident. Her parents heard the news on the radio and remained indoors until Tanya's return. Military police soon drove into the area and removed people to a distant shelter. At the shelter, medical authorities interviewed everyone and placed Tanya in a group of persons who had been heavily exposed and who would be monitored for signs of radiation sickness. Ten days later Tanya's granulocyte count had fallen below 0.1×10^9/L. An international medical team started her on GM-CSF.

Questions

1. What is the source of human GM-CSF?

2. Has GM-CSF proven useful for treating patients with radiation sickness?

3. What other diseases are considered treatable with GM-CSF?

4. What are the side effects of GM-CSF treatment?

Discussion

Recombinant human GM-CSF has been generated from both prokaryotic and eukaryotic cells. The copy DNA was synthesized from GM-CSF mRNA from T cells. *Escherichia coli* is a bacterial source of GM-CSF after being infected with a plasmid carrying the genome. The recombinant protein has 127 amino acids.

GM-CSF has had only partial success in treating persons exposed to radiation. In Brazil eight persons who were exposed to ^{137}Cs in a radiotherapy unit, received this monokine. Four of these had serious bacterial infections at the time therapy was initiated and died within a few days. The remaining four persons survived. After receiving the GM-CSF, the granulocyte counts increased significantly within a few days, and in as little as 12 hours in some individuals.

Clinical trials with GM-CSF have been applied to such diverse conditions as acquired immunodeficiency syndrome (AIDS), aplastic anemia, bone marrow transplantation, and advanced malignancy. The AIDS patients in one group experienced a significant rise in the number of granulocytes but only a slight increase in monocytes. The patients with aplastic anemia also responded to the therapy but this was temporary and cell counts fell when treatment ceased. Of 43 patients with myelodysplastic syndrome, many responded with increased granulocytes, and some with increased mononuclears. Again, these were transient findings, albeit dose-related responses. Patients with advanced cancers responded with increased white blood cell counts, but this response did not alter their cancerous state. Bone marrow transplant patients benefited the most from GM-CSF treatment. The monokine accelerated the return of circulating granulocytes and monocytes.

Numerous side effects plagued these clinical trials. Fluid retention, fever, myalgia, headache, skin rash, diarrhea, and bone pain have been recorded. These effects may be minimized in future trials by adjusting the dose and route of injection. GM-CSF is effective and, if these side effects can be overcome, continued therapy will be possible, which will overcome the transient response to this monokine seen in most patients.

GLOSSARY

---

activated macrophage   A macrophage from antigen-sensitized or otherwise stimulated animal.

alveolar macrophage   An aerobic macrophage of the lung.

antigen processing   The preservation of epitopes and the elimination of other portions of antigens by macrophages.

antigen presentation   The offering of epitopes to T cells by macrophages and certain other MHC class II–positive cells.

APC   Antigen-processing or -presenting cell.

basophil   A blood granulocyte whose granules release histamine during anaphylactic reactions.

chemotaxis   Attraction of leukocytes or other cells by chemicals.

colony-stimulating factor   Products that stimulate the maturation of white blood cells from their precursors.

CSF   Colony-stimulating factor.

dendritic cell   A nonphagocytic, antigen-presenting cell.

eosinophil   A white blood cell that contains cytoplasmic granules with an affinity for acid dyes.

Fc receptor   A cell receptor for the Fc portion of an immunoglobulin.

granulocyte   A collective term for leukocytes that have pronounced granules in their cytoplasm.

hydroxyl radical   A toxic form of oxygen produced by phagocytes; ·OH.

IL-1   Interleukin 1.

integrin   A family of proteins that promote cell adhesion.

interleukin   A hormonelike agent produced by leukocytes that acts on other leukocytes.

interleukin 1   A monokine that activates T cells and B cells.

Kupffer's cell   A macrophage of the liver.

Langerhans' cells   Antigen-presenting cells found in the skin.

macrophage   Tissue or blood phagocytes, 20 to 80 μm in diameter, containing lysosomes, vacuoles, and partially digested debris in their cytoplasm.

monocyte   White blood cell, 12 to 30 μm in diameter, with rounded nucleus; precursor to macrophage.

monokine   A protein elaborated by a monocyte or macrophage that acts on other host cells, especially leukocytes.

myeloperoxidase   An enzyme in lysosomes that aids intraphagocyte killing.

neutrophil   A leukocyte with granules that are not predominant in their affinity for acid or basic dyes.

opsonin   An agent such as an antibody that attaches to a cellular or particulate antigen and prepares it for phagocytosis.

phagocytosis The engulfing of cells or particulate matter by leukocytes, macrophages, or other cells.

polymorphonuclear neutrophilic leukocyte (PMN) A white blood cell with a granular cytoplasm and multilobed nucleus that is very active in phagocytosis.

singlet oxygen A toxic form of oxygen produced by phagocytes; $^1O_2$.

superoxide radical A toxic form of oxygen produced by phagocytes; $\cdot O_2$.

tuftsin A chemotactic tetrapeptide derived from a gamma globulin.

tumor necrosis factor α **(TNFα)** A protein from macrophages that is lytic for some tumor cells.

CHAPTER 3

◆

The Lymphocytes: Part 1
B Lymphocytes

The capture of antigen by macrophages can be totally independent of any influence of the antigen upon the macrophage. Admittedly antibody on the FcγR of the macrophage may assist in phagocytosis, but this antibody is not synthesized by the macrophages; it comes from lymphocytes. It is this same antibody produced by the lymphocyte that permits the lymphocyte to be described as an antigen-specific cell. There are *two major types of lymphocytes known as the B and T cells, and a third type called the* **null cell, natural killer (NK), or large granular lymphocyte (LGL).** The B cell produces antibody but the T cell also produces a special receptor for antigen. Both antibody and the T-cell receptor react with a single epitope of the antigen. The B cell sheds its antibody into the blood where it is responsible for humoral (circulating) immunity. The T cell does not secrete its receptor and participates only in the cell-mediated aspects of immunity. The null cells are not antigen specific, and react indiscriminately with their targets.

As lymphocytes, these cells obviously share many features, several of which are described in this chapter. In addition, special characteristics of the B lymphocytes and null or LGL cells are presented here, to be followed by a

51

description of T cells in the subsequent chapter.

The description of B cells focuses on the several discernible stages of their maturation, reflected by the acquisition of surface markers and the ability to synthesize immunoglobulins. Later the influence of interleukins on B-cell transformation to plasma cells is described. How antigens and mitogens affect the primary and secondary antibody responses is followed by a description of the hybridoma technique to conclude the chapter.

The Three Sets of Lymphocytes

LYMPHOCYTE MORPHOLOGY

The lymphocytes represent 30% of all white blood cells in the healthy adult. These cells range from 7 to 12 μm in diameter and are further characterized by a **large round nucleus** surrounded by a small fringe of **relatively agranular cytoplasm** (Fig. 3–1). The nucleus may have a single indentation, and the nuclear chromatin is often distributed irregularly in linear clumps, giving the appearance of a wagon wheel. LGL cells, which represent 1% to 5% of the lymphocytes, are slightly larger and

more granular than the B and T cells (Table 3–1).

The life span of lymphocytes differs markedly according to their class. B lymphocytes have a short life span, possibly no more than 1 week. The life span of T cells is measured in months or years.

All cells circulating normally in the blood are derived from stem cells that originate in the bone marrow, as described in Chapter 2. Most of these cell types are mature when they enter the blood; they are the end cells of their line. This is not true of monocytes, which are able to enter tissues and transform into macrophages. Neither is this true of lymphocytes, which undergo modification in the primary or central lymphoid organs after they leave the bone marrow and blood. This modification is most easily observed in birds, which have both a thymus and a bursa of Fabricius.

THE BURSA OF FABRICIUS

In humans, the B lymphocyte leaves the bone marrow as a cell already in the later stages of its transition to maturity. In fowl this is not the situation. *The avian B cell must pass through the bursa of Fabricius* before it is fully ma-

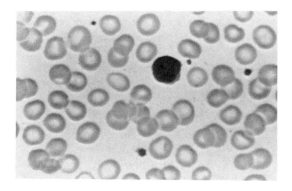

Figure 3–1. The central dark staining cell is a typical lymphocyte displaying its scant cytoplasm and large nucleus. (See color figure after Table of Contents.)

Table 3–1
MAJOR FEATURES OF THE THREE LYMPHOCYTE POPULATIONS

Characteristic	B Cells	T Cells	LGL Cells
Stem cell origin	Bone marrow	Bone marrow	Bone marrow
Maturation site	Bursa of Fabricius in fowl, bone marrow in mammals	Thymus	None
Percent of circulating lymphocytes	25%–35%	65%–75%	1%–5%
Major morphologic features	7 to 12 μm, large nucleus, smooth cytoplasm	Like B cells	More granular cytoplasm
Physiologic function	Immunoglobulin formation	Interleukin production	Natural cell killing via perforins and granzymes

ture. The bursa is subdivided into lobes or follicles separated by connective tissue. In these follicles, the B lymphocytes, so named because of the influence of the bursa, acquire an imprint that will allow them to respond to antigen by a transformation to plasma cells and secretion of antibody.

Mammals lack a bursal organ and the search for a single organ that functions as the bursal equivalent has been frustrating. Several gut-associated lymphoid tissues (GALT) have been suggested as bursal substitutes; these include the appendix, tonsils, and Peyer's patches. When experimental immunologists need a source of mammalian B cells, bone marrow is chosen, and these cells behave just like B cells from avian species. It is now accepted that *mammalian B cells need no phase outside bone marrow to function as mature cells.*

THE THYMUS

Lymphocytes destined to function as *T cells in humans or in avian species must be modified in the thymus.* The human thymus weighs 15 to 20 g at birth and may reach 40 g by puberty, after which it gradually atrophies. The thymus is subdivided into a series of lobules or follicles, much like the bursa. In these follicles, the T (thymic) lymphocytes collect and mature (Fig. 3–2). Here the T lymphocytes lose certain surface markers (proteins) and acquire or express others. These surface markers are most easily recognized by their specific antibodies, so it is equally appropriate to refer to them as surface antigens. Far more importantly, however, these T cells acquire unique properties that enable them to respond

---

MEMORY CHECK 3–1

◆

B lymphocytes

1. Are responsible for immunoglobulin synthesis
2. Are imprinted in the bursa of Fabricius in fowl
3. Mature in human bone marrow
4. Are functionally distinct from T cells and LGL cells
5. Are antigen specific

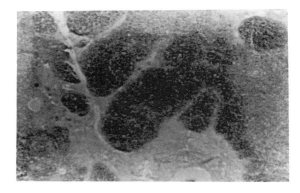

Figure 3-2. Notice the many lobes that house the lymphocytes in the thymus. (See color figure after Table of Contents.)

to antigens in a different way than do B cells. In fact, there are several T-cell subsets, each of which responds in a slightly different way to antigen. These will be described further in the next chapter.

After being influenced by the bursa or thymus, the B and T cells reenter the blood and are distributed throughout the body. These cells tend to accumulate in the **peripheral lymphoid tissues**.

PERIPHERAL LYMPHOID TISSUES

The lymph nodes and spleen are the principal peripheral lymphoid organs, but other soft organs, including lung, kidney, tonsil, and appendix, also contain a significant population of lymphocytes. These secondary lymphoid tissues are already functional at birth, thus rendering the animal immunocompetent from that time on. In lymph and lymph nodes the B cells represent about 25% of all the lymphocytes. Spleen and tonsils are balanced with nearly equal numbers of B and T cells. *The lymphocyte population of the blood is dominated by T cells, with the B cell contribution rarely exceeding 30%.* Lymphocytes in the thoracic duct are nearly 100% T cells.

Within these peripheral lymphoid organs, specific homing regions for the T and B cells can often be observed (Fig. 3-3). In lymph nodes and spleen, the B cells tend to inhabit the cortex and the T cells localize in the medullary sinuses. This selected distribution of T and B cells was confirmed by studying thymectomized animals, bursectomized chickens, or patients with selected immunodeficiency diseases (see Chapter 8). Antisera to the specific B- and T-cell markers have been used to determine this distribution.

When seen in the blood on their way from the bone marrow to the bursa or thymus, or as they leave those tissues to circulate, the lymphocytes of the B-

---

MEMORY CHECK 3-2

T lymphocytes

1. Are responsible for cell-mediated aspects of the immune response
2. Are imprinted in the thymus
3. Collect in distinct regions of the peripheral lymphoid tissue
4. Are distinct from B cells and LGL cells
5. Are antigen specific

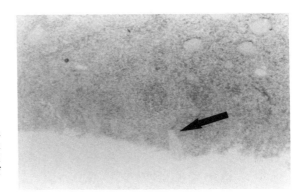

Figure 3-3. This preparation from a human spleen reveals a cluster of lymphocytes in a spherical structure known as a germinal center. (See color figure after Table of Contents.)

and T-cell sets are morphologically indistinguishable.

B-Cell Ontogeny

Although B cells may be morphologically indistinguishable from T cells, their functional differences are significant. These functions depend upon their ability to express different genes. The life history of these cells is interpretable by the appearance and/or loss of proteins that these genes regulate. Such markers of B cells are described here, and those of T cells are found in subsequent chapters.

Different stages of B-cell maturation have been given different names by different authors. It must be remembered that there is a plethora of surface proteins on the B-cell surface. The appearance of a new marker may be important to some observers who deem it necessary to establish a new intermediary in cell differentiation. That very same marker may be ignored by other observers who are focusing on the larger picture of B-cell development.

During fetal life human B-cell differentiation occurs in the liver; in adult life this occurs in the bone marrow. In avian species the bursa is an additional

tissue with a great influence on the B cell.

THE STEM CELL

The earliest recognizable lymphocytes of *both B- and T-cell lineage have the enzyme* **terminal deoxynucleotide transferase (Tdt)**. The stem B cell is recognized by the presence of **Ir gene products**—the DP, DQ, and DR proteins. These MHC proteins are also found on macrophages.

THE PRE-B CELL

The earliest change in a stem cell that places it in the B-cell lineage and separates it from other cells is a reordering of the genes involved in immunoglobulin synthesis (Fig. 3-4). Details of this process are described in Chapter 5, and only a capsule description is presented here. The simplest immunoglobulin molecule is composed of two identical heavy (large) peptide chains and two identical light (small) peptide chains. The heavy chain is encoded by four genes: V, D, J, and C. These genes are located distant from each other in the stem cell, but when this cell moves further into the B-cell lineage *it places the*

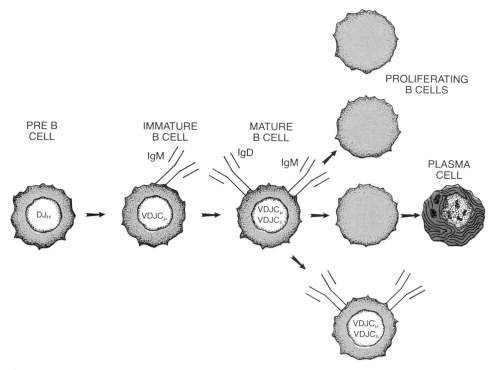

Figure 3–4. Progression of the B cell from its earliest stem cell stage to a plasma cell is shown here, with recordings of its genetic and surface protein adjustments. Notice that one of the earliest events is the formation of the immunoglobulin heavy chain, designated VDJC in the diagram. The terminal cell is a plasma cell.

D and J genes next to each other. This is followed by the *addition of the V gene.* The last step is the addition of the C gene, which is necessary for the synthesis of the H chain of IgM. Because all the genes are now aligned, *the H chain (μ chain) appears in the pre-B cell cytoplasm.*

THE IMMATURE B CELL

Light Chain Gene Rearrangement

In its long pathway to synthesis and secretion of immunoglobulins, the next step in B-cell maturation is *alignment of the light chain genes.* Three genes are used here—the V, J, and a C

gene for the light chain. These V and J genes are different from those used for the heavy chain described previously. Once again in their original position, these genes are not in sequence, but as the pre-B cell matures, the V and J genes are repositioned next to each other. This is followed by addition of the C gene.

Now the light chain genes are transcribed and translated to provide the peptide needed to pair with the μ chain. But two heavy chains and two light chains linked into a four-peptide protein represent only one of five such units needed to form the complete IgM. *This incomplete IgM is not secreted.* It has a sequence of hydrophobic amino acids in its amino end that locks it into the lipids of the cell membrane. This surface, or **sIgM**, is the first immunoglobulin made by the cell, albeit in an incomplete state. Notice that this occurs normally and does not represent a response to contact with antigen.

Immunoglobulin D

The step usually used to reflect the last stage of the immature B cell or the first stage of the mature B cell is the capability to *synthesize IgD*. Only traces of IgD can be found in what some authorities describe as the immature cell, but this quantity increases sharply in the cell level recognized as the mature B cell. Even *when engaged in IgD synthesis the cell does not cease IgM synthesis*. The genetic explanation for this is provided in Chapter 5, but it is of interest because it represents the solitary phase in the life of a B cell when it will make two different antibodies simultaneously.

An interesting aspect of this duality of immunoglobulin production is that *the antigen-combining parts of the IgD and IgM are the same*. This is part of the molecules controlled by the VDJ portion of the heavy chain and the VJ portion of the light chain. Because of the specificity of this part of an antibody molecule for a single epitope it has been given the special name **idiotype**. IgM and IgD are idiotypic proteins. These proteins serve as receptors for antigen offered by macrophages or other APC.

THE MATURE B CELL

The mature B cell now expresses both IgM and IgD on its surface in addition to the DP, DQ, and DR class II MHC proteins. By this stage, the Tdt enzyme has been lost. In its earlier stages of development certain proteins of unknown function such as CD10 have

been transiently present. Other markers not directly associated with the functional maturation of the B cell as an immunoglobulin-producing cell have also appeared.

Fcγ Receptor

A protein rarely found on T cells but found on the earliest recognized B cell is a receptor for IgG. This receptor binds to the heavy or γ chain of IgG. Moreover, it binds to a special section of the γ chain known as the Fc fragment. Hence, it is called Fcγ receptor, or FcγR. *The FcγR molecule is present on all later stages of B-cell development*. There are FcγR molecules on macrophages as well.

Complement Receptors

Four different proteins have been identified as complement receptors (see Chapter 6 for details). *Complement receptor 1 (CR1) and CR2 are both present on B cells*. CR1 (CD35) and CR2 (CD21) each preferentially bind C3b and its further degradation products. C4b of the complement system is also bound to these receptors. The function of CR1 on B cells is not known. *CR2 is the gateway used by the Epstein-Barr virus to enter B cells*. It may also have a role in immunoregulation of B cells.

Other Proteins

Other proteins are found on B cells. **MHC class I proteins** are found on pre-B cells. A number of CD markers appear at different times during maturation, including **CD11c, 19, 20, 23 (the Fcε receptor), CD45,** and numerous others. The function of many of these proteins is not known. Proteins that are useful in identifying neoplastic lymphocytes (leukemia) are the **B4 and**

CALLA (CD10) proteins discussed in Chapter 10.

MEMORY CHECK 3–3

◆

In B-cell ontogeny

1. The stem cell is undifferentiated

2. The pre-B cell rearranges its heavy chain genes

3. The immature cell produces a surface IgM

4. Mature cells produce IgM and IgD

5. Numerous surface markers—FcγR, CR, MHC class II proteins, and others—appear on the cell surface

---

The B-Cell Response to Antigen

CAPPING

After coating itself with IgM and IgD, the B cell is prepared to receive antigen. Combination of antigen with the immunoglobulin occurs at widely separated foci on the cell surface. (This can be determined by using fluorescent microscopy and an antigen that is labeled with a fluorescein dye.) Later the *antigen-antibody complexes coalesce to form an aggregate*, which, seen in profile on the perimeter of the cell, *gives the appearance of a cap*—the capping phenomenon. The antigen is then interiorized.

BIOCHEMISTRY

This contact with antigen catalyzes a series of enzyme transformations seen also in other activated cells—macrophages, neutrophils, T cells, and mast cells, to name a few. These changes include the *degradation of phosphatidylinositol 4,5-bisphosphate to several less-phosphorylated intermediates, the influx of Ca²⁺ into the cell, and the activation of protein kinase C.* It is not clear how these adjustments in cell metabolism are linked to B-cell differentiation into plasma cells. Nevertheless, the resting B cell is stimulated to enter the G1 phase of the cell growth cycle. At this stage, *the cell is influenced by T-cell–derived interleukins* to continue through S and G2 phases of the growth cycle and becomes a plasma cell.

INTERLEUKINS AFFECTING B CELLS

Interleukins produced by macrophages and T cells regulate several aspects of B-cell metabolism. Seldom are these interleukins limited to interaction with B cells, but other cell targets for these leukohormones are not considered here (Table 3–2).

Interleukin 1

Interleukin 1 (IL-1), secreted by macrophages, is described in Chapter 1 as a key agent in the activation of T cells, but IL-1 is also a growth factor for B cells.

Interleukin 2

The first T-cell interleukin to be described, interleukin 2 (IL-2) was originally called the **T-cell growth factor (TCGF)**, a peptide that cooperated with antigen to stimulate T-cell proliferation. **IL-2** is a 15,000-Mr protein that also contributes to B-cell metamorphosis into plasma cells. A receptor for IL-2 on T cells has been intensively studied

Table 3-2
INTERLEUKINS AFFECTING B CELLS

Agent	Cell Source*	Mr	Function
IL-1	Macrophages	15,000	T-cell but also B-cell growth factor
IL-2	T cells	15,000	T-cell growth factor but aids B-cell shift to plasma cell
IL-3	T cells	19,000	Uncertain (maturation?)
IL-4	T cells	20,000	B-cell stimulatory factor; promotes IgE synthesis
IL-5	T cells	13,000	B-cell growth factor; promotes IgA synthesis
IL-6	T cells	26,000	B-cell stimulatory factor 2; aids plasma cell formation

*Many cells produce interleukins; only the dominant producing cell is listed.

because this receptor, known as the Tac antigen, is present only on T-activated cells.

Interleukin 3

Interleukin 3 (IL-3) was originally defined as a T-cell product that *induces the expression of the* **enzyme 20 α steroid dehydrogenase (20 α SDH),** an enzyme believed to be a marker of mature T cells. It is now agreed that *the enzyme is present in other cells,* both mature and immature, and that a pronounced expression of 20 α SDH may follow exposure to other proteins, particularly GM-CSF and M-CSF. IL-3 now appears to have a multi-CSF function, and it is described in that context in Chapter 2.

Interleukin 4

Activated T cells secrete a 20,000-Mr protein that stimulates the growth of B cells **(B-cell–stimulating factor, or BSF1)** and is also active on T cells, granulocytes, and mast cells. **IL-4** may be produced only by one of the two subsets of T helper cells. *IL-4 is important in regulating the switch to IgE formation and in the expression of MHC class II proteins.* The latter is important in fostering B- and T-cell cooperation in the immune response.

Interleukin 5

The T cell that produces IL-4 also produces **IL-5.** IL-5 has several synonyms including **T-cell–replacing factor (TCRF) and B-cell growth factor II.** IL-5 is a peptide of only 13,000 Mr that promotes the conversion of B cells to IgA-synthesizing plasma cells.

Interleukin 6

B-cell–stimulating factor 2 (BSF2) and interferon β2 (IFN β2) are synonyms of IL-6, another T-cell peptide of low molecular weight (26,000 Mr). IL-6 is apparently *most active in the later stages of B-cell transformation* to plasma cells.

Interleukin 7

A recently derived seventh interleukin **(IL-7)** has been isolated from bone marrow and thymus stromal cells. This 25,000-Mr glycoprotein acts on early (those still lacking surface IgM) **but not mature B cells** as a growth stimulator. It is also a growth stimulant for immature—but not mature—T cells.

Interleukin 8

A monocyte-derived peptide of approximately 75,000 Mr that serves as a **chemotaxin for T cells,** has been labeled interleukin 8 **(IL-8)**. Its effect on B cells is uncertain.

Interleukin 9

Interleukin 9 **(IL-9)** was originally known as **T-cell growth factor III**. It stimulates the growth of **activated T cells** but has little effect on resting state T cells. IL-9 is a 36,000-Mr glycoprotein of which the protein accounts for only 14,150 Mr. It is secreted by CD4$^+$ T cells.

Interleukin 10

A B-cell–derived product that causes **proliferation of immature T cells** in a cooperative role with other interleukins has been renamed interleukin 10. **IL-10** induces T-cell growth but not T-cell maturation.

The role of several of these newly described interleukins on B-cell growth and maturation is yet to be determined; they are included here to make the discussion of interleukins complete.

PLASMA CELLS

The plasma cell is about the same diameter as its progenitor B cell and has a similar, large, rounded nucleus. Its cytoplasm, however, is unlike the featureless B-cell cytoplasm. *The plasma cell has an extensive rough endoplasmic reticulum, the ribosomal depository typical of cells actively engaged in protein synthesis.* The protein, of course, is immunoglobulin. Unlike the earlier cells, plasma cells not only synthesize immunoglobulins but also secrete them. However, a single plasma cell does not secrete all structural forms of immunoglobulin. The process of immunoglobulin class switching locks the plasma cell into production of a single immunoglobulin.

CLASS SWITCHING

Class switching requires that the plasma cell select a heavy chain C gene to which it is committed for the remainder of its life. Some cells will choose between IgM and IgD but others will change to IgG, IgA, or IgE. Moreover, for IgG and IgA one of the subclasses will be selected. Some *plasma cells, affected by IL-6, will make IgG1, whereas others, influenced by IFNγ, will make IgG2. IgA production is influenced positively by IL-5 and IgE by IL-4* (Fig. 3–5).

Thus, *the only antigen-driven phase in B-cell maturation is the simultaneous conversion to plasma cells and class switching.* This is influenced by lymphokines produced by T cells in the response to TD antigens.

MEMORY CHECK 3–4

The B-cell response to antigen

1. Begins with antigen capping and interiorization
2. Involves biochemical changes in phosphatidylinositol and a cellular influx of calcium
3. Requires the assistance of numerous interleukins from T cells
4. Results in a conversion to a plasma cell
5. Locks the plasma cell into production of a single molecular form of immunoglobulin

---

The Response of B Cells to Mitogens

Agents that initiate cell proliferation and differentiation are termed **mitogens**. B cells are sensitive to a number

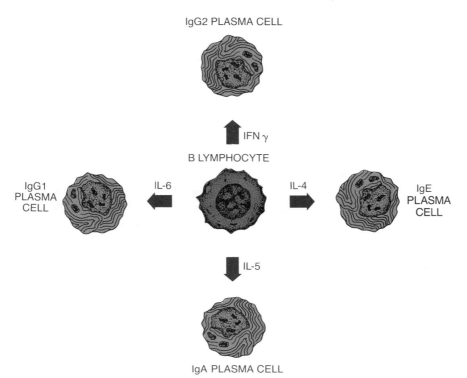

IgG2 PLASMA CELL

IFN γ

B LYMPHOCYTE

IgG1 PLASMA CELL   IL-6   IL-4   IgE PLASMA CELL

IL-5

IgA PLASMA CELL

Figure 3–5. Several interleukins influence the switch from the B cell to the immunoglobulin-secreting plasma cell.

of these agents from such diverse sources as kidney beans, bacteria, and T lymphocytes (Table 3–3). The mitogens from T cells are more typically referred to as interleukins, whose activity is best demonstrated as a cooperative endeavor with antigen to promote antibody synthesis.

LIPOPOLYSACCHARIDE (LPS)

Lipopolysaccharide (LPS) is a surface structure of most gram-negative bacteria generally described as its O, or somatic, antigen. There are slight variations in the structure of LPS in the cell wall of different bacteria, but all LPS

Table 3–3
MITOGENS AFFECTING B CELLS

Agent	Source	Mr
Lipopolysaccharide	Gram-negative bacteria	About 4000
Protein A	Strains of *Staphylococcus aureus*	42,000
Pokeweed mitogen	*Phytolacca* species	32,000
IgM	B cells	950,000
Phytohemagglutinin A	*Phaseolus* beans	115,000–140,000

molecules have a common structure consisting of a lipid, lipid A, linked to a polysaccharide core and immersed in the lipids of the cell membrane. From the polysaccharide core additional sugars provide the antigenic specificity characteristic of an individual bacterial cell. LPS is a toxin, the endotoxin of the bacterial cell that is released upon its death. The toxic activity of LPS resides in the lipid A portion of the molecule.

Also *present in the lipid A portion of LPS is its mitogenic property.* LPS is primarily a stimulant of B lymphocytes, and T cells are relatively unaffected. Typical of the properties of several mitogens, *LPS stimulates all B cells (is polyclonal)* regardless of their antigen specificity. Many different antibodies are produced as a result of this activation.

PROTEIN A

On the surface of 80% of all human isolates of *Staphylococcus aureus* there is a 42,000-Mr protein that reacts with the Fc portion of immunoglobulin G. This protein, protein A, has four combining sites for IgG. Many B cells have IgG on their surface, and this IgG is then bridged by protein A. This linkage of two surface molecules with a single ligand activates the B cell. Again, *protein A is a polyclonal B-cell stimulant.*

ANTI-IgM

Antibody to IgM on the B-cell surface is considered one of the most natural of the "artificial" stimulants. Antigen, as the cell stimulant through sIgM, is duplicated by anti-IgM. Once again, it is the combination of anti-IgM with two IgM molecules that is responsible for its activity. Anti-IgD could be used for this purpose, but anti-IgM is easier to prepare because of its more abundant antigen source.

OTHER MITOGENS

Pokeweed contains a protein that can be purified and used to activate both B and T cells. Pokeweed mitogen is considered to be *a lectin and to react with specific saccharides on the B-cell surface,* but these sugars have not been fully identified. **PHA, or phytohemagglutinin,** from red or yellow kidney beans, also activates both B and T cells. N-acetyl-D-galactosamine is the receptor for PHA. **Phorbol myristate,** a tumor-inducing lipid, is an interesting mitogen because it mimics one of the products of phosphatidylinositol metabolism that is formed after antigen stimulation of B cells.

MEMORY CHECK 3-5

The mitogen
1. LPS is a polyclonal B-cell mitogen
2. Protein A activates only B cells bearing IgG on their surface
3. Anti-IgM stimulates immature B cells
4. Pokeweed activates both B and T cells
5. Phorbol myristate activates via a mechanism similar to that of antigen

---

Immunoglobulin Response

The elaboration of immunoglobulins into the blood is clearly a complicated process involving macrophage process-

Table 3-4
COMPARISON OF THE PRIMARY AND SECONDARY
IMMUNOGLOBULIN RESPONSES

	Primary	Secondary
Time after antigen to detect immunoglobulin	5–15 days	2–4 days
First immunoglobulin detected	IgM	IgM and IgG
Major immunoglobulin	IgM and IgG	IgG
Titer achieved	Low	High
Duration of titer	Short	Long

ing and presentation of antigen, induction of interleukin synthesis by T cells, and the conversion of B cells into antibody-secreting plasma cells. The appearance of immunoglobulins in the blood falls into one of two kinetic patterns, depending upon whether it is the first (primary) or a subsequent (secondary) exposure to antigen (Table 3–4).

THE PRIMARY RESPONSE

Approximately *5 to 14 days after exposure to an antigen,* immunoglobulins that react specifically with that antigen can be detected in the blood. The synthesis of these globulins begins almost immediately after delivery of the antigen, but the initial few molecules are difficult to detect with the methods available. Moreover, residual antigen combines with these first antibody molecules to form immune complexes, which cloak the immunoglobulin with antigen. This makes the detection of antibody tenuous unless special methods are used to free the antibody molecules from the antigen.

Following the initial lag, a steady increase in the serum concentration (titer) of antibody can be observed. *The antibody titer reaches a peak and then declines.* The kinetics of this will vary according to the nature, quantity, and route of antigen injection; the health and responsiveness of the immunized person; the sensitivity of the testing methods; and whether or not adjuvants are used (Fig. 3–6).

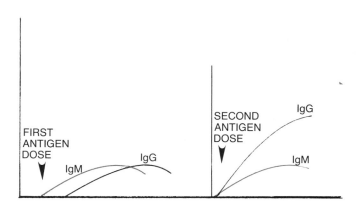

Figure 3-6. A comparison of the primary and secondary immunoglobulin responses illustrates the dominance of IgM in the former and IgG in the latter.

THE SECONDARY RESPONSE

When a second injection of antigen is given after a primary response has been observed, the antibody titer follows a quite different time frame from that initially observed. The **booster or secondary response** has in its beginning *a brief negative phase* in which the antibody titer decreases as the antibody molecules complex with the newly injected antigen. *Thereafter, an accelerated outpouring of antibody* into the blood causes a sharp increase in titer. This *elevated titer is much higher* than in the primary response and persists longer. This booster response *can be repeated periodically* to hold the antibody titer in an elevated condition.

Differences in the contribution of IgM and IgG to the primary and secondary (anamnestic) responses are responsible for the kinetics of the responses. The IgM and IgG contributions following the primary injection of antigen are similar in quantity, though IgM may appear a little earlier than IgG. In the anamnestic response, IgM again appears quickly but does not exceed the quantity seen in the primary response. In contrast the IgG titer becomes 10- to 100-fold greater than in the primary response. Because of the biologic half-life of only 8 days for IgM, its titer decays rapidly. In contrast, IgG has a half-life of 29 days, and since it is the dominant globulin in the booster response, the secondary curve has a protracted decay time.

Other than the fact that the booster effect can increase antibody levels well above the quantity that might be needed for resistance to tetanus, diphtheria, whooping cough, and so on, there are other important features to this response. Foremost is that the booster response can be reinitiated many times, even months or years after a primary series of antigen injec-

tions. Consequently, a person who has allowed his or her immunization program to lapse can recover a high level of immunity often after a single booster injection of antigen. Unknown periodic encounters with antigens of infectious organisms in nature often serve to hold the antibody titers in an elevated state. Although serious allergic reactions may follow subsequent injections of fluid antigens into a person, the immunizing agents used in human medicine have been highly purified and field-tested to prevent such occurrences.

MEMORY CHECK 3-6
◆

In the immunoglobulin response

1. IgM is the first antibody found in the blood
2. A lag of 5 to 15 days follows exposure to antigen before antibody is detectable
3. IgG is described as the anamnestic antibody
4. The titer in the anamnestic response is higher and of greater duration than in the primary response
5. Adjuvants are useful in prolonging the response to antigen

---

GERMINAL CENTERS

The serum antibody response to injections of antigen mirrors the unseen cytologic events in progress within lymphoid tissues. B-cell germinal centers in the cortical regions of lymph nodes and spleen begin to appear as the antigen injections are repeated. *These germinal centers contain a mixture of macrophages and T cells, with B cells in transition to becoming plasma cells.* Each clone of cells represents the progeny of a single B cell which has responded to a single antigenic determinant in the antigen. Memory cells appear that keep the individual primed for an anamnestic response upon a new encounter with antigen.

ADJUVANT EFFECTS

The immunoglobulin response is significantly improved by the inclusion of adjuvants in the immunizing program. Many successful adjuvants are emulsifiers that form an emulsion with antigen and from which the antigen is slowly released. This protracted release mimics what would be accomplished by regular daily boosters with small quantities of antigen. Adjuvants that precipitate or insolubilize antigens function in the same manner but may also improve antigen processing. Oil emulsions, calcium phosphate, calcium hydroxide, and alum are examples of delayed-release adjuvants. LPS, beryllium salts, vitamin A, and mycobacteria act directly upon lymphocytes either as physiologic stimulants or by trapping and holding these cells in lymph nodes where they are in close contact with other important cells. Owing to the toxicity of LPS and to granuloma formation provoked by beryllium and mycobacteria, these are not used in human medicine.

B-Cell Hybridomas

Immunization of an intact animal draws many structural forms of antibody into the blood. When all possible variations in antibody chemistry are considered, 3000 to 4000 different molecular forms of antibody that react with a single epitope of the antigen could be produced. Because most antigens contain several epitopes, each antigen stimulates many plasma cell clones, each responsive to a single epitope and able to produce just one molecular form of antibody. *An antiserum thus reflects a polyclonal plasma cell response.*

Manipulation of B cells in vitro can result in a monoclonal antiserum. This is possible through the **hybridoma technique of Köhler and Milstein**. This technique requires the use of a malignant plasma cell (plasmacytoma or myeloma cell) because this transformed cell will grow well in culture (Fig. 3–7). This cell is then fused with a B cell from an immunized animal. A B cell is unable to grow in culture. During fusion the chromosomes of the cells become mixed. This gives the capability of growth in culture from the plasmacytoma and antibody production from the B cell to this hybrid cell. B cell–B cell hybrids produced during fusion cannot grow, and myeloma–myeloma hybrids are poisoned by components in the medium. The hybridoma cells can grow because the B cells contribute enzymes that detoxify the medium and because they now have the growth properties of the plasmacytoma. *Because the hybridoma is derived from a single B cell, its antibody is restricted to a single molecular form—that is, it is a monoclonal antibody.* Monoclonal antibodies have been very useful in determining the number and location of epitopes on an antigen. They are also useful in analytic quantitative serology because a hybridoma-derived antibody, unlike a polyclonal antiserum, is always the same and does not vary according to time of immunization and antibody harvest.

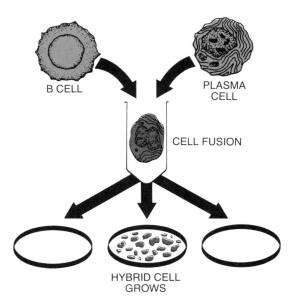

B CELL

PLASMA CELL

CELL FUSION

HYBRID CELL GROWS

Figure 3-7. The ability to harvest a hybridoma cell that is producing an antibody to a single epitope of an antigen depends upon the ability to combine cell growth ability and antibody synthesis from separate cells into the hybridoma.

Large Granular Lymphocytes

The lymphocyte ignored heretofore in this discussion is the **large granular lymphocyte (LGL)**, known also by its synonyms **null cell** and **natural killer (NK) cell**. These cells vary in the distribution of their cell markers at different stages of development or are a true mixed population. Some authors have asserted that all LGLs are not NKs.

Nevertheless, these cells usually *have the unique* **NK1 surface protein** *and the* **asialoganglioside GM1**. LGLs may have FcR for IgG, CD2 that reacts with sheep erythrocytes and LFA-3, and adherence molecules CD11a and CD18. Many interleukins—IL-2, IL-3, IFN, and others—activate these cells.

LGLs behave as natural killer cells on their first encounter with foreign cells, including transplanted cells, tumor cells, or self-cells that have become infected with an intracellular parasite. *LGLs discharge their granules*

upon contact with their target. As these granules dissolve, several proteins bind to the target. The most cytotoxic of these is **perforin**, which creates a hole in the target cell membrane. Other potential contributors to death of the target include seven proteases called **granzymes**. Perforin is of interest because it is chemically like one of the complement molecules that dissolves cell membranes. Recently it has been shown that antibodies to granzymes protect target cells against lysis.

References

del Guercio, P and Cruse, JM (eds): B Lymphocytes: Function and regulation. S Karger, Basel, 1989.

Hamblin, AS: Lymphokines. IRL Press, Oxford, 1988.

Kipps, TJ: The CD5 B cell. Adv Immunol 47:117, 1989.

Kishimoto, T: Factors, receptors, and signals for B lymphocyte activation. Prog Allergy 42:280, 1988.

Kishimoto, T and Hirano, T: Molecular regulation of B lymphocyte response. Annu Rev Immunol 6:485, 1988.

Marchalonis, JJ (ed): The Lymphocyte: Structure and Function, ed 2. Marcel Dekker, New York, 1988.

Takatsu, K: B-cell growth and differentiation factors, Proc Soc Exp Biol Med 188:243, 1988.

Trinchieri, G: Biology of natural killer cells. Adv Immunol 47:187, 1989.

Vitetta, ES, et al: Cellular interactions on the humoral immune response. Adv Immunol 45:1, 1989.

Weigle, WO: Factors and events in the activation, proliferation, and differentiation of B cells, CRC Crit Rev Immunol 7:285, 1987.

QUESTIONS AND ANSWERS

1. The earliest feature that identifies a lymphocyte as a B cell is
    A. The rearrangement of immunoglobulin heavy chain genes
    B. The rearrangement of immunoglobulin light chain genes
    C. Its appearance in the bursa of Fabricius (or its mammalian equivalent)
    D. The expression of class II MHC proteins on its surface
    E. The expression of class I MHC proteins on its surface

Answer A

The pre-B cell in the bone marrow first identifies itself as of the B-cell lineage by synthesizing μ chains, the heavy chain of IgM. This is followed by formation of the light chain. These two steps, unlike the acquisition of MHC class I and II proteins, are specific for B cells. The B cell that enters the bursa of Fabricius is already beyond the pre-B stage.

2. The transformation of a mature B cell to a plasma cell
    A. Can be accomplished by anti-IgM
    B. Is the natural role of antigen
    C. Requires IL-6 from T cells
    D. Does not alter the antigen specificity of the cell as class switching occurs
    E. All of the above

Answer E

Anti-IgM most closely resembles antigen because it reacts with the antigen receptor. Both answers A and B are correct. B-cell differentiation factor (IL-6) is necessary for plasma cell formation. Once a B cell expresses the capacity to bind to an epitope, it does not deviate from the specificity that its antigen receptor has expressed.

3. Which of the following is *not* true of the booster response?
    A. The titer of IgG exceeds that of IgM.
    B. It cannot be repeated multiple times.
    C. The lag phase is short compared with the primary response.
    D. The antibody titer remains high for a longer time than after the primary response.
    E. Germinal centers that develop contain a large population of plasma cells.

Answer B

The production of large amounts of IgG (answer A) requires the conversion of memory and B cells to plasma cells (answer E) during the anamnestic response.

This IgG appears quickly (answer C) and, since IgG has a 29-day half-life, it maintains an elevated antibody titer (answer D). Answer B is wrong—the booster response can be repeated numerous times during a person's life.

4. The presence of a well-developed endoplasmic reticulum in nonphagocytic mononuclear cells clustered in a germinal center suggests that the cells are
   A. T cells
   B. B cells
   C. Memory cells
   D. Plasma cells
   E. Null cells

Answer D

Neither T nor B cells are highly active in protein synthesis and do not contain much, if any, rough endoplasmic reticulum. Likewise, memory cells are essentially resting, nonsynthetic cells that cannot be recognized morphologically. Null cells may be found in lymphoid tissues but are not expanded in germinal centers. Their cytoplasmic granules are varied in function and structure.

5. The T-cell interleukin, especially required for the conversion of a mature B cell to a plasma cell, is
   A. IL-1
   B. IL-2
   C. IL-4
   D. IL-5
   E. IL-6

Answer E

Although most interleukins are pleiotropic, the primary role of IL-6, with its synonym of B-cell differentiating factor (BCDF), is to cause the B-cell–to–plasma-cell transformation. IL-2 is the T-cell growth factor, IL-4 is a B-cell stimulating factor, and IL-5 is a B-cell growth factor. IL-1 is not a T-cell product; it is produced by monocytes and macrophages.

Case Study: Immunoblastic Disease

Tom, a 29-year-old man, had been treated with aspirin and steroids for the past 7 years to control rheumatoid arthritis. During a routine annual medical examination, he was found to have extensive, peripheral lymphadenopathy. Splenomegaly, hepatomegaly, and a mediastinal mass were noted on further physical examination. Peripheral blood counts and differential were normal, as were serum protein and immunoglobulin levels. Liver function test results were abnormal. A lymph node biopsy revealed large (16 to 25 μm) cells with a basophilic-staining cytoplasm, many of which were undergoing mitosis. Because these were classified as lymphoid tumor cells, therapy was initiated immediately.

Questions

1. What is the nature of the lymphoid cell seen in this case?

2. What forms of lymphoid cell neoplasia must be considered here?

3. What are the differential diagnostic features of an immunocytologic nature?

4. What is the therapy for these diseases?

Discussion

Immunoblasts, the cells seen in this patient, are large cells ranging to 25 μm in diameter. They have an abundant cytoplasm and many ribosomes but little endoplasmic reticulum. They stain well with basic dyes such as pyronine. These cells normally arise from lymphocytes after an antigenic or mitogenic stimulus (ie, they are lymphocytes in an active state of cell growth that cannot progress to the plasma cell stage).

Immunoblastic proliferation is observed in several clinical settings. Patients with autoimmune diseases such as rheumatoid arthritis or lupus erythematosus may display an abnormal number of immunoblasts in their peripheral blood, but these are usually considered nonmalignant unless found widespread throughout lymphoid organs. Another nonmalignant condition that presents atypical lymphocytes is infectious mononucleosis. Among the malignancies, Waldenström's macroglobulinemia, Burkitt's lymphoma, acute lymphoid immunoblastic leukemia, immunoblastic sarcoma, and reticulosarcoma all have abnormal-appearing lymphoid cells. Although the therapy for these conditions varies somewhat from one to the other and depends on both the stage of the malignancy and the physician's preference, a combination of cytotoxic drugs such as methotrexate, cyclophosphamide, and vincristine with irradiation and surgery is common. The patient presented here was diagnosed as having immunoblastic lymphosarcoma (ILS) and treated with cyclophosphamide, irradiation, and surgery.

The cell in ILS is easily confused with that found in Burkitt's lymphoma. Both are heavily pyroninophilic. Burkitt's cells have exclusively B-cell characteristics and demonstrate the Epstein-Barr virus genome. ILS cells may express either B- or T-cell markers, or neither; therefore, the use of immunocytologic methods is not always contributory to the diagnosis, although such tests as those for cell-bound IgM antibody or IgD antibody, or both, should be conducted.

GLOSSARY

B cell   A lymphocyte that matures in the bursa of Fabricius or its mammalian equivalent.

bursa of Fabricius   A cloacal organ in fowl where the immunoglobulin-producing B cells mature.

capping phenomenon   The movement of dispersed antigens on the surface of the B cell to a single locus.

central lymphoid tissue   Bone marrow, thymus, and bursa of Fabricius.

class switching   A shift of IgM-IgD–synthesizing B cells to the synthesis of only one of IgG, IgM, IgA, IgD, or IgE.

GALT   Gut-associated lymphoid tissue.

interleukin 1   A monokine that activates B and T cells and stimulates B-cell proliferation.

interleukin 4   A T-cell product that stimulates B-cell proliferation, also known as B-cell growth factor.

interleukin 5   A T-cell product that stimulates B cells to become IgA-synthesizing plasma cells.

interleukin 6   A T-cell product that stimulates B-cell differentiation into plasma cells.

mitogen   An agent that stimulates cell mitosis.

plasma cell   The end cell of B-cell differentiation that is an active immunoglobulin-synthesizing cell.

CHAPTER 4

◆

The Lymphocytes: Part 2
T Lymphocytes

As will be recalled from the introductory section of the last two chapters, primitive cells in the fetal liver and bone marrow are the first recognizable cells of the lymphocyte lineage. Those cells that are destined to become T cells are endowed in the thymus with unique abilities that separate them from B cells. Upon their departure from the thymus, the adult T cells reenter the blood, pass through tissues, and collect in the lymphatic system, much as do the B lymphocytes. The circulatory path is completed when the T cells enter the thoracic duct and then the circulatory system, and begin another cycle.

In this chapter, the maturation of T cells after they leave the bone marrow is correlated with the new surface proteins these cells produce. The influence of hormones produced in the thymus on this process is also described. These surface markers are useful in classifying T cells according to their four major subsets—the helper, delayed-type hypersensitivity, cytotoxic, and suppressor cells. Each of these T-cell types produces a receptor that allows it to respond to antigen, and each produces interleukins specific for its own T-cell type.

In the final paragraphs of this chapter, the sensitivity of lymphocytes to immunosuppressive agents is described. This discussion is integrated with the natural control of the immune response via feedback inhibition and the idiotypic network.

T-Cell Ontogeny

T-cell development, like that of B cells, has been determined by the migration of these cells to the thymus and other organs from the bone marrow. Particularly in the thymus the appearance, sometimes transiently, of novel surface proteins is used to gauge the maturity of the cell. The T-cell pathway begins in the seventh week of gestation when cells recognizable as *T-cell precursors can be found in the human fetus. These cells are Tdt positive* and are later found in the bone marrow. Between the seventh and fourteenth weeks of gestation critical *events in the thymus mark the T cells* as different from other lymphocytes. These thymocytes begin to express characteristics shared with other cell lines, and eventually of unique T-cell markers.

EARLY CORTICAL THYMOCYTES

When the T cells first arrive in the thymus they tend to collect in the cortical region of the gland (Fig. 4-1). They may already express the CD7 and

CD38 proteins. **CD7** *is not specific for T cells*, it is also found on NK cells and some cells of the myeloid series. Although *CD7 persists through all later maturation stages, its function is not known* (Table 4-1). Likewise, CD38 is not unique to T cells, being found on plasma cells and myeloid cells as well. These early thymocytes will also produce CD5, CD9, and CD10. CD5 is found on all normal T cells, and on some malignant B-cell lines. CD9 is not specific for T cells; it is found on early B cells. **CD10** *is the common acute lymphoblastic leukemia antigen* (**CALLA**) found at different stages of malignant transformation in both T and B cells. *The first unique T-cell marker to appear is the CD2 protein, followed by* **CD3** (Fig. 4-2).

The CD2 Protein

The CD2 protein is a 50,000-Mr glycoprotein originally known as the **sheep red blood cell receptor**. Adhesion of T cells to sheep erythrocytes (T cell rosetting) was an early technique used to enumerate T cells, and to purify them from B cells. A more natural function of **CD2** *is as a receptor for* **leukocyte functional antigen 3 (LFA-3)**, *also known as* **CD58**. LFA-3 is present on thymic epithelial cells and leukocytes. Binding of T cells to leukocytes facilitates the transfer of IL-1 and antigen when the LFA-3-positive leuko-

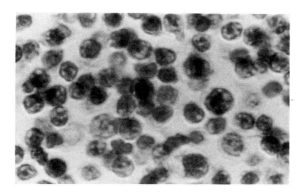

Figure 4-1. In the thymus, a dense population of lymphocytes—largely T cells—is detectable in tissue specimens. (See color figure after Table of Contents.)

Table 4–1
SELECTED CD PROTEINS PRESENT ON LYMPHOCYTES

CD Protein	Distribution	Function
CD7	T cells, LGL, and others	Unknown
CD5	T and B cells	Uncertain
CD2	T cells	Receptor for LFA-3
CD3	T cells	Cooperates with TCR
CD4	T cells	Recognize class II MHC protein
CD8	T cells	Recognize class I MHC protein
CD10	T and B cells	Common acute lymphoblastic leukemia marker
CD25	T and B cells, monocytes	IL-2 receptor

cyte is a macrophage. It is believed that adhesion of the young T cell to the cortical thymic epithelium serves to concentrate the T cells at the source of thymic hormones needed for their maturation. Some of these thymic hormones are discussed subsequently.

The CD3 Protein

A second protein, **CD3**, soon appears on these cortical thymocytes. This protein is a complex of three peptides: γ of 25,000 Mr, δ of 20,000 Mr, and ϵ of 20,000 Mr. Two additional peptides are believed to be a part of this complex. Initially *it was believed that CD3 was* *the T-cell receptor* for antigen, but this concept was denied by the observation that all sources of CD3 were structurally identical. Since this lacked agreement with the diversity of structure needed to give the antigen receptor selectivity, this idea was discarded. Further study indicated that *CD3 was intimately associated with the antigen receptor and functioned as a signal transducer* to the interior of the cell.

The CD3 peptides are closely interlaced at the foot of a dimeric protein that forms at about the same time as CD3. This new protein is the *antigen receptor for T cells* (Fig. 4–3). There are, in fact, two different forms of this

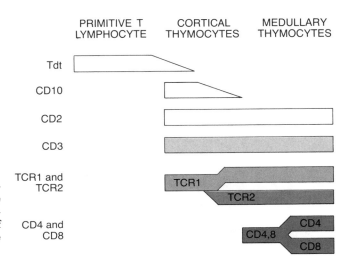

Figure 4–2. Numerous cell surface proteins are present on the T-cell surface. This diagram relates the appearance and loss of several surface markers to the stage of T-cell development.

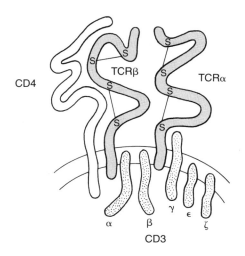

CD4

TCRβ

TCRα

γ ε

α   β   ζ

CD3

Figure 4–3. Details of the CD3-TCR association are indicated in this illustration. Notice that the CD3 protein consists potentially of five separate peptides, and the TCR protein of two peptides.

receptor. The *earliest to appear is* **TCR1**, *a dimer of the* γ *and* δ *peptides.* Slightly *later, on a separate population of cells,* **TCR2** appears. TCR2 is chemically similar to TCR1 but is composed of two different peptides, α and β. The TCR2-positive cells also express the CD4 and CD8 proteins.

MEDULLARY THYMOCYTES

In the medulla, the dually CD4- and CD8-positive cells now segregate into singly CD4- or CD8-positive cells. This division is approximately 65% CD4 and 35% CD8 (Table 4–2).

CD4-Positive Cells

The CD4 molecule is approximately 55,000 Mr and is found, with some exceptions, on T cells that interact with macrophages, and B cells, both of which express MHC class II proteins. **CD4** *is thought to engage with the class II protein on the antigen-presenting cell* so that, like the CD2–LFA-3 system, the antigen message and IL-1 are inescapably passed to the T cell. Antibodies to CD4 interfere sharply with this interaction. These *CD4-positive T cells are of two separate subsets—the* **helper (or T$_H$) cells** *and those that participate in* **delayed-type hypersensitivity (T$_{DTH}$ cells)**.

Table 4–2
IMPORTANT T-CELL MARKERS

CD Protein	Mr	Function
CD2	50,000	Ligand for LFA-3 and sheep erythrocytes
CD3	γ25,000	Cooperative transducer with TCR
	δ20,000	
	ε20,000	
CD4	55,000	Class II recognition aid on T$_H$ and T$_{DTH}$ cells, HIV receptor
CD8	32,000 dimer	Class I recognition aid on T$_C$ and T$_S$ cells
IL-2R	33,000 Mr polymerizes	Receptor for IL-2, synonym of Tac antigen
TCR1	γ ≈ 40,000 Mr	Antigen receptor
	δ ≈ 40,000 Mr	
TCR2	α ≈ 40,000 Mr	Antigen receptor
	β ≈ 40,000 Mr	

The CD4 protein is the entryway for the virus that causes AIDS. Replication of the virus within the helper T cell destroys the role of this cell in the immune response.

CD8-Positive Cells

The CD8 molecule is about 33,000 Mr and readily polymerizes in solution. In lower animals, two peptides are a part of CD8 but as yet only one human CD8 peptide is known. **CD8-positive T cells,** *like the CD4 T cells, are also divisible into two groups*—**the suppressor (T_S) and cytotoxic (T_C) cells.** T_C cells are also known as cytotoxic lymphocytes (CTL) or cytotoxic T cells (CTC). *CD8-positive cells interact with cells that present antigen in the context of MHC class I proteins.* Again, like CD4, CD8 is believed to cement the T cell with class I–positive cells. The assignment of human CD8-positive cells as cytotoxic cells is a useful convenience, even though it is known that human CD4 cells may also be cytotoxic. The separation of functions of CD4 and CD8 cells is more constant in lower animal species.

MEMORY CHECK 4–1
◆

The development of T cell(s)

1. Into mature T cells is accomplished in the thymus
2. Markers CD2 and CD3 in the thymic cortex is the first expression of specific T-cell proteins
3. Antigen receptors TCR1 and TCR2 occurs in the cortical-medullary transition period
4. In the thymic medulla leads to the functional division of CD4-positive and CD8-positive cells.

INFLUENCE OF THYMIC HORMONES

Under the influence of cellular and molecular forces, the immature T cell undergoes maturation and differentiation within the thymus. Several **regulatory peptides (hormones)** are potentially involved in this transformation, including thymosin, thymopoietin, thymulin, and several others.

Thymosins

Thymosin α1 is one of the most active of 20 or more proteins extracted from the thymus and collectively labeled as thymosins. Among the activities of thymosin α1 are stimulation of the CD2 concentration on T cells, increasing T-cell sensitivity to concanavalin A, restoring T-cell activities to T-cell–deficient mice, and increasing the number of helper T cells. Additional thymosins α7 and β4 may supplement the α1 peptide.

Thymulin

A small peptide only 859 Mr, either concentrated or synthesized in Hassall's corpuscles of the thymus, is a second potential thymic hormone. This peptide, **thymulin**, inhibits the development of suppressor T cells, increases other T-cell activities in T-cell–deficient animals, and increases the number of cells that respond to concanavalin A.

Thymopoietin II

The Tdt-positive progenitors of T cells lose this enzyme when exposed to **thymopoietin.** This hormone of 5562 Mr is a product of the thymic epithelium. Thymopoietin induces the synthesis of characteristic surface proteins of T cells, and as such must be considered a thymic hormone.

Other Thymic Peptides

A few additional peptides found in the blood or in thymus extracts have been purified sufficiently to distinguish them from the aforementioned peptides. Thymic humoral factor, thymic replacing factor, and other thymosins are within this group of potential T-cell maturation factors. Although many of these hormones have been isolated from mouse or bovine thymus, few studies have been made with human tissues.

The T-Cell Receptors

The antigen receptor on T cells was originally known as the Ti protein. This receptor consisted of two peptides —the α and β peptides. Subsequently, a second variation of the antigen receptor was recognized on T cells and its peptides were designated the γ and δ peptides. Because this second receptor appeared earlier in T-cell ontogeny, it became known as T-cell receptor 1 (TCR1) and the α/β receptor became TCR2. Variations in the structure of these proteins provide antigen specificity to the T cells.

TCR PEPTIDES

The four peptides α, β, γ, and δ are closely related structurally. Each is a glycoprotein of approximately 40,000 to 50,000 Mr. Each is a structure whose *amino acid sequence is compartmented into discrete domains.* The **constant (C) domain**, so named because its sequence is essentially identical within all α chains, within all β chains, and so forth, is itself divisible into three regions. The carboxy terminal 5 to 15 amino acids are its cytoplasmic tail, after which progressing toward the cell exterior there is a transmembrane re-

gion of approximately 20 to 30 amino acids. The largest sector of the C domains usually exceeds 90 amino acids, within which *a disulfide loop of about 60 to 70 amino acids is regularly present.*

The next major segment of the TCR is the variable domain, but prior to that domain there is a small sector of 40 to 60 amino acids, usually subdivided *into the* **D and J segments**, *which may or may not incorporate one or more* **N regions**. The N regions are small areas where nucleotide excisions vary the number of amino acids that span this region. The sum of D, J, and N is to provide a link between the C and variable domains. These also provide a unique specificity to each peptide since the *D, J, and N, regions are inconstant in amino acid sequence* from one specimen to another.

The D-J-N bridge is followed by *a region of the greatest amino acid diversity* from one peptide to another, and is logically described as **the variable (V) domain**. The V domain is always about 100 amino acids in length and includes a disulfide bond loop of about 60 amino acids. This V domain is a critical domain that provides antigen specificity

---

MEMORY CHECK 4–2

The T-cell receptor

1. That appears first is the TCR1, γ/δ receptor
2. That appears second is the TCR2, α/β receptor
3. Has specific domains of constant and variable amino acid sequence
4. Variable domain consists of D, J, N, and V regions
5. Is a member of the immunoglobulin superfamily

to the TCR proteins. As mentioned, it is assisted in this by variations in the D, J, and N sequences.

The structure of the TCR proteins is reminiscent of that seen in the immunoglobulins with their major V and C domains. The TCR proteins are placed with a number of other proteins (Chapter 5) in the immunoglobulin supergene family.

T-CELL DIVERSITY

The capability of the total T-cell population in an individual to recognize an enormous number of antigenic specificities is easily calculated from a few basic assumptions. If the α peptide is formed from a supply of 60 V and 40 J domains, the product is 2400. Then presume the β peptide is varied by approximately 30 V domains, 2 D domains, and 12 J domains, for a total of 720 variations. The α/β chain product is 2400×720 or 1.7×10^6 variations. The addition of γ/δ possibilities extends this number to about 10^{15} epitope specificities. Though these calculations are hypothetical, if accepted as valid estimates, they explain our ability to respond to a huge number of epitopes.

TCR GENES

The T-cell receptor genes for the α and β peptide are located on human chromosome 14, the same chromosome on which the immunoglobulin H chain genes are situated. Chromosome 7 houses the genes for the β and γ peptides. The latter genes are slightly less complex than those for the other two peptides.

The β gene consists of a sequence of a variable (V), joining (J), and constant (C) gene sequence in which the J-C gene pair is duplicated but in sequence (Fig. 4–4). The number of V genes probably exceeds 30. Each J gene is believed to have as many as six variations. $C_{\beta 1}$ and $C_{\beta 2}$ are the sole forms of the C gene.

The γ peptide is derived from a V-J-C sequence in which a single C, at least three J, and an unknown number of V genes contribute. A second human γ

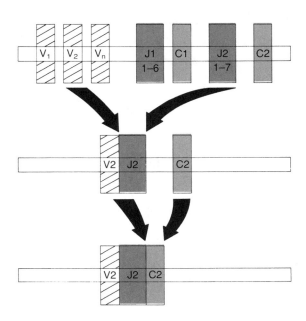

Figure 4–4. The β peptide of the T-cell receptor is created from the selection of a single V gene from a pool of V genes and a J gene–C gene tandem set. The V gene is first moved to the J of a J-C gene pair, and the V-J pair is moved adjacent to the C gene.

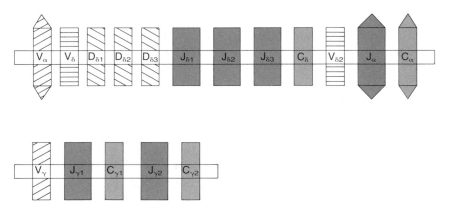

Figure 4–5. The upper sequence shows the gene arrangement for the α and δ peptides of the T-cell receptor. Notice that the genes of one peptide are interrupted by genes of the other peptide sequence. The lower scheme is the genetic arrangement for the γ peptide.

gene has been identified in which the C gene is duplicated.

The *α and δ genes are of genetic interest because they are interspersed with each other* (Fig. 4–5). The sequence begins with the V_δ and V_α genes, followed by three D_δ and three J_δ genes, and the C_δ gene. A second V_δ gene then precedes the J_α and C_α gene. The position of the expected D_α gene(s)

is uncertain. It is still uncertain how many V-gene variations exist.

In order for the two peptides to be synthesized, *the genes for a single peptide must be translocated to form either the V-D-J-C or the V-J-C sequence* with the concomitant removal of introns and unwanted genes. In this gene relocation, the α and γ V and J genes are juxtaposed prior to addition of the C gene. For the β and δ genes, D-J intermediates are formed first, followed by sequential addition of the V and C gene. These rearrangements are among the earliest events in T-cell ontogeny. The biochemical process involved is the same as that used to describe gene alignment of immunoglobulin genes. In accordance with the historically earlier description of immunoglobulin gene shuffling, the details of this and an explanation of the 7/9 and 12/23 rule are included in the next chapter.

MEMORY CHECK 4–3

TCR gene(s)

1. Are needed for each of the V, D, J, and C domains of the TCR proteins

2. For the α and δ peptides are intermixed on human chromosome 14

3. For the β and γ peptides are in separate regions of human chromosome 7

4. Are not sequential in the primitive T cell but are aligned in mature cells

5. Alignment is by the 7/9 and 12/23 rule also used to align immunoglobulin structural genes

---

T-CELL ACTIVATION AND DELETION

The CD3 protein is synthesized in fetal life more or less in phase with the formation of TCR. The CD3 peptides are located more deeply in the cell membrane lipids and may function as a transmitter (after TCR combination with antigen) to enzymes within the cell interior that initiate cell proliferation. The biochemical scheme of this activation is common to that of other activated cells—that is, alterations in phosphatidylinositol metabolism, calcium uptake, and protein kinase activation.

The biochemical explanation remains uncertain, but during thymic life T cells that would ordinarily respond to self-antigens are inactivated. It has been hypothesized that the immature T cell that contacts self-antigens in the thymus undergoes apoptosis, a condition of programmed cell death that cannot be halted. Whatever the true mechanism, *deletion of self-directed T cells* occurs during early thymic development and minimizes the opportunity for autoimmune disease.

INTERLEUKIN RECEPTORS

Some of the surface proteins on T cells serve special functions as receptors for the interleukins but only the IL-1 and IL-2 receptors have been well characterized.

Interleukin 1 Receptor

Interleukin 1, a key product of macrophages, is responsible, with antigen, for the activation of T cells (Fig. 4–6). The **IL-1 receptor (IL-1R)** is present as an 80,000-Mr protein found in rather low numbers: approximately 250 molecules per T cell. Figures as high as 5000 molecules per cell have been reported, and this discrepancy in numbers is partially attributable to the cells examined and their stage of activation. This receptor binds both IL-1α and IL-1β.

Interleukin 2 Receptor

A novel protein that discriminates activated T cells from those not yet exposed to antigen or IL-1 was initially labeled the **Tac protein**. Subsequently this molecule became recognized as the **IL-2 receptor**. IL-2 is synthesized by T_{H1} cells and has both an endocrine

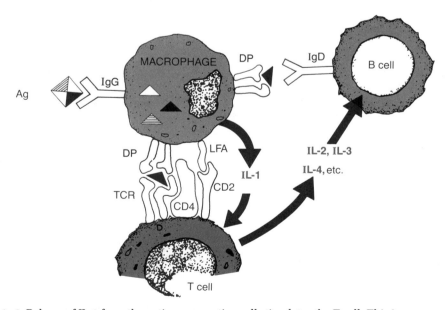

Figure 4–6. Release of IL-1 from the antigen presenting cell stimulates the T cell. This is a companion event to the transfer of antigen and CD2–LFA-3 interaction. The T cell subsequently elaborates interleukins that promote antibody synthesis. This illustration emphasizes the interrelationship of macrophages, T cells, and B cells in the immunoglobulin response.

(it stimulates other T cells) and an autocrine function (it is self-stimulating). IL-2R numbers per cell are low (about 200) before activation but increase to 4000 to 12,000 after T-cell activation. IL-2R has a basic size of 33,000 Mr, but extensive glycosylation elevates it to 55,000 Mr.

T-CELL VARIETIES

It has already become apparent that there are many differences among T cells. These differences depend upon their level of maturation, the influence of hormones, the activation state, the presence of surface proteins, and other factors. An extremely important division of T cells is between those that are CD4-positive and MHC class II protein–dependent and those that are CD8-positive and MHC class I–dependent. The former group includes the helper and delayed-type hypersensitivity T cells; the latter group contains suppressor and cytotoxic T cells (Table 4–3).

HELPER T CELLS

Helper T cells *are characterized as possessing the CD4 protein and a TCR that recognizes antigen presented in the context of the class II MHC protein.* TH subsets designated as T_{H1} and T_{H2} have been identified in mice and are assumed to exist in other mammals. These cells can be distinguished by the array of interleukins that they secrete. Interleukins assist the B cell in different stages in its transition to the plasma cell, but, equally important, they also stimulate subpopulations of T cells.

T_{H1} cells are noted for their *secretion of IL-2 and IL-3.* As described in the previous chapter, IL-2 participates principally as a T-cell growth stimulant. It is this property that labels these CD4 cells as helper T cells. IL-3 is a maturing factor for T cells and other cells, drawing them from their early immature life stage to that of more mature cells. These activities are necessary to provide a supply of T cells and to generate expansive clones of all sub-

Table 4–3
FEATURES OF THE MAJOR T-CELL POPULATIONS

T-Cell Population	Key CD Marker	Function
Helper T cell (T_H)	CD4	1. Aids B cells in antibody formation 2. Aids all other T cells 3. T_{H1} subset secretes IL-2, IL-3, IFNγ, and GM-CSF 4. T_{H2} subset secretes IL-3, IL-4, and IL-5
Delayed-type hypersensitivity T cell (T_{DTH})	CD4	1. Secretes macrophage chemotaxin 2. Secretes macrophage migration inhibitory factor
Cytotoxic T cell (T_C or CTL)	CD8	1. Destroys cells with foreign surface antigen 2. Secretes lymphotoxin (tumor necrosis factor β)
Suppressor T cell (T_S)	CD8	Inhibits other T cells via suppressor factor secretion

sets of T cells that can react with antigen.

T_{H1} *cells also secrete IFNγ and GM-CSF;* the latter supports an emerging population of phagocytic cells. IFNγ has numerous functions, including a stimulation of B-cell proliferation—especially those B cells secreting IgM and IgG. T_{H1} cells are probably identical to T_{DTH} cells, and there is some evidence that IFNγ may be important in delayed-type hypersensitivity.

The T_{H2} *subset secretes* a different population of lymphokines. *IL-3, IL-4, and IL-5 are the major interleukins* that affect B cells. All three of these cause B-cell proliferation. IL-4 stimulates IgE synthesis but inhibits IgM and IgG synthesis. IL-5 stimulates IgM, IgG, and IgA synthesis.

Shared features of T_{H1} and T_{H2} are IL-3, GM-CSF, IgM, and IgG production (Table 4–4).

Interferons

An interferon was first discovered when it was shown that animals with a viral infection had in their blood a nonantibody, low-molecular-weight peptide that would protect other ani-mals from the viral infection. In fact, the interferon lacked antigen specificity and would protect against many unrelated intracellular parasites beyond the inducing virus. Subsequent studies revealed that there are **three major interferons (IFNs):** $α$, $β$, **and** $γ$. These interferons are biochemically similar, while possessing individually unique properties.

Interferon $α$. Interferon $α$ is a T-cell product found in more than 20 subtypes based on slight differences in amino acid sequence. This protein is a glycosylated peptide of about 18,000 Mr. Antigen-, mitogen-, and dsRNA-stimulated T cells secrete IFNα, but this is not an exclusive property of these cells since fibroblasts and others also may produce this protein. *A major function of IFNα is to inhibit viral replication and to slow cell proliferation,* including that of tumors (Chapter 10). In addition, IFNα stimulates the expression of MHC class I and II proteins and FcγR on macrophages and NK cells.

The biochemical basis of these activities is not fully explained but the antiviral property is ascribed to a *degradation of ATP to form 2′5′-oligoadenylate polymers. This may stimulate an endo-*

Table 4–4
DIFFERENTIATION OF T_{H1} AND T_{H2} CELLS

Characteristic	T_{H1}	T_{H2}
CD4 positive	+	+
CD8 positive	−	−
IL-2 production	+	−
IFNγ production	+	−
IL-3 production	+	+
IL-4 production	−	+
IL-5 production	−	+
GM-CSF production	+	+
Stimulate IgE synthesis	−	+
Stimulate IgG and IgM synthesis	+	+
Delayed-type hypersensitivity role	+	−

nuclease that cleaves RNA, thereby slowing cell growth and retarding viral replication.

Interferon β. Two forms of IFNβ are known. IFNβ1 and β2 are approximately 20,000 Mr, are not glycosylated, and are produced by fibroblasts and other cells, including macrophages, T and B cells, and so on. IFNβ2 is synonymous with IL-6, discussed earlier. Many nonviral agents can induce IFNβ1 synthesis.

The major effects of IFNβ1 are the same as described for IFNα. This is explainable in part through the use of a common receptor for both IFNs. This activated receptor, regardless of its ligand, stimulates only one set of responses.

Interferon γ. The third IFN, though also possessing antiviral activity, is separable from the other two on the basis of chemistry and function. IFNγ is sensitive to acid pH and uses a different cell receptor than the α and β molecules use. It is produced dominantly by T_{H1} cells in response to many mitogens and antigens. This prompted the description of *IFNγ as an immune interferon* or as an *immunoregulatory interferon.*

Among the properties of IFNγ, supporting its cytoregulatory role, is its stimulation of NK cells, its induction of macrophage-activating factor synthesis, its ability to enhance MHC class II gene expression, and its ability to increase the density of IL-2R on T cells.

DELAYED-TYPE HYPERSENSITIVITY T CELLS

T_{DTH} cells cannot at present be distinguished from T_{H1} cells. During the delayed-type hypersensitivity reaction, these cells secrete interleukins that adjust the histologic appearance of the reaction site. Among these interleukins are macrophage chemotaxin, macrophage migration inhibitory factors, and macrophage-activating factor (IFNβ).

Macrophage Chemotaxin

Reexposure to antigen of a previously sensitized T_{DTH} cell initiates the elaboration of **macrophage chemotaxin**. This attracts monocytes and macrophages into the hypersensitivity reaction site. The histologic appearance of the DTH site is much different from that seen in other hypersensitivity reactions, which are usually dominated by granulocytes. The macrophage chemotaxin is responsible for this.

The biochemical characterization of this chemotaxin is still incomplete. A peptide of about 12,500 Mr, it is heat-stable at 56°C for 30 minutes. It has been confused with interferons in the past and its exact identity is still not known.

Macrophage Migration Inhibitory Factor

A T-cell–derived product that arrests the motility of macrophages after their attraction by the macrophage chemotaxin is the **migration inhibitory factor (MIF)**. The biochemical nature of this molecule too is obscure. It appears to be a peptide of approximately 32,500 Mr but MIF activity has been once again ascribed to IFNγ and other peptides.

Macrophage-Activating Factor

Macrophage-activating factor (MAF) is identical to IFNβ, as described earlier.

CYTOTOXIC T CELLS

Human T$_C$ cells are not as conveniently placed relative to the CD4 and CD8 proteins as are the T$_C$ cells of lower animals. Although it is still convenient to consider human T$_C$ cells as CD8 positive, some CTLs are CD4 positive.

T$_C$ *cells are activated by antigen offered with class I MHC protein.* IL-2 from T$_{H1}$ cells is necessary for T$_C$ proliferation after engagement with antigen via its TCR. CD2 binding to LFA-3 assists in this process.

Cellular targets for T$_C$ include host cells expressing a novel surface antigen as a result of an intracellular infection. Consequently, T$_C$ cells are an important component of our defense against viral, certain bacterial, certain fungal, and certain animal parasite infections. These cells are cytodestructive for tumor cells, most or all of which possess novel antigens associated with their malignancy. Transplanted tissues are also subject to attack by T$_C$ cells.

The biochemical basis for T$_C$ destruction of cellular targets is based on their ability to discharge **perforins and granzymes** similar or identical to those released by LGL cells described in the previous chapter. They may also secrete a special toxin, the lymphotoxin (LT).

Lymphotoxin

Exposure of T cells to antigens or mitogens causes secretion of **lymphotoxin (LT), also known as tumor-cell necrosis factor β (TNFβ)**. LT is similar in structure and activity to TNFα, an important secretory product of macrophages, as described in Chapter 2.

LT is a protein of about 18,000 Mr that readily polymerizes in solution. This accounts for its description in multiples of 18,000 to 20,000 up to 200,000 Mr. The importance of LT in the cytolytic destruction of CTL targets is currently in dispute. This is in part because of the probability that human CTLs represent a heterogeneous population, some using LT and some using other lytic agents. Those supporting LT as a true lysin also cite the presence of perforin (cytolysin) and granzymes in CTLs. These same cytotoxic agents are found in NK cells, as described in Chapter 3.

SUPPRESSOR T CELLS

A second subset of CD8-positive T cells that responds to the growth hormones of the T$_H$ cells is the suppressor or T$_S$ cell. Recently the true nature of this cell and its interaction with accessory proteins on antigen-presenting cells has come under serious question. The dispute focuses on the nature of the I-J character, an antigen stated to be the interactive determinant of T$_S$ and antigen-presenting cells, both being I-J positive. The I-J protein and its genetic origin have escaped description.

Nevertheless, a functional T$_S$ cell does exist even if it is not easily placed among the total T-cell population.

These cells can be transferred from immunotolerant animals to demonstrate immune unresponsiveness in a recipient that is later exposed to the same antigen used to induce the T_S donor cells (ie, the T_S cell is antigen specific). T_S cells are considered important in controlling T_H cells so that the immune response does not continue unchecked.

T-suppressor factors have been described. These are thought to activate a sequence of suppressor cells — T_S, T_{S_2}, and T_{S_3}, with this last cell being the effector T_S cell. Clearly more experimentation is needed to clarify the status of human T_S-cell activity.

MEMORY CHECK 4 – 5

◆

The CD8-positive T cells include

1. MHC class I–restricted T_C cells
2. MHC class I–restricted T_S cells
3. T_C cells that destroy target cells via perforin, granzyme, and lymphotoxin secretion

---

T-Cell Response to Mitogens

T cells show a different spectrum of sensitivity to mitogens than B cells. These mitogens attach to polysaccharides in the T-cell membrane, a characteristic of many lectins, and induce the cell to go through a growth cycle. In this cycle, the lymphocytic characteristics are retained; there is no differentiation equivalent to the plasma cell in the B-cell line.

CONCANAVALIN A

An extract of the jack bean *Canavalia* contains a 100,000-Mr protein, **concanavalin A (ConA)**, that binds to the surface of both B and T cells. The receptors for this protein are mannopyranosides or glucopyranosides. The B cell remains inert after ConA binding, but the T cell enters a phase of cell growth and division. *This mitogenic surge in T cells mimics its response to antigen* (ie, the T cell begins to secrete interleukins). This has been useful in the isolation of lymphokines from antigen-free culture media and in following biochemical changes in T cells associated with activation.

PHYTOHEMAGGLUTININ A

An extract of the red or yellow kidney bean has the ability to agglutinate erythrocytes and to function as a *mitogen for both B and T cells* in some species. The active principle in this extract, **phytohemagglutinin A (PHA)**, is a protein in excess of 100,000 Mr and binds to acetylgalactosamine residues on the mammalian cell surface.

POKEWEED MITOGEN

The active ingredient in extracts of the pokeweed is a small protein of 32,000 Mr. A receptor for **pokeweed mitogen (PWM)** is present on both T and B cells. *PWM is useful in activating mixed populations of these cells* and has proved useful in evaluating immunocompetence in cases of suspected immunodeficiency. If the T cells or B cells, or both, do not respond, then an immunodeficiency can be suspected.

Immunosuppression of T and B Cells

When there is a failure to note an immune response that is unassociated with prior treatment with antigen (ie, immune tolerance), a state of immunosuppression exists. Both B and T cells are sensitive, often more so than macrophages, to irradiation and cytotoxic drugs. Because B and T cells are often in discrete anatomic clusters, they are readily subject to surgical removal. Immune inadequacy after these treatments is considered a secondary immunodeficiency in contrast to primary genetic immunodeficiency (Chapter 8).

CHEMICAL SUPPRESSION

Used primarily to halt or moderate the growth of neoplastic tissue, cytotoxic drugs are often very effective in suppressing the immune response because lymphocytes and phagocytes are among the cells most sensitive to these compounds. Cytotoxic drugs are chemically classified as folic acid analogs, purine or pyrimidine analogs, or alkylating agents. In addition, the anti-inflammatory corticosteroids are im-

munosuppressive. Various combinations of these agents are used to combat transplant rejection.

Corticosteroids

Chemical modifications of the basic structure of the **adrenocortical hormones** are legion (Fig. 4–7). These have been formulated to preserve the anti-inflammatory nature of these compounds and to eliminate their undesirable side effects, especially their propensity to cause edema (Cushing's syndrome). The human lymphocyte is less sensitive to the steroidal drugs than are those of other species which may actually lyse in the presence of therapeutic concentrations. A therapeutic dose of steroids in humans produces a transient lymphopenia, but this is self-correcting within 24 hours. Although B-cell numbers are decreased, the largest effect of steroids is upon T cells. Blood monocyte numbers

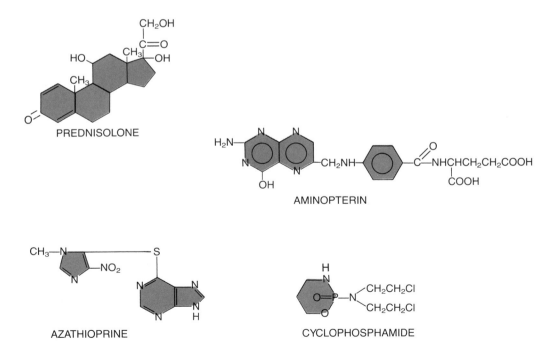

Figure 4–7. Examples of each of the four major chemical immunosuppressive groups—corticosteroids, folic acid analogs, purine analogs, and pyrimidine analogs—are shown.

are also transiently decreased after steroid injections. Because of the transitory nature of these changes, *long-term therapy with steroids is required to demonstrate a decrease in immunoglobulin levels.*

Folic Acid Analogs

Folic acid is a dietary precursor to tetrahydrofolic acid, which is an important coenzyme required for the transfer of the one-carbon units. One-carbon units are needed for the synthesis of the purines, which are incorporated into DNA and RNA. Although methotrexate and aminopterin are not as widely used now as previously, both of these **folic acid analogs** *arrest the growth of lymphocytes by inhibiting the synthesis of nucleic acids and thus of proteins.* Consequently, B- and T-cell replication is prevented and they cannot express their adaptive functions of immunoglobulin and lymphokine production.

Purine and Pyrimidine Analogs

The **purine and pyrimidine analogs** are currently among the most widely used immunosuppressive drugs. Frequently, the compound employed is a *simple structural mimic of the purine or pyrimidine* base per se, as in the thio-substituted compounds (6-thioguanine, 6-mercaptopurine) or as in 5-fluorouracil. Certain other modifications, exemplified by azathioprine, apparently aid entrance of the compound into lymphocytes, after which the compound is hydrolyzed to free the altered base. **Substituted nucleosides** in which the natural ribose or deoxyribose is replaced with another pentose (cytosine arabinoside), or in which an altered purine or pyrimidine is coupled with the natural pentose, are very active cytotoxins. Bromodeoxyuridine

and iododeoxyuridine are examples of the latter.

Alkylating Agents

Difunctional alkylating agents can attach to two $-NH_2-$, $-OH-$, or $-SH-$bearing compounds. In this manner, **alkylating agents such as cyclophosphamide** *can unite two strands of DNA or form a DNA-DNA complex or form other unions that are not salvageable by normal cell repair mechanisms. Proteins can also be linked covalently to each other or to DNA or RNA. The result of these reactions is a blockade of synthetic processes needed for cell growth and function.*

Miscellaneous Chemical Agents

A vast number of natural and synthetic products have been investigated for their immunosuppressive potential. Only a few of these have proved useful. The plant alkaloids vincristine and vinblastine are used to inhibit tumor growth and transplant rejection. One of the most used agents is **cyclosporin A**, a fungal product that failed as an antibiotic but that was found to have a highly specific toxicity for T cells. The unnamed product FK506 is similar to cyclosporin A in its fungal origin and selective activity for T cells not yet activated by antigen and IL-1.

RADIATION

The use of x-rays as an early cytotoxic approach to the control of neoplastic growth soon revealed x-irradiation to be a potent immunosuppressant. Although subpopulations of lymphocytes vary in their radioresistance, lymphocytes are far more sensitive to x-rays than are structural cells.

IMMUNOGLOBULIN

Two separate rationales led to the use of immunoglobulins as immunomodulators. The first of these was that passive immunization against an antigen to which a person was soon to be exposed should bind the antigen, speed its elimination from the body, and lessen or prevent an active immune response. Close attention to details is necessary in this technique because under certain circumstances immune complexes may form that would stimulate the immune response. If antibody exceeds antigen in these immune complexes, then the desired inhibitory result is achieved, but when the reverse occurs an adjuvant effect is observed. Immune complexes may even deposit on blood vessel walls, in the glomerulus, or elsewhere, where they will cause tissue destruction.

Feedback Inhibition

The most dramatic example of specific immunoglobulin modulation of the immune response is seen in the control of hemolytic disease of the newborn due to the Rh antigen. Maternal sensitization to the Rh antigens can result in the production of IgG, which then transmigrates the placental barrier and reacts with fetal erythrocytes that bear the Rh antigen. This causes serious hemolytic episodes, even death, of the fetus or newborn child. Because sensitization of women to the Rh antigen occurs most frequently during delivery, *the administration of anti-Rh sera at the time of birthing* has been employed to control this alloimmune disease. The ability of this antibody to deny antibody synthesis in the mother has been termed **feedback inhibition**. This may function through a stimulation of T_S cells.

Idiotypic Network

A second possible explanation of how the passive administration of antibody can downgrade the response to an antigen is related to a theory of immune control called the **idiotypic network**. This is a second method, in addition to the role of T_S cells, for the natural control of the antibody response.

When an antibody is released into the blood from plasma cells, in a sense this is the first time the individual has been exposed to the antibody. Previously, the antibody was a captive of the mature B cell. This circulating antibody now appears to other B cells as a new antigen, never before encountered. Consequently, these B cells are converted to plasma cells and secrete an *antibody that reacts with the first antibody*. Because the second antibody reacts with a structural region of the first antibody known as its idiotope, *the second antibody is called an* **anti-idiotypic antibody**. However, the anti-idiotypic antibody, because of its novelty, stimulates an anti-anti-idiotypic antibody. This process continues ad infinitum.

The capacity of each anti-idiotypic antibody to react with its predecessor in the chain reduces the concentration of that antibody in the blood. This idiotypic network of antibody interaction is a natural control mechanism for the antibody response, always holding it within physiologically sound limits. The passive administrations of antibody may simply trigger a vigorous idiotypic control network.

Antilymphocyte Sera

The third rationale suggesting the possibility of immune response regulation by immunoglobulin is based on the knowledge that antisera to cellular antigens are often cytotoxic in the presence of complement. By using human lymphocytes as the antigen for some lower animal species **an antilymphocyte serum** *can be prepared that will destroy lymphocytes* when infused into a human subject. Without an effective population of lymphocytes, an immune response is not possible. The most common practical application of this is the administration of anti-T-cell sera (ATS), or its globulin fraction (ATG), to patients receiving tissue transplants. Because the rejection of grafted tissue is primarily a reflection of T-cell function, this is a logical, though not an antigen-specific method, to control the immune response.

MEMORY CHECK 4 – 6

Immunosuppression of T and B cells

1. Is possible with a wide array of cytotoxic drugs
2. By passive administration of antibody may operate by either feedback control or the idiotypic network
3. Is possible with antilymphocyte sera

References

Brenner, MB, Strominger, JL, and Krangel, MS: The $\gamma\delta$ T cell receptor. Adv Immunol 43:133, 1988.

Clevers, H, et al: The T cell receptor/CD3 complex: A dynamic protein ensemble. Annu Rev Immunol 6:629, 1988.

Folkes, BJ and Pardoll, DM: Molecular and cellular events of T cell development. Adv Immunol 44:207, 1989.

Hedrick, SM: Specificity of the T cell receptor for antigen. Adv Immunol 43:193, 1988.

Kourilsky, P and Claverie, J-M: MHC-antigen interaction: What does the T cell receptor see? Adv Immunol 45:107, 1989.

Kupfer, A and Singer, SJ: Cell biology of cytotoxic and helper T-cell functions. Annu Rev Immunol 7:309, 1989.

Mosmann, TR and Coffman, RL: Heterogeneity of cytotokine secretion patterns and functions of helper T cells. Adv Immunol 46:111, 1989.

Mosmann, TR and Coffman, RL: TH1 and TH2 cells: Different patterns of lymphokine secretion lead to different functional properties. Annu Rev Immunol 7:195, 1989.

Parnes, JR: Molecular biology and function of CD4 and CD8. Adv Immunol 44:265, 1989.

Paul, NL and Ruddle, NH: Lymphotoxin. Annu Rev Immunol 6:381, 1988.

Raulet, DH: The structure, function, and molecular genetics of the γ/δ T cell receptor. Annu Rev Immunol 7:175, 1989.

Smith, KA: The interleukin 2 receptor. Adv Immunol 42:165, 1988.

Townsend, A and Bodmer, H: Antigen recognition by class I-restricted lymphocytes. Annu Rev Immunol 7:601, 1989.

vonBoehmer, H: The developmental biology of T lymphocytes. Annu Rev Immunol 6:309, 1988.

Yednock, TA and Rosen, SD: Lymphocyte homing. Adv Immunol 44:313, 1989.

QUESTIONS AND ANSWERS

1. Which of the following is the best description of a TCR?
   A. It is found only on CD4$^+$ cells.
   B. It is composed of three proteins: α, β, and γ.
   C. It reacts with antigen and an MHC protein.
   D. It reacts with unprocessed antigens more firmly than with processed antigen determinants.
   E. It is found on macrophages and T lymphocytes.

Answer C

Antigen receptors on T cells are of two types, and each consists of two peptides. TCR2 is formed from the α and β peptides, and TCR1 from the γ and δ peptides. Both CD4- and CD8-positive T cells contain TCR. TCR combines with processed epitopes plus either the MHC class I or II protein. Macrophages are antigen nonspecific and lack TCR.

2. Which of the following is *not* a major product secreted by T cells?
   A. IL-1
   B. IL-2
   C. IL-4
   D. IL-5
   E. γ interferon

Answer A

IL-1 is a major interleukin secreted by macrophages. All the other substances are secreted by T cells. T_{H1} cells secrete primarily IL-2, IL-3, and IFNγ. T_{H2} cells secrete primarily IL-4, IL-5, and IL-6.

3. Which of the following is a true statement?
   A. CD4 cells are outnumbered approximately 2:1 by CD8 cells in the peripheral blood.
   B. CD2 is a receptor for sheep erythrocytes and LFA-3.
   C. CD3 is a TCR.
   D. T cells respond better to haptens than do B cells.
   E. Cells of the B-cell lineage but not of the T-cell lineage are present in bone marrow.

Answer B

CD4 cells outnumber CD8 cells by approximately 2:1, rather than the reverse as stated in answer A. Answer B is correct. CD3 is associated with but is not a TCR. B cells respond better than T cells to haptens. Pre-T cells emigrate from the bone marrow to the thymus, where they mature, and human B cells are also present in the bone marrow.

4. Which of the following is true of T$_{DTH}$ cells?
   A. They do not secrete lymphokines.
   B. They cannot be distinguished from other CD4-positive cells.
   C. They react with antigen plus MHC class I proteins.
   D. They have a shorter life span than plasma cells.
   E. None of the above.

Answer E

T$_{DTH}$ cells secrete MIF and a macrophage chemotaxin. They can be distinguished from other T cells by minor surface markers. When reacting with antigen, their TCR uses class II MHC proteins. Like other T cells, they have a longer life span than plasma cells. Answers A through D statements are false, which makes E the correct answer.

5. Which of the following is *not* considered a T-cell mitogen?
   A. Concanavalin A (ConA)
   B. Phytohemagglutinin A (PHA)
   C. Pokeweed mitogen (PWM)
   D. Lipopolysaccharide (LPS)

Answer D

All of the agents listed, except LPS, stimulate T cells. PWM also activates B cells, as does PHA.

GLOSSARY

CD1, CD2, CD3, and so on Cluster designation of surface proteins on T cells.

CTC Cytotoxic T cell.

CTL Cytotoxic T lymphocyte.

helper T cell A subclass of T cells (T_H) that aids in the activation of other T cells and B cells.

interferons (IFN) A series of three related lymphokines—α, β, and γ—the last having an immunoregulatory role.

lymphotoxin (LT) A cytolytic protein produced by T_C cells, identical to TNFβ.

macrophage chemotaxin A chemotaxin produced by T_{DTH} cells.

macrophage migration inhibitory factor (MIF) A product of T_{DTH} cells that arrests macrophage motility.

rosetting The adsorption of sheep erythrocytes to T cells.

suppressor cell A subclass of T cells (T_S) whose function is opposite that of T_H cells.

Tac An antigen on activated T cells that serves as the IL-2 receptor.

T_C Cytotoxic T cell.

TCR A T-cell receptor for antigen—either TCR1 (γ/δ) or TCR2 (α/β).

T_{DTH} A T cell that participates in delayed-type hypersensitivity reactions.

T_H Helper T cell.

thymic hormones Products of the thymic epithelium, such as thymosin, thymopoietin, and so forth, needed for the maturation of T cells.

TNF β Tumor necrosis factor β derived from T_C cells.

T_S Suppressor T cell.

TSF T-cell suppressor factor.

CHAPTER 5

◆

The Immunoglobulins

The antigen-specific products of plasma cells, the antibodies, more descriptively referred to as immunoglobulins, share many structural features. Yet within these structures there are variations that enable the immunoglobulins to be distinguished from each other and provide the specificity for the antigen with which they react. These characteristics are considered in this chapter. The **five immunoglobulins are designated IgG, IgM, IgA, IgD, and IgE**, where "Ig" refers to immunoglobulin and the additional letter refers to some distinguishing property of that particular immunoglobulin. These five antibody molecules are present in the blood plasma, and **a secretory form of IgA** is found in milk and saliva, and in bronchial, intestinal, vaginal, and other secretions. Special **membrane-bound forms of IgM and IgD** are also described in this chapter. The genetic origin of these immunoglobulins is presented in the final section of the chapter.

The individual peptides that constitute these immunoglobulins are described in detail in this chapter. A consideration of these chemical details shows the relationships of these peptides to each other, illustrates how minor differences affect the biologic function of the immunoglobulin, and reveals how antibody can be produced in vivo. The section on immunoglobulin genetics is of value because it was through a study of antibodies that the dogma of "one gene—one protein" was broken.

Immunoglobulins as Four-Peptide Units

The chemical structure of the immunoglobulins has a common theme through all their blood and secretory forms. The Nobel prize–winning studies of Edelman deduced that the immunoglobulin foundation was a construct of four disulfide-linked peptides. Modest variations in these peptide chains confer specificity on each immunoglobulin.

The structure of each immunoglobulin is based on a union of four peptides to form a larger protein. *Two of the peptides are of low molecular weight* (22,000 Mr) and are known as the **light (or L) chains**. The *two larger peptides,* **the heavy (or H) chains**, vary in size from one immunoglobulin to another. The smallest of the H chains is 55,000 Mr, the largest 75,000 Mr. It is on the basis of differences in the H chains that the five major antibodies are distin-

guished. The H chains are designated as γ, μ, α, δ, ϵ, and these identify the immunoglobulin classes, or isotypes, as IgG, IgM, IgA, IgD, and IgE, respectively. The two H chains in an individual immunoglobulin molecule are identical and are linked to each other by one or more interchain disulfide bonds. The L chains in a single immunoglobulin molecule are also identical, but just as the H chains may differ from one antibody to another, so also may the L chains. In this instance, the variation is less because there are only two types of L chains, the κ and λ chains. Disulfide bonds unite the H chains with the L chains to create the four-chain molecule (Table 5–1).

THE LIGHT CHAINS AS BENCE JONES PROTEINS

The amino acid sequences of the L and H chains are known. Naturally this determination was simpler for the L chains because of their lower molecular weight. The sequencing of the L chain was simplified by the discovery that **L chains and Bence Jones proteins are identical**. Bence Jones proteins are

Table 5-1
CHARACTERISTICS OF THE IMMUNOGLOBULIN PEPTIDES*

Peptide	Mr	Allotypes	Disulfide Loops	Chromosome
Light chains				
κ type	22,000	Km 1, Km 2, Km 3	2	2
λ type	22,000	None	2	22
Heavy chains				
γ chain	55,000	Gm	4	14
α chain	55,000	IgA2m(1)	4	14
		1gA2m(2)		
μ chain	75,000	—	5	14
δ chain	63,000	—	4	14
ϵ chain	73,000	—	5	14

*See Table 5–3 for J chain and secretory component.

found in the blood or urine, or both, of most patients with **multiple myeloma**, a disease that can be considered a plasma cell neoplasm, or a plasmacytoma. These neoplastic plasma cells frequently fail to produce H chains, which causes a surplus of L chains. These Bence Jones L chains are excreted in the urine, from which they are easily purified free of other proteins. This is also facilitated by the curious nature of the Bence Jones protein to be soluble at room temperature, to precipitate at 60°C to 80°C, and to become soluble again as the temperature is raised farther. The sequencing studies of Bence Jones proteins revealed that two types existed that were only slightly different from each other; this conclusion was also reached from studies of the Bence Jones proteins as antigens. These types are designated the **κ- and λ-type L chains**.

κ Chains

Kappa chains consist of 214 amino acids, of which the carboxy terminal in most samples is cysteine. Disulfide bonding between this cysteine and a cysteine in an H chain is the mechanism of their linkage. κ chains contain four other cysteine residues that are linked to form two internal disulfide bonds. The first of these occurs at positions 21 and 86, creating an amino acid bridge of 65 amino acids. The second disulfide group bridges cysteines at positions 135 and 194. The exact amino acid positions of these bonds may vary from one L chain to another as a result of amino acid additions or deletions. The presence of disulfide bonds that span roughly 60 amino acids is one feature that has permitted a grouping of many proteins under the heading of immunoglobulin supergene family. This is discussed in a later section.

λ Chains

Lambda chains differ only slightly from κ chains. Shared characteristics include the complement of 214 amino acids and five cysteines—one for interchain linkage with the H chain and four for intrachain disulfide linkages. The internal disulfide bonds in λ chains are in virtually the same relative positions as in κ chains.

L-Chain Allotypes

κ and λ chains, because of their close similarity, would meet the definition of allotypic proteins, except that they are derived from completely separate rather than allelic genes. *The structural gene for κ chains is on human chromosome 2, whereas the gene for the λ chain is on human chromosome 22.*

Three allelic forms **(allotypes) of the κ chain** have been identified. These *are designated as κ* **marker (Km) 1, Km 2, and Km 3**. These κ markers represent special epitopes that provide an antigenic specificity for the allotype. For example, an antibody versus κ chain Km 1 would react with all κ chains because they share several antigenic traits, but the reaction would be greatest with Km 1 because it represents a supplementary epitope that Km 2 and Km 3 lack. These allotypes de-

---

MEMORY CHECK 5–1

Immunoglobulin light (L) chains

1. Are 22,000 Mr
2. Are the same as Bence Jones proteins
3. Are either of the κ or the λ type
4. Of the κ type have three allotypes: Km 1, Km 2, and Km 3
5. Contain five cysteines

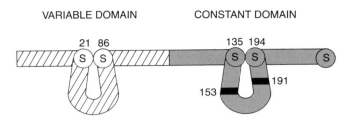

Figure 5-1. Both the κ and λ light chains are divisible into variable and constant amino acid sequence domains, and each domain has a disulfide loop of approximately 60 amino acids. The κ chain illustrated expresses the Km markers by amino acid substitutions at positions 153 and 191.

pend upon amino acid substitutions at positions 153 and 191. These are Val/ Leu, Ala/Leu, and Ala/Val for Km 1, Km 2, and Km 3, respectively (Fig. 5-1).

Allotypic variation of λ chains apparently does not exist. Nonallelic markers Ke, Oz, and Mcg arise because of gene duplication on chromosome 22 and the selection of one or another of these genes for synthesis of the λ chain.

THE HEAVY CHAINS

The H chains of the immunoglobulins differ from each other more than do the L chains. This is reflected by significant differences in their molecular weight, their oligosaccharide content, their stability to heat and reducing agents, their ability to bind to cells, and additional properties. Nevertheless, there are similarities in the arrangement of the H and L chains, as emphasized in the next section.

Isotypes (Classes)

These differences in the nature of the heavy chains just mentioned provided the criteria for establishing the five immunoglobulin isotypes. These H chains are γ, μ, α, δ, and ε, respectively, for isotypes IgG, IgM, IgA, IgD, and IgE. The major features of these five isotypic H chains are presented in later dis-

cussions of the complete immunoglobulins. Generally the H chains are molecules of 55,000 to 75,000 Mr. In the typical immunoglobulin each H chain is linked to an L chain by a single disulfide bond, but there is an important exception in IgA. *The H chains are joined to each other by multiple interchain disulfide bonds.* The number of these varies from 2 to 14, but their position is relatively constant—near the center of the H chain. Intrachain disulfide loops of approximately 60 amino acids are repeated four or five times in each immunoglobulin. Additional cysteines are present near the carboxy terminals of IgM and IgA. These are necessary as sites for binding the additional peptides found in these isotypes. Polysaccharide side arms are attached to H chains but not to L chains, thus placing all immunoglobulins among the glycoproteins.

Subclasses

IgG and IgA exist in forms termed **subclasses**. The major structural difference in the **four IgG subclasses** is in the number of disulfide bonds that join the two H chains. IgG1 and IgG3 have two such bonds, IgG2 has four, and IgG3 has 15. These four IgG subclasses also use two different systems of L-H chain bonding. In IgG1 this disulfide bond is usually at or near L chain position 213 and links to essentially the same position in the H chain. For IgG2, IgG3, and IgG4 the L chain cysteine 213 is linked to the H chain cysteine at position 110.

IgA1 is much like IgG1 except for the use of the α heavy chain rather than the γ chain. In **IgA2**, the L chains are joined to each other by disulfide bonds, but this L-L pair associates with the H chains via electrostatic rather than covalent bonds. The H chains are joined together through typical disulfide bonds.

H-Chain Allotypes

Allotypic variants also exist within the IgG and IgA populations. These allotypic differences depend upon antigenic differences related to amino acid substitutions in specific regions of the H chain. These γ **markers (Gm)** *are unequally distributed among the IgG subclasses,* with IgG3 having approximately half of the total. In several instances, the amino acid sequences responsible for the allotype have been identified. Gm 1 is determined by a sequence of Asp Glu Leu at positions

356 to 358 in IgG1. Gm 17, also in IgG1, relies on a Lys at position 214. If this amino acid is replaced by Arg, then Gm 3 is created.

Allotypes do not exist in IgA1, only in IgA2. The two forms of IgA2 are A2m(1) and A2m(2).

THE IMMUNOGLOBULIN FRAGMENTS

The Nobel prize – winning studies of Porter, who used papain to digest immunoglobulins, was instrumental in identifying the critical antigen-combining sites in antibody molecules. Porter's studies also identified the region in antibody molecules that were responsible for cell-binding interaction with complement and other functions. Subsequently, pepsin was used to produce slightly different digestion products of the antibody molecule, which confirmed the earlier studies with papain.

Papain Digestion

Enzymatic digestion of the four-chain unit of immunoglobulin G with papain nicks an identical peptide bond in each of the two H chains and produces **one Fc fragment and two Fab fragments**. These fragments were named to reflect their ease of crystallization **(Fc)** and their antigen-binding **(Fab)** properties. Each Fab fragment consists of an entire L chain and approximately half (the amino terminal half) of the H chain. The Fc fragment consists of the carboxyl half of the two H chains united by one or more disulfide bonds. Because each of the fragments is approximately 50,000 Mr, the total immunoglobulin structure of 150,000 Mr is accounted for by the Fc and duplicate Fab fragments. This reinforces the knowledge that intact IgG molecule

---

MEMORY CHECK 5 – 2
◆

Immunoglobulin heavy (H) chains

1. Vary from 55,000 to 75,000 Mr
2. Determine the immunoglobulin isotype (class) as IgG, IgM, IgA, IgD, or IgE
3. Of IgG create its four subclasses
4. Of IgG have numerous Gm allotypes
5. Are not linked to light chains in IgA2
6. Of IgA2 have two allotypes — A2m1 and A2m2

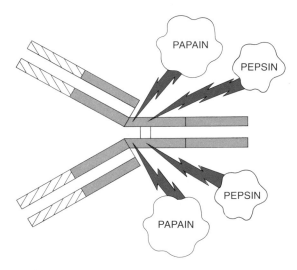

Figure 5–2. The cleavage sites of papain to produce two Fab fragments and an Fc fragment are compared with pepsin cleavage which produces F(ab′)$_2$ and Fc′.

binds two molecules of antigen (Fig. 5–2).

Pepsin Digestion

Pepsin proteolysis results in cleavage of the H chain at a different position than in the case of papain proteolysis. Pepsin cleavage produces only two fragments, one of which is slightly smaller than the Fc fragment and is designated the **Fc′ fragment**. The other fragment is similar to two joined Fab units but differs by having a little more of each H chain (the reason that Fc′ is smaller than Fc). It is termed the **F(ab′)$_2$ fragment**. The Fc or Fc′ fragments contain the regions that enable the immunoglobulin to attach to host cells (macrophages, B cells, and eosinophils), depending upon the antibody class. The Fc or Fc′ regions also activate the complement system when the Fab ends of the molecule have reacted with antigen.

THE IMMUNOGLOBULIN DOMAINS

Within the L and H chains are sections or domains that are quite similar to each other. This similarity applies not only within L or H chains but between them as well.

Variable Domains

All *L chains can be considered as constructed of two halves of equal size, each of 107 amino acids*, for a total of 214 amino acids. *The first 107 amino acids from the amino terminal end vary extensively in sequence from one L chain to another, so much so that this region is referred to as the **variable domain of the L chain (V_L)**. These first amino acids from the amino terminus of H chains also vary from each other in amino acid content and sequence, and are called the V_H domains (Fig. 5–3).

Because the L chain contains a portion of the antigen-binding site, it must be in the V_L region. Likewise, the antigen-reactive site in the H chain resides in its V_H domain.

Constant Domains and Hinge Region in H chains

Amino acid sequencing of the remainder of the L and H chains revealed a continuation of the domain system. This system differs in the L and H chains. The 107 amino acids that fol-

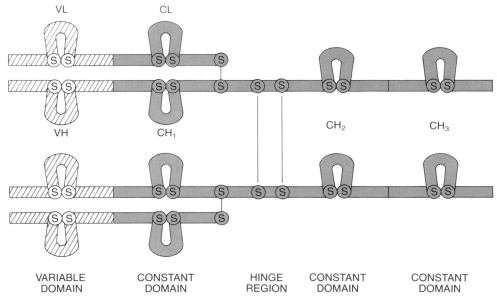

Figure 5–3. Using IgG as reflective of the four-peptide structure of the immunoglobulins, the relative size of the L and H chains, the presence and location of V and C domains, the location of disulfide loops, and the L-L and H-H chain bonding can be noted. The hinge region is the area in which the H chains are joined to each other.

MEMORY CHECK 5–3

Immunoglobulin

1. Fab fragments each contain one antibody-binding site

2. F(ab′)₂ fragments each contain two antibody-binding sites

3. Fc and Fc′ fragments are responsible for cell binding and complement activation

4. Domains have a variable or constant sequence of approximately 107 amino acids each

5. L chains have one V and one C domain

6. H chains have one V and three or four C domains

7. Hinge regions indicate the site of H to H chain linkage.

---

low the V_L domain have a similar amino acid content and sequence as the same region in other L chains and are appropriately designated the **constant domain of the light chain (C_L)**. Each L chain has one V and one C domain. Following the V domain in H chains there are either three or four C domains, depending upon the immunoglobulin class.

Because of their large size, less than half the total amino acid content of the H chains is contained in the V_H and a single C_H domain. The next sequence of amino acids, extending from amino acids 220 through 235 in IgG1, is known as **the hinge region**. This is the region *where the H and H chains are linked together*. The size of the hinge region varies considerably from one immunoglobulin to another. The hinge region of IgG3 is nearly eight times larger than that of IgG1. Thereafter, progressing toward the carboxyl end of the H chain, two more constant domains appear, each again containing about 110 amino acids. Because of the presence of several C domains in H chains, it is necessary to number them C_{H1}, C_{H2}, and C_{H3}. IgM and IgE differ from this model by having a fourth C_H domain.

The Immunoglobulin Supergene Family

All the domains, whether they are V or C, share several features. Each contains approximately 110 amino acids and a 60-to-65 amino acid loop between two cysteines. Each has its ends arranged in the typical α helix of proteins with its central area held in a β pleated sheet dominated by hydrophobic amino acids. Here the amino acids are held in a plane, do not twist at the peptide bond, and create a shelf or cleft known as the immunoglobulin cleft. Within the V domains these clefts are considered the docking sites of antigen between the V_L and V_H domains.

This commonality of structure extends beyond the immunoglobulins to an array of other proteins, many of which have important functions in the immune response. Not all of them have a true **V domain** in the sense of amino acid sequence variability, but this region has the α helix–β pleated sheet arrangement and disulfide loop. Most of these molecules have a **C domain** that has little, if any, diversity in its amino acid make-up from one specimen to another. These proteins include CD2, CD3, CD4, CD7, CD8, CD28, TCR, MHC class I, MHC class II, leukocyte functional antigen 3 (LFA-3), the receptor for IgG (FcγRI), and approximately 15 additional proteins. These are grouped under the umbrella term, **immunoglobulin supergene family** (Table 5–2). These proteins may have an ancestral genetic relationship but are known currently to arise from separate genes (Fig. 5–4).

Several members of the supergene family interact with each other in the immune response. TCR reacts with the class I and class II MHC proteins; IgG reacts with FcγRI, CD4 and CD8 also react with the class I and class II MHC proteins, and CD2 binds to LFA-3.

Table 5-2
SELECTED MEMBERS OF THE IMMUNOGLOBULIN SUPERGENE FAMILY

Supergene Member	Mr	Function
Immunoglobulins	150,000–950,000	As antibody, numerous activities
CD2	50,000	Binds LFA-3, cell adhesion
CD3	65,000	Associated with TCR
CD4	55,000	Binds MHC class II protein, receptor for the acquired immunodeficiency syndrome (AIDS) virus
CD7	—	Unknown
CD8	33,000, dimeric	Binds MHC class I protein
CD28	—	Unknown
TCR	40,000, dimeric	T-cell receptor for antigen
MHC class I	45,000	Transplantation antigen
MHC class II	30,000, dimeric	Immune response protein
LFA-3	55,000	Binds CD2, cell adhesion
FcγR1	72,000	Reacts with IgG

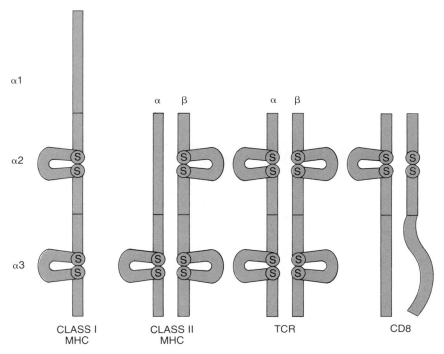

Figure 5–4. Only four members of the immunoglobulin supergene are illustrated, which shows how slight are the variations in their structure.

Hypervariable Domains

Variations in the amino acid sequences of the V_L and V_H domains have already been cited as the means by which antigen specificity is created in an antibody. The variation of amino acid substitutions at a single position in a V domain varies considerably from one immunoglobulin molecule to another. For example, position 8 might be occupied by only three different amino acids in 10 different immunoglobulins, whereas position 35 might use 10 different amino acids. Position 35 can then be described as a hypervariable position.

In V_L *domains three* **hypervariable (HV) regions** *have been identified as positions 30 to 35, 50 to 55, and 95 to 105. Three hypervariable regions are recognizable also in H chains at essentially the same positions as they occur*

in L chains. Because these amino acid groups are found only in the V domains it was originally conceived and later demonstrated by experimentation that these created the antigen-binding sites.

The regions between the HV domains are referred to as the framework regions (FR), in contrast to complementarity determining region, a synonym for HV (Fig. 5–5).

Idiotype

Since the antigen-binding site of each antibody differs from that of another antibody, the HV regions represent a totally unique set of amino acids. In some instances these groupings create an antigenic determinant site, which can be identified by using an immunoglobulin as an antigen to immunize an animal. If the resulting antibody is spe-

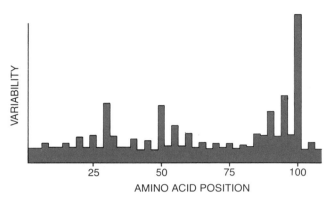

Figure 5–5. Variability in the number of amino acids present in a light chain clearly identifies the three HV regions when plotted as a bar graph.

cific for the original immunoglobulin and does not react with others, in all probability *the HV region has functioned as an epitope.* When this is the case, *that epitopic site is called an* **idiotope** *and the molecule is an* **idiotypic molecule**. An antibody directed against this molecule is an anti-idiotypic antibody.

Accessory Proteins

Two additional proteins, the joining (J) protein and the secretory component (SC), are found in a secretory IgA. All IgM molecules have the J chain but do not have SC (Table 5–3).

J CHAIN

IgA present on mucosal tissues and in milk, spermatic fluid, saliva, and other secretions differs in chemistry from serum IgA by the addition of the **J and SC proteins, and is referred to as secretory IgA**. The J protein is a 15,000-Mr molecule rich in aspartic acid (16%) and containing five cysteines. Two of these cysteines are used to establish disulfide bridges with two of the standard IgA molecules. In this way, the J chain forms a dimeric IgA. J chain in IgM forms a pentameric molecule consisting of five of the four-peptide units. J chain bridges two of the IgM units and the remainder cross-link with each other. Unique enzymes may be required to have the J chain ratio to immunoglobulin monomers differ in IgA and IgM.

SECRETORY COMPONENT

A protein of approximately 75,000 Mr first isolated from secretory IgA was erroneously believed to be the critical molecule that enabled this form of IgA

Table 5-3
CHARACTERISTICS OF IMMUNOGLOBULIN ACCESSORY PROTEINS

Protein	Chemistry	Mr	Function
J chain	Rich in aspartic acid	15,000	Links units of polymeric immunoglobulins
Secretory component	Rich in glycine	75,000	Protects IgA against proteolysis, unproved secretory function

to transport itself across mucosal surfaces. Even though SC may not be instrumental in secretion, its ability to coil around the hinge region and around C_{H2} and C_{H3} domains *protects secretory IgA against destruction by digestive enzymes* found in secretions. Unlike J chain, SC is synthesized in glandular cells near mucosal borders. The IgA doublet carrying J chain contacts the glandular cell, accepts SC, and is discharged into the alimentary canal, the respiratory tract, and so forth.

MEMORY CHECK 5-4
◆

Immunoglobulin(s)

1. Have three hypervariable domains in the L chain
2. Have three hypervariable domains in the H chain
3. Idiotypes are antigenic determinants associated with the HV domains
4. Of the immunoglobulin supergene family have a V-C domain structure
5. J chains are present in IgM and IgA
6. SC is found in secretory IgA

The Immunoglobulins

IMMUNOGLOBULIN G

IgG is approximately 150,000 Mr, based on a size of 22,000 Mr for each L chain and 55,000 Mr for each H chain. This immunoglobulin represents about 75% to 85% of all immunoglobulin in the sera of adults. It is present at a concentration of 1250 ± 500 mg/dL of adult serum. When reference is made simply to gamma globulin or to antibody, IgG is the molecule intended. IgG is also noted for its long half-life of approxi-

Table 5-4
PROPERTIES OF IgG

Physico-Chemical Properties

Molecular weight	150,000
Electrophoretic mobility	γ
Carbohydrate content (%)	2.5–4
Resistance to —SH reagents	High
Concentration (mg/dL of serum)	1275 ± 500
Amount of serum immunoglobulins (%)	75–85
Half-life (days)	25–35
Rate of synthesis (mg/kg of body weight/day)	28

Biologic Properties

Passes the placental barrier, except for IgG3
Best anamnestic antibody
Good neutralizing antibody
Subclasses except IgG4 activate the complement system

mately 29 days, longer than that of any other immunoglobulin. It is also synthesized at a greater rate than other immunoglobulins. These factors contribute to its dominance in sera (Table 5–4).

The IgG subclasses are unequally present in serum, usually at a ratio of 7 : 2 to 1 : 0.05 for subclasses 1 through 4, respectively. Likewise, the κ and λ chain varieties of IgG are in unequal proportions at about 66% κ and 33% λ. Allotypic Gm markers are also unequally distributed among the IgG subclasses.

The quantity of IgG present in serum is not the only feature that indicates its importance. IgG also serves several important biologic roles:

1. It is the only immunoglobulin able to *pass the placental barrier* and convey the mother's immunities to her unborn child.
2. IgG is the most *significant anamnestic antibody*.
3. Antibodies of the IgG class *are very avid; they bind very tightly to*

the antigen with which they react. This is important in immunity against toxins and infectious agents, which are unable to free themselves from IgG and cause disease.

4. Some subclasses of IgG *function with the complement system*, thus stimulating the chemotactic response of phagocytes.

5. IgG on the surface of an antigen *acts as an opsonizing antibody* through its reaction with Fc receptors on macrophages (see Chapter 2).

IMMUNOGLOBULIN M

IgM is a macroglobulin of nearly 1,000,000 Mr. IgM is known as the gamma M or beta 2M immunoglobulin, as its position in the electrophoretic profile usually bridges the gamma and the beta regions. Immunoglobulin M is found in low concentration in normal serum at a level of about 125 ± 45 mg/dL. This represents about 5% to 10% of the total immunoglobulin in the normal adult. This low quantity is a reflection of a short half-life of about 9 to 11 days and a low rate of synthesis at 5 to 8 mg/kg of body weight per day (Table 5 – 5).

This huge *IgM molecule is composed of five of the basic four-chain units plus J chain.* Further adding to the size of IgM is the content of four rather than three CH domains in the H chain, each of which is about 75,000 Mr. About 10% of the weight of IgM is present in the form of polysaccharide. The L chains may be either κ or λ type. IgM is sensitive to dissociation by sulfhydryl-reducing reagents such as 2-mercaptoethanol. When dissociated, five IgM subunits are formed, each consisting of two L and two H chains. These do not retain all the serologic activities expressed by the larger IgM because they dissociate readily from antigen.

Table 5-5
PROPERTIES OF IgM

Physico-Chemical Properties

Molecular weight	950,000
Electrophoretic mobility	Fast γ–slow β
Carbohydrate content (%)	10
Resistance to —SH reagents	Low
Heavy chain constant domains	4
Concentration (mg/dL of serum)	125 ± 45
Amount of serum immunoglobulins (%)	5 – 10
Half-life (days)	9 – 11
Rate of synthesis (mg/kg of body weight/day)	5 – 8

Biologic Properties

Produced early in B-cell ontogeny
Produced early after antigenic exposure
Responds well to polysaccharide antigens
Little anamnestic response
Fails to pass the placental barrier
An excellent agglutinating antibody
An excellent cytolytic antibody when complement is present

IgM contributes significantly to immunity by *reacting well with the polysaccharide antigens on the outer surface of pathogenic bacteria and by advancing phagocytosis.* IgM is a *powerful activator of the complement system* that can kill bacterial cells by cytolysis.

A unique membrane form of IgM is present on immature B cells where it functions as an antigen receptor. The heavy chain of membrane IgM is structurally like serum IgM except that it has a few additional hydrophobic amino acids at the end of the H chains to enable insertion into the B-cell outer membrane. This IgM is also incomplete in a structural sense because it consists of only two L chains and two H chains.

IMMUNOGLOBULIN A

Immunoglobulin A in serum is reported to have a size of 160,000 Mr, but this is only partially true. Almost 20%

of serum IgA is present in polymeric forms. *Two IgA subclasses are recognized—IgA1 and IgA2—the latter of which has no disulfide bonds between its L and H chains. IgA1 has a longer hinge than IgA2. Two allotypic forms of IgA2 are recognized: A2m(1) and A2m(2). The secretory form is the third structural variation of IgA.* IgA is the second most populous immunoglobulin in sera at a level of about 225 ± 55 mg/dL. More than three fourths of this is IgA1. It has a half-life of only 6 to 8 days and is synthesized at about the same rate as IgM (Table 5–6).

Attachment of J chain to secretory IgA (and to serum IgM) is accomplished through disulfide bonding with the Fc regions of the α and μ chains, respectively. During synthesis, the attachment of J chain to secretory IgA precedes the addition of secretory component because J chain is synthesized in plasma cells and SC is not (Fig. 5–6).

The biologic importance of serum IgA is uncertain. It does not pass the placental barrier nor activate the complement system. Persons who are deficient in IgA have a modest increase in their incidence of infectious disease, especially of the sinopulmonary tissues. This is largely due to the absence of secretory IgA and the prominent role

of IgA in bathing the mucosal surfaces and preventing contact of infectious microorganisms with the underlying cell surface.

IMMUNOGLOBULIN D

The recognition that a myeloma protein was not structurally related to IgG, IgM, or IgA led to the description of a fourth immunoglobulin, IgD. The ear-

Table 5-6
PROPERTIES OF IgA

Physico-Chemical Properties	
Molecular weight	160,000*
Electrophoretic mobility	Fast γ–slow β
Carbohydrate content (%)	10
Concentration (mg/dL of serum)	225 ± 55
Amount of serum immunoglobulins (%)	5–15
Half-life (days)	6–8
Rate of synthesis (mg/kg of body weight/day)	8–10

Biologic Properties
Does not react with the complement system
Secretory type exists
Does not pass the placental barrier

*Polymeric forms exist.

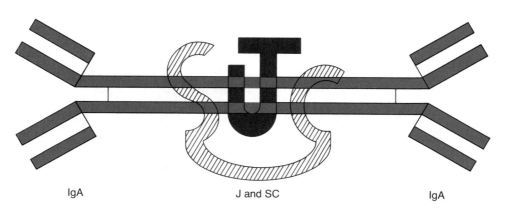

IgA   J and SC   IgA

Figure 5–6. Two molecules of IgA are linked by one molecule of J chain and one of secretory component to form secretory IgA.

lier failure to recognize IgD as a normal component of serum was due to its scarcity in normal serum. IgD is now accepted as a minor component of the immunoglobulin fraction, being present at only 3 mg/dL, which is less than 1% of the serum immunoglobulins. IgD has a molecular weight of 180,000. It is constructed of either κ or λ light chains joined to δ heavy chains. The latter have a molecular weight of approximately 63,000 owing to an extended hinge region, which explains why IgD exceeds IgG in molecular weight. IgD has a very short half-life of only 2 to 3 days, and a very low rate of synthesis (Table 5–7).

Although IgD is scant in serum and quantitatively may be insignificant, antibody activity in IgD versus tetanus toxoid, poliomyelitis virus, blood group antigens, and other antigens has been detected. A membrane form of IgD is found on the surface of B cells where it operates with IgM as an antigen receptor. Membrane IgD has a few extra amino acids in its Fc domains that enable insertion in the B-cell membrane.

IMMUNOGLOBULIN E

IgE is discussed in Chapter 12.

MEMORY CHECK 5–5

◆

Important general statements about the immunoglobulins include the following:

1. IgG is the most protective.
2. IgM is a good activator of the complement system.
3. Secretory IgA may be more important in immunity than serum IgA.
4. The role of IgD in immunity is uncertain.

Myelomas and Hybridomas

Elucidation of the structure of the immunoglobulins depended upon the availability of a source of pure immunoglobulins or portions thereof. To a large extent this requirement was met when it was discovered that the L chains of immunoglobulins were antigenically related to Bence Jones proteins in the blood, or urine of patients with multiple myeloma, or both. Multiple myeloma was recognized as a special form of cancer in which sheets of plasma cells could be found in the lymphoid organs and bone marrow. In addition to an excessive secretion of L chains, some plasmacytomas secreted the complete immunoglobulin molecule. Because of the large population of these cells in the cancerous growths, large quantities of these myeloma proteins appeared in the blood. The **myeloma proteins, known as M components**, were soon *identified as complete immunoglobulin molecules, and be-*

Table 5-7
PROPERTIES OF IgD

Physico-Chemical Properties	
Molecular weight	180,000
Electrophoretic mobility	Fast γ
Carbohydrate content (%)	12
Concentration (mg/dL of serum)	3
Amount of serum immunoglobulins (%)	<1
Half-life (days)	2–3
Rate of synthesis (mg/kg of body weight/day)	0.4
Biologic Properties	
Present on immature B cells	
Protective function uncertain	

cause of their abundance became the source of early information about the structure of immunoglobulins. Moreover, the M component was usually a single structural form of an immunoglobulin because the myeloma was of a single clone of B cells. These structural studies were further facilitated by the availability of inducible plasmacytomas in mice, which provided a second source of pure immunoglobulins.

All of our fundamental knowledge about the structure of the immunoglobulins has been supported by the Nobel prize–winning development of the hybridoma technique by Köhler and Milstein. **Antibody-producing hybridomas** *are produced by fusing a myeloma cell with a spleen cell (B cell)* from an animal immunized with an antigen of choice (Fig. 5–7). The myeloma cells have the unrestricted growth properties of cancer cells and can be easily perpetuated in culture. Spleen cells cannot be so easily perpetuated. Fusogenic chemicals such as polyethylene glycol are used to labilize the cell membranes of these two cells held together in a mixed culture. When the fusogen is withdrawn and the cells separate, some cells contain nuclear elements of both parents. These cells retain the growth behavior of the myeloma and the antibody-secreting property of the spleen cells.

By the use of a selective growth medium containing hypoxanthine, aminopterin, and thymidine (HAT medium), growth of the parent myeloma cell is inhibited so they do not contaminate growth of the hybridoma cells. Of course, the original spleen B cells still cannot grow. By cell dilution procedures it is possible to recover a single, antibody-producing hybrid that is then perpetuated until a large clone of antibody-producing cells is available (see Fig. 3–7).

One problem with this simple approach is that some cells will retain the M protein antibody-producing capacity of the myeloma cell and add the spleen B-cell capability. To avoid the prospect that two antibodies will be produced by the hybridoma, a mutant myeloma cell unable to produce antibody is used in the fusion. From this source, a monoclonal antibody can be secured in substantial amounts (100 μg/mL of culture fluid) for use in structural or other studies. A **monoclonal antibody** *is one derived from a single clone of antibody-producing cells.* The monoclonal antibodies are specific for a *single* antigenic determinant of the original antigen. This contrasts with polyclonal antibodies found in sera that arise from multiple clones of antibody-producing cells that react with different epitopes. By manipulating the

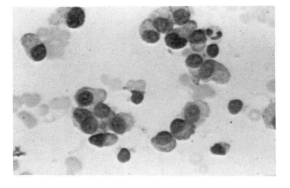

Figure 5–7. This cluster of malignant plasma cells is typical of those seen in malignant myeloma. (See color figure after Table of Contents.)

hybridoma cell, it is possible to study immunoglobulin genetics (eg, to identify which chromosomes carry the structural genes for the L or H chains, to provide DNA for an immunoglobulin of a specified isotype, and so on).

Immunoglobulin Genetics

The genes for the κ, λ, and the H chains of all immunoglobulin isotypes are located on human chromosomes 2, 22, and 14, respectively. The genetic dogma that a single structural gene dictated the structure of a complete peptide was challenged by Dreyer and Bennett, who hypothesized that an immunoglobulin light chain could be constructed from a vast array of V genes and a single C gene. They suggested that a V gene could be selected and moved next to a C gene to form the DNA exon needed to form the L chain. This would provide the antigen specificity (V gene variation) demanded by an array of antibody molecules and would prevent the uneconomic duplication of the C genes. Ultimately it was proved, predominantly by the 1986 Nobel laureate Tonegawa, that numerous V genes did exist, and when the cell began to produce antibody, it selected a V gene and translocated it proximal to the C gene. From the V-C DNA, transcription formed the messenger RNA, from which the protein was translated. This system applies equally to the L and H chains but with the addition of two new genes, J and D, needed to complete the synthesis of the variable domains.

LIGHT CHAIN GENES

These gene arrangements, their translocations, and final structure are very similar for the κ and λ chains, with minor differences. Three genes, not simply a V and a C gene, situated on human chromosome 2, are required to construct the complete κ gene. One of these is the C gene that encodes the terminal 107 amino acids that constitute the C domain. A V gene encodes the bulk of the variable domain and is responsible for the first 90 amino acids. This stimulated a search for a third gene needed to encode the remaining few amino acids of the variable domain, which resulted in the discovery of the joining (J) gene. *The V gene encodes HV1 and HV2, and the J gene encodes HV3 (Fig. 5–8).*

In order to create the vast number of antigen specificities of κ chains, there must be a large number of V or J genes, or both, to combine with the C gene. The exact number of $V_κ$ genes is not known, but it is believed to be 200 or more. This contrasts with the number of $J_κ$ genes, of which five have been identified (one of these, however, is nonfunctional).

Thus, *an array of 200 or more V genes, plus four J genes, plus a solitary C gene, compose the κ L chain gene bank.* The sequence of these functional genes is V_1, V_2, V_3, V_n, and so on, J_1, J_2, J_3, J_4, and C.

The λ chain gene arrangement is similar to that for the κ chain. V genes encode the first 90 amino acids of the variable domain, but rather than having a single C gene the λ L chain has four functional C genes. Each of these is linked to a J gene. There are also pseudo-J genes that are inactive. The *functional lambda gene sequence is V_1, V_2, V_3, V_n (JC_1), (JC_2), (JC_3), (JC_4).*

The device by which V genes are positioned next to the λ J-C genes or the κ J genes is based on excision of the undesired, intervening genes by an endonuclease, followed by ligation of the cut in the DNA strand. *Errors in ligation are responsible for the very high variability at or near position 103 in*

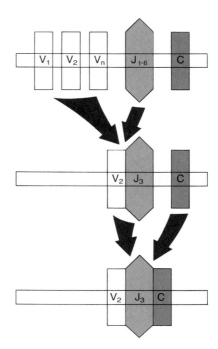

Figure 5–8. Of the genetic selections necessary to complete an L chain, first is the choice of one of many V genes to add to a J gene, of which there are only a few; later, a single C gene is added.

immunoglobulin chains. This alignment is aided by a system known as the **heptamer-nonamer, or 7/9 and 12/23, rule**. The heptamer is a seven-base sequence at the 3′ side of a V gene that is matched by a reverse sequence on the 5′ side of the J gene. Between these heptamers two reversed sequences of nine bases are placed. One of these is 12 bases and the other is 23 bases from the nonamer. Slightly less than 12 bases complete one turn in the DNA helix, and 23 bases constitute two turns in the helix. "Lollipop" or loop formation allows the nonamers and the heptamers to hydrogen bond with each other, simultaneously placing the 3′ end of the chosen V gene adjacent to the 5′ end of the J gene (or J-C gene pair) (Fig. 5–9). The undesired V and J genes are in the "lollipop." Cleavage and resealing of the DNA at the V-J gene intercept in κ chains forms the complete V-J-C construct because the C gene is in a direct reading frame after the J genes. In λ chains, the J-C pair is

already aligned. In H chains, the D-J genes are first positioned next to each other, followed by the V and C genes.

HEAVY CHAIN GENES

The genes for all immunoglobulin isotypes are located on human chromosome 14. The C_H genes are in the following order: μ, δ, $\gamma 3$, $\gamma 1$, $\gamma 2$, $\gamma 4$, ϵ, α (Fig. 5–10). Each of these genes includes the number of C_H domains needed for its immunoglobulin plus hinge region codons. These C_H genes are preceded by genes for the variable domain. This domain is encoded by three genes, rather than the two required for light chains. *Interposed between the V and J genes of H chains is a* **diversity (D) gene**. As might be expected, the V gene dominates the structure of the V domain. The D and J genes account for only 15 to 20 amino acids each.

The *initial step* in the assembly of

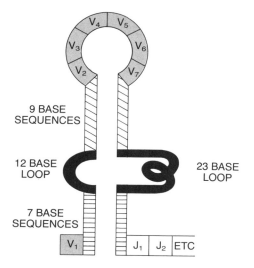

Figure 5–9. The alignment of the 7- and 9-base sequences separated by a 12-base and a 23-base loop of the ascending and descending arms is instrumental in positioning of the V and J genes.

these genes is a rearrangement in which *one of the four D genes is translocated to one of the six functional J genes.* (There are nine J genes in all, but three are nonfunctional.) This excision of the undesirable D and J genes is accomplished by the 7/9 and 12/23 rule. The assembly of the D-J gene pair is the first genetic event that identifies the B-cell progenitor cell. After this, one of the many V_H chain genes is moved to the D-J pair, again by application of the 7/9 and 12/23 rule. Now that the complete variable domain of the H chain is determined, the immature B cell produces a transcript that includes both the μ and δ H chain constant domain genes. By selective translation and processing of the master RNA transcript, either IgM or IgD is produced.

CLASS SWITCHING

It must be remembered that these choices are made before the B cell encounters antigen. The antigen-driven events include a cellular differentiation to become a plasma cell and to switch to a fixed class of antibody synthesis. Some cells stay locked in either IgM or IgD synthesis, while others select a different C_H gene by a process known as class switching. *Class switching does not use the familiar 7/9 and 12/23 rule.* It is not certain how class switching is accomplished. Between each of the C_H genes pentamers of GGGGT follow a series of GAGCT sequences. These appear to be the key switch sequences, but it is unclear how they effect a looping-out of the C_H genes that will be discarded. Some of

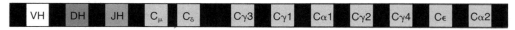

Figure 5–10. The sequence of the human C genes on chromosome 14 follow the V, D, and J genes. Pseudo C genes are not included in this drawing.

these sites may be hindered or enhanced by interleukins; IL-4, for example, is known to stimulate IgE synthesis. In any event, the cell selects its C domain gene and moves the V-D-J construct to it, to prepare for H chain synthesis.

MEMORY CHECK 5–6

Immunoglobulin

1. Genes for κ, λ, and H chains are on human chromosomes, 2, 22, and 14, respectively
2. V, J, and C genes determine L chain structure
3. V, D, J, and C genes determine H chain structure
4. D to J and V to DJ chain translocations follow the 7/9 and 12/23 rule
5. H chain switching is encoded by special switch sequences, not by the 7/9 and 12/23 rule

SECRETED AND MEMBRANE IgM AND IgD

Optional splice sites in the C genes for IgM and IgD account for the **secreted and membrane forms** *of these immunoglobulins.* The immature B cell selects the codon for the membrane form, the form that dictates an extended C_H tail of hydrophobic amino acids. The plasma cell makes the opposite choice.

References

Calabi, F and Neuberger, MS (eds): Molecular Genetics of Immunoglobulin. Elsevier, Amsterdam, 1987.

Day, ED: Advanced Immunochemistry, ed. 2. Wiley-Liss, New York, 1990.

Hames, BD and Glover, DM (eds): Molecular Immunology. IRL Press, Oxford, 1988.

Papadea, C and Check, IJ: Human immunoglobulin G and immunoglobulin G subclasses: Biochemical, genetic, and clinical aspects. CRC Crit Rev Clin Lab Sci 27:27, 1989.

Williams, AF and Barclay, AN: The immunoglobulin superfamily—domains for cell surface recognition. Annu Rev Immunol 6:381, 1988.

Zentivanyi, A, Maurer, PD, and Janicki, BW (eds): Antibodies. Plenum Press, New York, 1987.

QUESTIONS AND ANSWERS

1. A complete Bence Jones protein is
   A. An immunoglobulin L chain
   B. Composed of one variable and one constant domain
   C. Antigenic, and its antiserum would react with IgG
   D. A product of B lymphocytes or plasma cells, or both
   E. All of the above

Answer E

Bence Jones proteins are either κ- or λ-type L chains and, with rare exceptions, contain one V and one C domain. Because Bence Jones proteins are produced by plasmacytomas, they arise from plasma cells, but the oncogenic status of these cells does not preclude minor variations in the V or C domains of their protein product. An antibody to any portion of an immunoglobulin will react with the whole molecule.

2. In IgG
   A. Each H chain–L chain pair has its structural mirror image in the other half of the molecule
   B. Myeloma, the cells producing the IgG are known as hybridomas
   C. There are two H chain subclasses
   D. There are four L chain types
   E. All of the above

Answer A

In the basic four-peptide unit of the immunoglobulins a separation of the H chains from each other yields two identical H-L chain units. Answer A is correct; all other options are incorrect. IgG has four different H chain subclasses and two L chain types, not the reverse as suggested by answers C and D. Hybridomas are fused products, usually of a myeloma cell with another cell.

3. Four constant domains are present in the H chains of
   A. IgD and IgM
   B. IgA and IgM
   C. IgD and IgA
   D. IgM and IgE
   E. IgA and IgE

Answer D

IgM and IgE each have a fourth C_H domain in each H chain. IgD is of greater size than IgG because of an extended hinge region. The difference between the molecular weight of IgG4 and those of the other IgG subclasses is also due to a larger hinge.

4. Even a highly purified preparation of IgG will be distributed rather broadly, in electrophoresis, compared with albumin. This is because IgG

   A. In one individual has both κ and λ L chains

   B. Molecules may be produced by different plasma cells, and thus differ slightly from each other

   C. Directed against different antigens would have different amino acid compositions

   D. Molecules vary in their content of Gm determinants

   E. All of the above.

Answer E

Immunoglobulins of any isotype distribute themselves broadly because of their multiple variations in structure. These include different L chains, different Km markers, different Gm markers, and different constructions in their HV regions as they respond to different epitopes in the antigen.

5. The major cause of hypervariability at or near positions 103 and 104 in L chains is

   A. The alternate choices of switch sequences to link the J gene and the C gene

   B. Infidelity of endonuclease scission and ligation of the DNA strand

   C. A failure of the 7/9 and 12/23 rule to remove undesired J genes

   D. Faults in the D-J gene alignment

   E. An unusual switch sequence placed just before the C gene of the L chain

Answer B

Switch sequences are used to select the proper C gene for H chains rather than L chains; therefore, answers A and E are erroneous. Answer D is also incorrect because D genes are found only in H chains. As far as is known, the 7/9 and 12/23 rule applies to all V and J genes, and the erroneous inclusion of an extra J gene would create a truly aberrant antibody. This leaves answer B as the correct choice.

Case Study: Multiple Myeloma

Harry, a 53-year-old postal deliveryman, stepped down from his truck and felt his lower leg snap. A housewife nearby called an ambulance and Harry was transported to the hospital. X-ray examination located the break but also revealed extensive coinlike lesions in the bone. The physical examination revealed enlarged lymph nodes in the cervical, axillary, and groin areas. The hemoglobin level was 12.4 g/dL, the white blood cell count was 9200/mm³, and the serum bilirubin was increased. Urinalysis was 1+ for protein. Serum protein electrophoresis indicated a possible polyclonal gammopathy of the IgG and IgA classes. Total serum protein levels were normal. Bone marrow aspiration and quantitative immunoglobulin determinations were ordered.

Questions

1. What is the probable nature of the proteinuria?

2. How does the total serum level remain normal with a concurrent polyclonal gammopathy?

3. How can a polyclonal gammopathy be suggested only from serum electrophoresis?

4. What is the preferred procedure for immunoglobulin quantitation?

Discussion

The coin lesions seen on x-ray examination were an important clue to the diagnosis of multiple myeloma. In this disease, the proliferation of plasma cells in the bone marrow may erode local areas of bone. Weakening of the bone then allows even very modest stresses to result in a fracture.

Bence Jones protein was the cause of the proteinuria. This was determined by the thermal response of this protein in acid media. To test for Bence Jones protein, it may be necessary to acidify the urine to pH 4.5 with dilute acetic acid. The exact temperatures at which precipitation and dissolution will occur vary from specimen to specimen; some Bence Jones proteins do not dissolve at 100°C. The frequency of Bence Jones protein in the urine of myeloma patients varies from as low as 30% to as high as 88%. This wide range is undoubtedly caused by differences in technique (acidity of urine), protein concentration, and temperature criteria. The electrophoresis of 5- to 10-fold concentrated urine has done much to improve the urinary identification of Bence Jones protein. Systematic investigation of Bence Jones protein indicates an incidence in urine in excess of 50%. The Bence Jones protein is frequently the only protein in the urine, where it is situated in the electrophoretic position occupied by the gamma globulins. It is a light chain of the immunoglobulins and may exist in dimeric or polymeric forms.

As an aside, it is interesting that the name of Sir Henry Bence Jones has been perpetuated by this protein. Bence Jones was a clinical pathologist who recognized the protein in a urine sample supplied by Dr. Dalrymple. A second physician, Dr.

Watson, later cared for the patient. The names of the patient and the two attending physicians have fallen into obscurity.

Polyclonal and monoclonal M components do not necessarily disturb the total gamma globulin concentration of the serum; in fact, hypogammaglobulinemia is seen in 12% of all patients with myeloma. One interpretation of this is the normal plasma cells have been inhibited by cells of the plasmacytoma. Serum electrophoresis may identify the class of the hypogammaglobulinemic as well as the hypergammaglobulinemic protein. Simple serum electrophoresis will often distinguish an IgG myeloma from the others. Mixed IgA and IgM proteins will appear in nearly the same electrophoretic position and obscure the identification of the condition as a polyclonal disease. IgG with either IgA or IgM is more easily identified, although whether the second protein is A or M is often difficult to decide. This distinction has been made from semiquantitative immunoelectrophoretic determinations with specific antisera against IgG, IgA, and IgM tested against the myeloma serum of normal and diluted strength. If the serum IgG and IgA are no longer detectable with specific antisera tested against diluted serum, but the IgM is, then the indication is that the myeloma is of the IgM class. Radial quantitative immunodiffusion tests and nephelometry are now preferred because they are more sensitive and quantitative. In the patient described, this test recovered 3.2 g/dL of IgG and 0.6 g/dL of IgA. Normal values should approximate 1.3 g/dL for IgG and 0.3 g/dL for IgA; thus, the patient had a combined IgG and IgA myeloma.

GLOSSARY

---

allotype　A characteristic not shared by other proteins controlled by an allelic gene.

antibody fragment　A portion of an antibody molecule created by enzymatic digestion.

Bence Jones protein　An immunoglobulin L chain found in the urine and blood of myeloma patients.

C_{H1}, C_{H2}, C_{H3}, and C_{H4}　Regions of the H chains of immunoglobulins that have constant amino acid sequences.

C_L　The constant amino acid sequence in an immunoglobulin light chain.

class switch　The change from producing IgM and IgD to the production of other immunoglobulins.

constant domain　The C_H and C_L regions of immunoglobulins.

D gene　Diversity gene.

diversity gene　A gene that regulates the structure between the V and J gene contributions to an H chain.

Fab fragment　The antigen-binding fragment of an immunoglobulin, two of which are produced after papain digestion.

$F(ab')_2$ fragment　Two Fab fragments plus an additional segment of an H chain produced by pepsin digestion of an immunoglobulin.

Fc　The remainder of the H chains after removal of the two Fab fragments from an immunoglobulin.

Fc'　The fragment remaining after removal of the $F(ab')_2$ fragment from an immunoglobulin.

FR　Framework region.

framework region　The region in the V domains between the HV regions.

H chain　The heavy, isotype-determining chain of an immunoglobulin.

hinge region　A region in an H chain near the site of papain or pepsin cleavage.

HV　Hypervariable region.

hybridoma　The fusion product of a myeloma cell with a B cell.

hypervariable domain　A section of intense amino acid sequence variation in a V domain.

idiotope　An antigenic site created in the HV region of an immunoglobulin.

immunoglobulin supergene family　A family of proteins with V and C domains similar to that present in immunoglobulins.

isotype　Synonym of antibody class and dependent upon the nature of the H chain in an immunoglobulin.

J chain　A polypeptide that joins the units in polymeric immunoglobulins, ie, secretory IgA or IgM.

J gene   Joining gene.

joining gene   A gene that specifies the structure of a sequence immediately prior to C_L or C_{H1}.

L chain   The light chain, either κ or λ, in an immunoglobulin.

SC   Secretory component.

secretory component   A protein found in secretory IgA.

switch sequence   A DNA sequence that separates the H-chain C genes.

V domain   Variable domain.

variable domain   A region of variable amino acid sequence.

CHAPTER 6

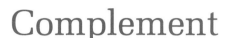

Complement

The complement system consists of a series of proteins in the blood. The complement proteins amplify the biologic effects of antigen-antibody reactions and uncover protective functions hidden in these proteins. These functions can also be recruited by combination of the complement molecules with oligosaccharides instead of serologic reactions. Before these protective functions can be released, each succeeding complement component is enlisted into a cascade by an earlier component. The complement proteins are essentially inert until converted into a biologically active molecule by an earlier component. These proteins and their activities are subject to control by a series of circulating and cell-bound regulators. In this chapter the complement cascade, the biologic properties emanating from it, and their control are described.

In order to explain the basis for these many activities of the complement system it is necessary to examine the chemistry of the individual components. This is first described for the classic pathway—the antibody-dependent pathway. In this scheme, the early complement components C1, C4, C2, and C3 are naturally considered first, and followed by a description of the membrane attack complex composed of C5 through C9. Subsequently, the molecules of the alternative complement pathway are considered.

Two important sections follow this biochemical section of the chapter: (1) A discussion of the several biologic activities emanating from complement, and (2) a lengthy description of the many naturally occurring inhibitors or regulators of the complement system, a section closely tied to that on complement receptors.

General Properties of Complement

Several physicochemical properties enable the molecules of the complement system to be distinguished from immunoglobulins and interleukins. The **complement proteins are constitutive molecules** whose appearance in blood is unrelated to antigenic stimulation, whereas the interleukins and immunoglobulins are formed and secreted as an adaptive response to antigens. Many functions of the complement system are based on the proteolytic cleavage of parent molecules that release activation peptides. These peptides are often responsible for the major activities of complement. In contrast, antibodies and interleukins act as entire holoproteins. Some of the newly generated proteins of the complement system or their precursor molecules are *inactivated at 56°C for 30 minutes*, a treatment that has no effect on most immunoglobulins. After this treatment complement is said to be inactivated. The proteins of the complement system interact with each other in an interlacing molecular cascade, unlike immunoglobulins and interleukins that act as single units. The interactions of the complement molecules are regulated by inactivators or inhibitors in the blood. Similar regulatory molecules have not yet been described for interleukins and immunoglobulins. Finally, like the interleukins and immunoglobulins, a number of cell receptors assist in expressing the biologic properties hidden within the complement system (Table 6–1).

Table 6–1
GENERAL PROPERTIES OF THE COMPLEMENT SYSTEM

Property	Conditions
Stability	Inactivated at 56°C for 30 minutes
Activation	1. By IgG or IgM (classic pathway)
	2. Complex saccharides and polyionic compounds (alternative pathway)
Biologic activities	1. Chemotaxin in C5a
	2. Anaphylatoxins C3a, C4a, and C5a
	3. Enzyme activity in C1r, C1s, C3 convertase, C5 convertase, and factor D
	4. Cell lysis
Immunologic properties	1. Opsonization by C3b
	2. Immune adherence by C3b
	3. Immune lysis, all nine components required
	4. Used in complement fixation tests

Thus, the complement system is chemically unique and unrelated to the interleukins. However, a complement-immunoglobulin association does exist although this is limited to the serologic reaction of antibody with antigen that initiates that classic complement activation pathway. Free antibody does not activate the complement system; only antibody that has combined with antigen is able to do this. It is interesting that only IgM and IgG can activate the complement system — IgA, IgD, and IgE are all inactive. Of the IgG subclasses, IgG4 is inactive.

ACTIVATION PATHWAYS

The complement system is conveniently divided into two compartments, based on which way the system is activated. In the **classic activation pathway,** which is initiated by a serologic reaction, nine proteins, designated **C1 through C9,** participate. The serologic reaction must involve IgG or IgM; other immunoglobulin isotypes are inactive. In the **alternative activation pathway**, which is initiated by complex polysaccharides and not by antibody, components C1, C2, and C4 of the classic pathway are omitted and are replaced by three molecules unique to the alternative pathway. During activation of the complement system, several peptides are released that contribute to several important physiologic responses. These include edema, a universal part of the inflammatory response, and the chemoattraction of phagocytes to the site of complement activation — that is, where an antibody has reacted with an invading microbe. The peptides not released from the complement cascade remain attached to the antigen-antibody-complement complex. These proteins also participate in the immune response by

improving phagocytosis and by lysis of cellular antigens.

COMPLEMENT-DERIVED ACTIVITIES

Several remarkable activities are generated from complement. **Anaphylatoxins C3a, C4a, and C5a** — the activation peptides from their corresponding complement components — are all able to degranulate mast cells and basophils, releasing histamine, and producing edema and smooth muscle contraction. **C3b,** the residue of C3 after the removal of C3a, is an important **opsonin** that improves phagocytosis of foreign particles: bacteria, viruses, yeasts, and the like. **C5a is a chemotaxin** that attracts phagocytes to these infectious agents where C3b can express its opsonic role. Even if phagocytic destruction of a microbe does not occur via the functions of C3b and C5a, lysis of antibody-coated cells may follow the participation of the last complement molecule, C9. The gram-negative bacteria are very sensitive to this **immune lysis,** but the gram-positive bacteria, yeast, and molds are quite resistant. Unfortunately, if autoantibodies on the surface of sensitive host cells bind complement, the function of these cells may be impaired and expressed as an autoimmune disease.

NOMENCLATURE

The nomenclature used to describe the complement system can be confusing. When a complement protein is altered by an enzyme, the protein is said to be activated. However, if one now tries to measure all the complement proteins as they exist in their natural state, this altered protein cannot be found. Now it is said that complement has been inactivated. **Complement activation and inactivation** refer to the same thing, one from the viewpoint of a new activity, the other from a loss of a parent molecule.

Complement fixation is an ancient term that is still encountered, especially in serology. It refers to the binding of complement to an antigen-antibody complex. All nine of the classic cascade proteins do not bind to the antibody; the earlier components of the cascade may, but the late-acting molecules bind to the earlier participants.

As already indicated, complement-derived peptides are designated by letters: C3a, C3b, and C5a are examples. This should not be confused with the standard biochemical lettering system for peptides in multipeptide proteins —C3α, C3β, and so on. Some authors designate an activated molecule by placing a bar over its designation, as in $\overline{C1s}$.

MEMORY CHECK 6 – 1

◆

Complement

1. Consists of a series of normal blood constituents
2. Can be activated by either the classic or alternative pathway
3. Activation by the classic pathway requires antigen and IgG or IgM
4. Activation by the alternative pathway is initiated by complex oligosaccharides
5. Activation is controlled by numerous regulator molecules
6. Activation generates numerous biologic activities important for health
7. Is inactivated by holding serum at 56°C for 30 minutes

The Classic Activation Pathway

The proteins of the complement system are best described according to their membership in the classic or alternative complement cascade.

When a serologic reaction takes place between either IgM or subclasses 1, 2, or 3 of IgG and an antigen in the presence of complement, the classic complement cascade is activated. During this process, each complement molecule reacts in its turn with the earlier part of complex. In this way, once the cascade has begun, despite the presence of inhibitors, it tends to go to completion. Each of the first five molecules is chemically changed by a proteolytic event that releases an activation peptide. New biologic properties are expressed in company with these chemical changes at each stage in the cascade. Components C6, C7, C8, and C9 join the complement reaction sequence without chemical change, and no significant new properties appear until C8 and C9 are added.

THE RECOGNITION UNIT — C1

Complement molecule C1 is called the recognition unit because it is the first complement molecule whose behavior is influenced by the antigen-antibody reaction: it now recognizes the antibody and binds to it.

Serologic Requirements

The proteins of the complement system are merely a part of the plasma proteins until a serologic reaction of antigen occurs with either IgG or IgM. Immunoglobulin subclasses **IgG1, IgG2, and IgG3** each have binding sites in both their C_{H2} and C_{H3} domains for the first unit of complement. IgG4 lacks these sites. Because of the rigidity of the C1 molecule, it cannot link to two sites in a single IgG molecule. C1 must bridge two IgGs before it can initiate the cascade. Because of the pentameric structure of IgM, multiple binding sites for C1 exist in a single antibody molecule. C1 binding to IgM occurs in its C_{H4} domains.

Of course, antigen-free IgG and IgM have no influence on the complement system. How the combination of these antibodies frees their C1 binding sites is uncertain.

The C1 Complex

C1 is a large molecule of approximately 750,000 Mr and is composed of the subunits C1q, plus two molecules of C1r and two molecules of C1s (Table 6–2). Calcium is essential to the maintenance of this trimolecular complex. Removal of this calcium by chelating compounds will block the classic pathway.

C1q is the largest part of the C1 triad at 400,000 Mr. Two molecules of C1r and C1s are held within the stems of the elongate bouquet of the tulip-shaped C1q peptides. Two of the six

"blossoms" of C1q react with antibody. Simultaneous with this binding, **C1r expresses a proteo-esterase activity** that was previously masked in a proenzyme form. The C1r enzyme appears to have only **C1s** as its substrate, which it then converts to an **active protease.** C1r and C1s are each 85,000 Mr and are split into unequal parts linked by a disulfide bond when transformed into enzymes. The smaller 27,000-Mr fragment is the enzymatically active portion in each molecule. Activated C1 is often referred to simply as $\overline{C1s}$ (Fig. 6–1).

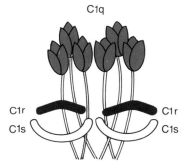

Figure 6–1. The C1 complex is composed of C1q, C1r, and C1s. C1q is a collection of six molecules formed from eighteen peptides. C1 has globular or tuliplike heads whose "stems" hold two molecules each of C1r and C1s.

Table 6–2
CHEMISTRY OF THE COMPLEMENT COMPONENT OF THE CLASSIC PATHWAY

Component	Mr	Serum Concentration (μg/mL)
C1q, r, s complex	750,000	70
C2	117,000	25
C4	196,000	400
C3	195,000	1600
C5	190,000	80
C6	120,000	65
C7	120,000	55
C8	150,000	55
C9	75,000	60

ACTIVATION UNIT

Three proteins, C4, C2, and C3, compose the activation unit. They participate in the order indicated rather than in numeric order because they were identified as individual proteins before their position in the cascade was determined. The phrase "activation unit" is used because each molecule releases a peptide in order to participate in the flowing complement system. Each parent molecule is akin to a proenzyme of a proenzyme-enzyme pair.

C4

C4 has its genetic origin in the MHC. The duplicate set of genes, C4A and C4B, each produces an active C4 molecule. The macrophage is the cell source of these C4 proteins which originate as the more structurally complex **pro C4** proteins. The pro C4 molecules are glycosylated single peptides that lose their leader (signal) sequence upon secretion from the macrophage. A serum protease clips the extracellular pro C4 in two places to create a three-chain protein held together by disulfide bonds. The molecule is now approximately 196,000 Mr.

As C4 in the blood contacts the heavy chain of C1s in the antigen-antibody aggregate, the enzymatically active C1s light chain cleaves the α chain of C4 on the carboxyl side of arginine 77. This releases C4a, a small peptide of 8750 Mr (Fig. 6-2).

C4a is an anaphylatoxin, a term that indicates that it can bind to tissue **mast cells** and basophils. This deranges the stability of these cells, forcing them to discharge their cytoplasmic granules. The histamine in these granules causes several aspects of the inflammatory response, most notably the contraction of smooth muscles. This alteration of the muscle cells of the blood vessels

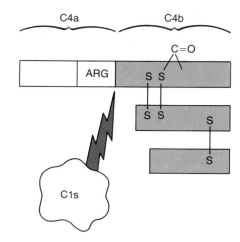

Figure 6-2. Splitting of C4 by C1s releases C4a and leaves C4b. The thioester grouping allows C4b to covalently link to antigen. A very similar cleavage occurs in C3 and C5 to release C3a and C5a. C3b has a thioester group, but C5b does not.

creates gaps that allow fluid to leak into the tissues, causing edema. To some extent this activity is controlled by **the anaphylatoxin inhibitor (AnaINH)**.

C4 is an interesting molecule because it has an **internal thioester bond** that spans Cys-Gly-Glu-Gln. Removal of C4a from C4 labilizes this construct, freeing a reactive acyl grouping. If this grouping reacts with antigen, the C4b residue serves as the building site for the next complement component. C4b does not normally bind to any part of the C1 trimer. Binding of C4b to antigen is regulated by the C4b-binding protein, factor H, and factor I as discussed later.

C2

C2 is a beta globulin of 117,000 Mr. Relatively little is known about C2 except that C1s splits it and removes C2b (34,000 Mr), a molecule that has kinin-like activity—that is, an ability to contract smooth muscle and cause edema.

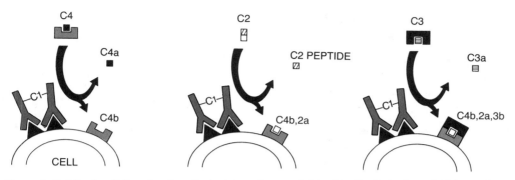

Figure 6-3. After two IgG molecules attached to antigen are bridged by C1, C4 is cleaved. C4b attaches to the antigen surface and C4a is freed as an anaphylatoxin. Subsequently, C2a is formed and binds to C4b. Then C3 is attacked to release the C3a anaphylatoxin. C3b attaches to the building C4b2a complex.

C2b may be the etiologic agent of hereditary angioneurotic edema (HANE), discussed below. C2a (70,000 Mr) binds to C4b on the antigen surface (Fig. 6-3).

The **C1s, C4b, C2a complex** is known as the **C3 convertase.** C3 convertase activity is still present after separating C1s from the other two components. This is accepted as evidence that C2a is the enzymatically active unit of the C3 convertase.

C3

C3 is a key intermediate in both the classic and alternative pathways of complement activation; thus its high concentration of 1600 μg/mL of serum is biologically important. The split products of C3, namely C3a and C3b, are important in several complement-derived activities. **C3a,** the molecule released by the action of the convertase on C3, is an **anaphylatoxin.** The remaining C3b attaches to C4b as the complement complex builds on the antigen. The attachment of C3b furnishes several biological properties to the complex. The complex is now **opsonized, prepared for phagocytosis,** and can bind to C3b receptors on macro-phages. This property of C3b is very important in immunity. Receptors for C3b on erythrocytes aid in the *removal of immune complexes* from the blood by transporting them to the spleen, where they are captured and degraded.

C3 has several parallels with C4. Like C4, it is conceived as a pro C3 synthesized by macrophages. The **pro C3** is altered after secretion to form a disulfide-linked dipeptide of 195,000 Mr. The C3a peptide of 9000 Mr removed by the C3 convertase, like C4a, is an anaphylatoxin. C3a has 77 amino acids of which the carboxyl terminal is arginine, just as in C4a. C3b also contains a **thioester group** that spans cysteine at position 1010 to glutamine at position 1014. This enables C3b to join the building complex by covalent association. Binding of C3b to the earlier components is important in continuing the cascade by creating the C5 convertase. *The C5 convertase is C4b, C2a, C3b,* with C2a being the catalytic source of the enzyme.

Failure of C3b to combine with the complex leaves it subject to proteolytic cleavage by several C3b regulating proteins. Factors H and I, and the membrane cofactor protein (MCP) form a series of degradation products when they digest C3b (see farther on).

THE MEMBRANE ATTACK COMPLEX

Of the remaining molecules in the classic activation pathway, only C5 undergoes enzymatic transformation in order to participate in the complement cascade. The remaining components aggregate with each other, eventually forming a hydrophobic macrocomplex that inserts into the outer membrane of cellular antigens, causing their lytic destruction. This membrane attack complex (MAC) consists of C5b, C6, C7, C8, and C9 (Fig. 6–4).

C5

Macrophages secrete a **pro C5** precursor molecule that is nicked by a serum protease to form C5, 190,000 Mr. C5 differs from C4 and C3 by lacking the thioester linkage. In addition, its C5a peptide is **doubly anaphylatoxic and chemotactic.** The C5a peptide of 11,500 Mr is much larger than C4a and C3a because of a substantial component of polysaccharide.

The C5a anaphylatoxin is rendered inert by AnaINH, which removes the carboxyl terminal arginine to create **desArgC5a,** but this does not destroy

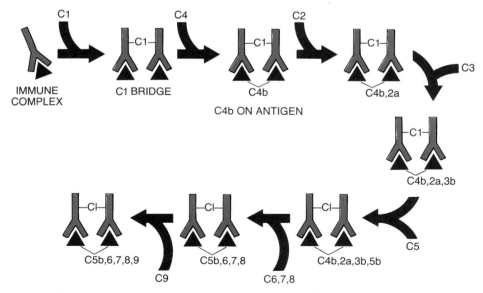

Figure 6–4. This shows the complete complement cascade by the classic activation sequence that ultimately causes cell lysis.

its **chemotactic property.** C5b, a relatively unstable molecule, becomes stabilized by combination with the later-acting components.

C6, C7, and C8

Without enzymatic change produced by the earlier enzymes in the classic pathway, C6 (120,000 Mr) binds to C5b in a 1:1 ratio. This causes the large protein complex to assume a more hydrophobic nature. This becomes especially pronounced upon the addition of C7, and the complex now attaches to lipids in the cell membrane of cellular antigens. C7, approximately the same size as C6, has a remarkable amino acid homology with C8 and C9, which may aid polymerization of these three components with each other. After C8 binds to C7, the complex C5b, C6, C7, C8 leaves C3b and embeds itself into the lipid bilayer. Sensitive cellular antigens now become "leaky" and slowly lose their cytoplasmic contents.

C9

Even though cells may become leaky when C8 enters the aggregate, true lysis requires the addition of C9. C9 is a small protein of 75,000 Mr; however, it self-aggregates to form complexes that average 15 C9 units. This aggregate forms in such a way that it is shaped like a **hydrophobic** tube that has a **hydrophilic core.** This tube penetrates both the exterior and interior margins of the lipid bilayer, and the soluble contents of the cell cytoplasm flow through this tube, resulting in cell lysis (Fig. 6–5). C9 is chemically related to a protein, **perforin,** that is secreted by LGL. As described earlier, LGL cells also cause a lytic attack on the host cell by boring holes through the lipid bilayer.

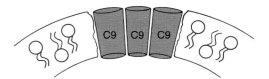

Figure 6–5. Polymerization of C9 and its penetration into the cell membrane creates pores that allow the cell cytoplasm to escape, thereby causing cell death.

MEMORY CHECK 6–3

◆

In the membrane attack complex

1. C5a anaphylatoxin and chemotaxin is produced
2. C7, C8, and C9 are chemically similar
3. The cells become "leaky" after the addition of C8
4. The cells are lysed after the huge complex of C5b, C6, C7, C8, and C9 penetrates the lipid bilayer
5. C9 is chemically related to the perforin of LGL cells

The Alternative Activation Pathway

GENERAL FEATURES

A key feature of the alternative pathway of complement activation is that the first three proteins of the classic activation pathway—C1, C4, and C2—and antibody do not participate in the molecular cascade. Activators of the alternative pathway catalyze the conversion of another series of normal serum proteins, factor B, factor D, and properdin (Table 6–3).

Formerly it was believed that properdin, a human serum protein first

Table 6-3
CHEMISTRY OF THE COMPLEMENT COMPONENTS OF THE
ALTERNATIVE PATHWAY

Component	Mr	Serum Concentration (μg/mL)
Factor B	93,000	200
Factor D	24,000	1
Properdin	184,000	20

described by Pillemer in 1954, was the first protein to function in the alternative pathway. For that reason the non-antibody pathway for the activation of complement has been called the properdin pathway. Currently it is accepted that properdin is the last of the molecules unique to the alternative pathway.

A major physical difference in the two mechanisms of complement activation is that the classic system results in cytolysis when the antigen is cellular. The alternative system does not progress on the surface of an antigen, it proceeds in solution. Cell lysis by the alternative pathway is an accident due to the unexpected deposition of the reagents on cells near the scene of complement activation.

THE ORIGIN OF C3b

C3b, or a C3b-like protein, is the first complement protein in the alternative pathway; it can be thought of as the recognition unit. It is believed that the unstable thioester bond in C3 periodically opens and closes to reform itself. If, instead of resealing upon itself, the C3 should bind to a polysaccharide or other agent known to catalyze the alternative pathway, then a C3b-macromolecule pair not unlike C3b attached

to antigen of the classic pathway would be formed. A polysaccharide is suggested here because the abundance of hydroxyl groups they contain could serve as the linkage groups for the thioester. Furthermore, complex oligosaccharides, lipopolysaccharide, teichoic acid, nucleic acids, and so on, are all known to be excellent activators of the alternative complement pathway.

THE ACTIVATION UNIT

Factor B

The molecule of the alternative pathway that binds C3b is factor B. **Factor B** of the alternative pathway is the *counterpart to C2* of the classic pathway. Both are proenzymes that become transformed into proteo-esterases. They are also essentially the same size. Factor B is slightly smaller at 93,000 Mr than C2 at 115,000 Mr. *The union of C3b with factor B creates a sensitivity in factor B to proteolysis by factor D.*

Factor D and the C3 Convertase

Factor D is a naturally occurring serum protease that clips a single Arg-Lys bond in factor B only when B is bound to C3b. Magnesium is a cofactor for this reaction that releases Ba (33,000 Mr) and leaves Bb (60,000 Mr) on C3b. C3bBb now has the ability to cleave C3; that is, **C3bBb** is *the C3 convertase of the alternative pathway*. As more C3b is produced, it binds to the C3bBb dimer to produce (C3b)nBb. This C3b-rich complex now acquires the C5-convertase activity necessary to continue the cascade into the remaining familiar C6, C7, C8, C9 proteins.

Properdin

The C3 and C5 convertases of the alternative complement pathway are unstable but become stabilized when they acquire properdin. **Properdin (P)**, a normal serum protein of 184,000 Mr, is needed to *stabilize the C3 convertase (and C5 convertase)* so that enough new C3b can be produced to form the C5 convertase (Fig. 6–6). The partici-

pation of C3b in an enzyme system that generates more C3b is termed the C3b-amplification cycle.

MEMORY CHECK 6–4

In the alternative complement pathway

1. A C3b-like molecule is the recognition unit
2. Factors B and D are the activation unit
3. C5, C6, C7, C8, and C9 are activated but function as a membrane attack complex purely by accident
4. The reactions occur in the fluid phase of the blood
5. Properdin stabilizes the C3 and C5 convertases

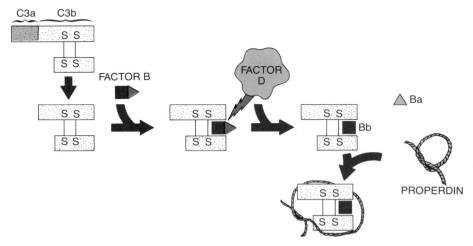

Figure 6–6. In the alternative complement pathway, C3b or a C3b-like molecule is produced from C3 and binds factor B. This exposes B to cleavage by factor D, which removes the peptide Ba. The remaining C3bBb is the C3 convertase. This convertase is stabilized by properdin. The addition of more C3b molecules forms the C5 convertase.

Biologic Functions of Complement

The stepwise description of the molecular events of classic and alternative pathways of complement do not give credit to the importance of new biologic activities that arise at each stage in the complement cascade. In the following paragraphs these biologic functions are described as they relate to health and disease.

LYSIS

The most dramatic of the complement functions is the termination of the classic pathway in **cell lysis.** Pathogenic bacteria of the **gram-negative type** are subject to **complement-mediated cytolysis**, and a combination of lysozyme and complement is deadly to gram-positive bacteria. Fungi, acid-fast bacteria, and many animal parasites are resistant to complement. Antibody and complement can also be destructive to host cells and are responsible for some forms of hemolytic anemia, granulocytopenia, thrombocytopenia, and lymphopenia.

ENZYMES

Numerous **new enzymes** are expressed in the two complement activation pathways, although no new enzymes appear in the MAC unit of the classic pathway. In its recognition unit, both **C1r** and **C1s** emerge as new trypsinlike proteases. C1s is not activated until altered by C1r.

C3 convertase activity is present in both the classic and alternative complement pathways. In the former, C3 convertase, activity appears after C2a enters the serologic complex. C2a is also critical to the **C5 convertase** of the classic pathway. Because C3 and C5 are very similar molecules, it is not unexpected that their cleavage is effected by the same enzyme.

In the alternative pathway, **Factor D** is a key enzyme that removes the activation peptide Ba from factor B. This does not occur until C3b has combined with factor B. The new complex C3bBb is the C3 convertase of the alternative pathway, and it is converted to a C5 convertase when it accumulates additional C3b from the amplification circuit.

ANAPHYLATOXIC ACTIVITY

An anaphylatoxin may be defined as a biologic agent that produces permeability changes in blood vessels that are inhibited by antihistamines. Anaphylatoxins degranulate mast cells and basophils, thereby causing the release of histamine from its storage site. In the complement system, there are three anaphylatoxins: **C4a**, generated by the action of C1s on C4; **C3a**, formed by the action of the C3 convertases on C3; and **C5a**, produced by the C5 convertases acting on C5 (Table 6–4). Anaphylatoxic C3a and C5a can be derived from the classic pathway when pathogenic bacteria combine with their antibody, or from the alternative pathway by bacteria or other infectious agents that have an external coat of polysaccharide either in their capsule or cell wall. A kinin is liberated from C2, but this is apparently different from the vasoactive peptides released by anaphylatoxins (Chapter 12).

CHEMOTACTIC ACTIVITY

Leukotaxins such as C5a induce the directional migration of leukocytes from an area of lesser concentration to

Table 6-4
SELECTED COMPLEMENT INHIBITORS AND INACTIVATORS

Inhibitor or Inactivator	Function
C1 INH	Inhibits the activated C1s complex
AnaINH	Is a carboxypeptidase; removes terminal arginine from C3a, C4a, and C5a
C4b-binding protein	Binds C4b
Factor H	Cleaves C3b
Factor I	Cleaves C3b and C4b

an area of higher concentration of the chemotaxin. In addition, a chemotaxin is apparently also liberated from the C5, C6, C7 maze, which is not identical to C5a, but the exact identity of this leukoattractant has never been elucidated and its existence is still putative.

OPSONIZATION

Opsonins are substances that modify the particle to be engulfed so that it is more easily ingested by the phagocytic cell. Chemotaxins stimulate the phagocytic cell to move toward the ingestible particle. Attachment of the complement peptides to antibody-sensitized red blood cells has been used to determine if these fractions participate in direct opsonization. The results indicate that no erythrophagocytosis occurs until **C3b** is attached. **Opsonization** is not further increased by addition of the late-acting components of complement.

IMMUNE ADHERENCE

If extraneous cells or particulate matter are present during a serologic reaction that includes complement, these cells will clump in a reaction known as **immune adherence** or serologic adhesion. This reaction has been rediscovered several times, but the term "immune adherence" seems now to be generally accepted. Immune adherence can be a sensitive detector of a serologic reation. The indicator particle may be a platelet, erythrocyte, leukocyte, yeast, heterologous bacterium, starch granule, or other entity. During the course of the agglutination reaction between the particulate antigen and its specific antibody, the indicator particles attach and cling to the antigen. Analyses with functionally purified components of complement affirm that C3 is the last in the complement series needed for immune adherence. Since C3a is released and C3b is attached to the antigen, it is clear that C3b is the key portion of C3 in this reaction. It is believed that immune adherence occurs on blood vessel walls in vivo, thereby favoring phagocytic destruction of microorganisms present in the blood.

MISCELLANEOUS ACTIVITIES

The addition of C1 stabilizes the antigen-antibody combination so that it is not easily dissociated. The apparent change in the affinity of the immunoglobulin for antigen is presumably caused by a readjustment in the ionic forces that hold the reactants together. The addition of C4 to antiviral immunoglobulins does more to neutralize infectivity of the virus than does the simple virus-antivirus combination.

The blood-clotting system in mammals, like the complement system, relies on the interaction of several different proteins that sequentially activate one another until in the final step fibrinogen is converted to fibrin by thrombin. It is not pertinent to review each of these steps here, but the initial step—the conversion of Hageman factor (factor XII) to activated Hageman factor—is important to the complement system. The serologic trigger that initiates Hageman factor activation in vivo is uncertain, but, once activated, it starts a series of reactions that involve several physiologic systems. The first of these is the clotting sequence just mentioned. The second is the formation of plasminogen activator from plasminogen proactivator. As its name indicates, plasminogen activator converts plasminogen to plasmin. Plasmin is a proteolytic enzyme that is indiscriminate in its choice of substrates. Plasmin will digest fibrin, thus creating a role for Hageman factor in both clot formation and clot dissolution. Plasmin will activate C1 and begin the entire complement cascade in the absence of any serologic reaction.

MEMORY CHECK 6–5
◆

Complement proteins contribute to

1. Cell lysis
2. New enzymes
3. Anaphylatoxins
4. Chemotaxis
5. Opsonization
6. Immune adherence
7. Complement fixation tests

Inhibitors and Inactivators of the Complement System

A multitude of biologic functions are associated with complement and the complement-derived peptides. Obviously biologic control devices have evolved to regulate these activities; otherwise, once initiated they would continue until the complement system was exhausted. For example, it is known that under the proper circumstances plasmin can activate C1. It would be detrimental to the immune defense system if plasmin generated during blood clotting were to begin an uncontrolled depletion of the complement system.

These control substances may digest and destroy the complement protein typical of inactivators or may bind and inhibit the protein. In the latter instance, the complement protein is not degraded. Unfortunately, in the complement system, the use of the terms "inactivator" and "inhibitor" is not faithful to their definition.

C1 INH

The first complement regulator to be described was **the C1 inhibitor (C1 INH)**, also called C1s INH because it inhibits the enzyme generated from C1s (and also C1r) rather than inhibiting the conversion of the proenzyme forms of C1r and C1s to their enzyme state. C1 INH is a protein of 90,000 Mr found in the α globulin fraction of normal serum (Table 6–4). Nearly 30% of C1 INH is in the form of polysaccharide and this may be important in its neutralization of C1s. The neutral C1s-C1 INH and C1r-C1 INH complexes are formed at a 1:1 ratio; that is, four molecules of C1 INH are needed to neutralize the two molecules each of C1r and C1s.

A genetic deficiency of C1 INH causes hereditary angioneurotic edema, which is discussed in Chapter 8.

FACTOR H

Factor H is another normal blood component that regulates the complement system. **Factor H,** previously known as the β1H protein, binds to either free or cell-bound C3b. In the first situation C3b is prevented from binding to antigen because it is enzymatically *digested by factor I, factor H serving only as a cofactor.* The cell-bound C3b cleavage is facilitated by complement receptor 1 (CR1).

FACTOR I

The destruction of C3b is not the only property of **factor I;** *it can also inactivate C4b.* Factor I consists of two peptides of 50,000 Mr and 40,000 Mr held together by a disulfide bond. The smaller unit is the protease. Digestion of C3b and C4b is assisted by factor H, and complement receptor 1 (CR1) participates in these reactions. Factor H is the primary assistant when factor I cleaves the α chain of free C3b or C4b, and CR1 is the assistant for factor I degradation of bound C3b or C4b (Fig. 6–7).

AnaINH

AnaINH is the abbreviation for the **carboxypeptidase** known as the anaphylatoxin inhibitor that removes the carboxyl terminal arginine from C3a, C4a, and C5a. It is an inactivator rather than an inhibitor. AnaINH is a large α globulin of 300,000 Mr. The des arginine derivatives are no longer active anaphylatoxins; however, desArgC5a is still chemotactic.

C4b-BINDING PROTEIN

An enormous serum protein measuring 600,000 Mr can combine with six molecules of C4b at one time because of a unique starfishlike structure of seven legs radiating from a central core. This C4b-binding protein (C4BP) blocks a continuation of the complement cascade. Factor I may be critical at this stage, cleaving C4b when held in the grasp of C4BP. C4BP is a member of a group of proteins termed the **regulators of complement activity (RCA proteins).** These proteins have their structural gene on **human chromosome 1** and contain a series of *consensus repeat sequences of 60 to 70 amino acids* (Fig. 6–8). *RCA members are C4BP, decay-accelerating factor (DAF), membrane cofactor protein (MCP), factor H, CR1, and CR2* (Table 6–5).

DECAY-ACCELERATING FACTOR

The C3 and C5 convertases of both complement activation pathways are subject to dissociation and inactivation by decay-accelerating factor **(DAF)**. This protein is found on the surface of several cell types including erythrocytes and granulocytes, but it is also found in a soluble form in the body fluids. The ability of DAF to separate C4b from C2a is responsible for the decay of the two convertases.

DAF is a protein of approximately 72,000 Mr. It is structurally related to

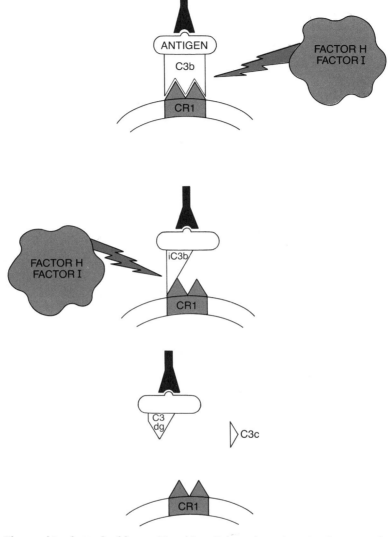

Figure 6-7. The combined attack of factors H and I on C3b produces inactive fragments from C3b and eventually dissociates it from the antigen-antibody complex.

factor H and C4BP by possessing consensus repeat sequences of 60 amino acids. Three other members of the RCA group found on cell surfaces are CR1, CR2, and MCP.

Deficiency of DAF leads to paroxysmal nocturnal hemoglobinuria (see Chapter 8).

MEMBRANE COFACTOR PROTEIN

A protein found on monocytes, granulocytes, and B and T lymphocytes appears to *cooperate with factor I* in its proteolysis of C3b and C4b and is aptly named **membrane cofactor protein**

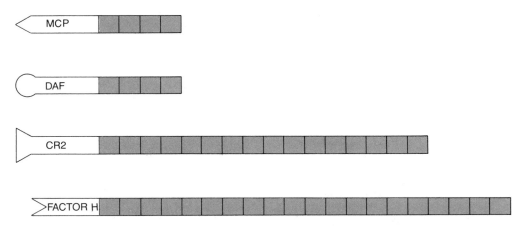

Figure 6-8. These figures reveal the consensus repeat structure of four complement receptors, varying only in the number of these segments and in the means by which they attach to the cell surface.

(MCP). The molecular weight of MCP varies from 50,000 to 70,000 Mr as the result of variable glycosylation.

HOMOLOGOUS RESTRICTION FACTOR

A novel protein on the erythrocyte surface that protects the cell against lysis by its own (homologous) source of complement is known as **homologous restriction factor (HRF)**. This protein is structurally related to C8 and C9, but it is unclear how this relates to its protective role.

S PROTEIN

A hydrophilic complex formed by the addition of S protein to C5b, C6, C7 *prevents* the developing complement complex from *embedding in the lipid bilayer* of the target antigen. **S protein, a synonym for vitronectin**, is an 80,000-Mr protein responsible for this activity.

Complement Receptors

Receptors are cell surface components that function as ligands for molecules normally in solution. Receptors for

Table 6-5
REGULATORS OF COMPLEMENT ACTIVITY (RCA) PROTEINS

Protein	Function
C4b-binding protein	Binds C4b
Factor H	Inactivates C3b, cofactor of factor I
CR1 (CD35)	Binds C3b; is Mac1 antigen on macrophages
CR2 (CD21)	Binds C3b; is Epstein-Barr virus receptor
DAF	Dissociates C3 and C5 convertases
MCP	Is a cofactor of factor I

several complement-related molecules, including the anaphylatoxins and C1q, have been described, but the receptors best understood are those for C3b and C4b.

CR1

Complement receptor 1 (CR1), also known as protein CD35, *is found on a broad spectrum of cells,* including monocytes, macrophages, polymorphonuclear neutrophils, eosinophils, B cells, T cells, and erythrocytes. This distribution suggests a wide variety of functions but, in fact, few are definitely known. Because CR1 binds C3b, a role as an opsonin is indicated for the CR1 found on phagocytic cells. This aids the antibody-dependent cell cytotoxic function of these cells. On B cells CR1 may be an immunomodulator. Erythrocyte CR1 is involved in the removal of soluble immune complexes from the circulation. All CR1 molecules are not the same size, ranging from 190,000 to 250,000. This is due to the variable inclusion of these long amino acid consensus repeat sequences common to the RCA group of complement regulators.

CR2

The **CR2 receptor** is found on B cells as a 140,000-Mr molecule that, like CR1, binds C3b. This molecule serves as the **receptor for the Epstein-Barr virus,** an agent that infects B cells, and one that is closely associated with Burkitt's lymphoma. *CD21 is a synonym for CR2.* The role of CR2 as a C3b binder is unknown, but the presence of CR2 on B cells hints at a role in the control of immunoglobulin synthesis.

CR3

The **CR3 receptor** is found on macrophages, LGL cells, and many others (including neutrophils, eosinophils, and dendritic cells). In molecular terms, CR3 is one of a series of molecules (the integrins described in Chapter 2) that have different α chains but share identical 95,000-Mr β chains. The CR3 α chain is 165,000 Mr; the β chain of lymphocyte functional antigen–1 (LFA-1) is 185,000 Mr. Glycoprotein 150/95 has a 150,000-Mr β chain. LFA-1 aids binding to T cells because of its pairing with CD2 on the lymphocyte. Glycoprotein 150/95 may be a complement receptor like CR3. *CR3 is the* **Mac1 antigen** also known as the M1 antigen on macrophages. CR3 binds to C3b and is important in antibody-dependent cell cytotoxicity and phagocytosis.

MEMORY CHECK 6 – 6
◆

Receptors or regulators of the complement system

1. May combine but not destroy a component; eg, C1 INH

2. May destroy a component by proteolytic digestion; eg, factor I

3. May be cell bound; eg, MCP, DAF, HRF

4. May be cell-free proteins; eg, factor H, factor I, AnaINH, C1 INH, C4BP, S protein

5. May share long consensus repeat sequences; eg, DAF, factor H, C4BP, CR1, CR2, MCP

6. May be found on several cell types; eg, CR1, CR3, MCP

Genetics of Complement

The chromosomal origin of all components of the complement system is not yet identified. As previously mentioned, several complement regulators grouped under the category of regulators of complement activity (RCA) share human chromosome 1 as the locus of their structural gene.

Human chromosome 6 is a key genetic unit because it houses the MHC class I and class II proteins. The class I proteins have a powerful control over the acceptance or rejection of tissue transplants. As described in an earlier chapter, the class II proteins are immunoregulatory molecules. The class III proteins of the MHC are C2, C4, factor B, TNFα, and TNFβ. The human C4 gene has been duplicated as C4A and C4B. Several allotypes of C2, C4, and factor B are known. This is not unique to these complement proteins, several others, including C3, also having multiple allotypic forms.

Genes for C1r and C1s are present on human chromosome 12. Their dual presence on a single chromosome, and their similar structure and function indicate a possible gene duplication.

Complement Fixation

As mentioned in the introduction to this chapter, the activation of the complement pathway can be described in several ways — complement activation emphasizes its catalytic aspects; complement inactivation indicates that complement is used or removed; and complement fixation suggests that complement is bound to the antigen-antibody system. The latter is only partially true; indeed, some of the most significant functions of complement are related to the fractions liberated during activation. But the term "complement fixation" is still preferred to describe the serologic tests in which an exact amount of complement is added to what is believed to be an antigen-antibody or **test system**. For example, a serum sample can be tested to determine whether it contains antibodies that will react with a specific antigen in the presence of complement. If this is true, the complement will be fixed into the serologic complex. This prevents the complement from reacting with the subsequently added indicator system. The **indicator system** consists of sheep red blood cells plus anti-red blood cell hemolysin. The red blood cells cannot be lysed by the antibody if complement is unavailable. Thus, one can determine if complement were fixed in the first antigen-antibody pair. If so, there is no hemolysis and the complement fixation test result is positive. In negative test results, hemolysis occurs. The complement fixation test is described more fully in Chapter 14.

References

Ahearn, JM and Fearon, DT: Structure and function of the complement receptors CR2 (CD35) and CR2 (CD21). Adv Immunol 46:183, 1989.

Law, SKA and Reid, KBM: Complement in Focus. IRL Press, Oxford, 1988.

Muller-Eberhard, HJ: The membrane attack complex of complement. Annu Rev Immunol 4:503, 1986.

Muller-Eberhard, HJ and Colten, HR: The complement system. Prog Immunol 6:267, 1986.

Reid, KBM: Activation and control of the complement system. Essays Biochem 22:27, 1986.

Ross, GD (ed): Immunobiology of the Complement System. Academic Press, Orlando, FL, 1986.

Whaley, K (ed): Complement in Health and Disease. MTP Press, Lancaster, PA, 1987.

QUESTIONS AND ANSWERS

1. The proteins of the complement system
   A. Number nine in both the classic and the alternative pathways
   B. Do not increase in concentration during immunization
   C. Can enter serologic reactions involving IgM or IgG but not IgE
   D. May be missing in some immunodeficiency conditions
   E. All of the above

Answer E

There are nine major proteins in both the classic and the alternative pathway. C1, C4, and C2 of the classic pathway are replaced by factors B, D, and properdin of the alternative pathway, respectively. Complement does not increase during immunization; its level may even decrease if it becomes bound into antigen-antibody complexes. IgE is not a complement-activating immunoglobulin, but IgM and IgG (with the exception of IgG4) share complement-activating activity. Immunodeficiency diseases such as HANE and DAF deficiency exist because of a loss of a complement regulator, but losses of C2, C3, and other complement molecules are known. Thus, all answers are correct.

2. Which of the following is not a cell surface (bound) regulator of the complement system?
   A. C1 INH
   B. DAF
   C. CR1
   D. CR2
   E. MCP

Answer A

C1 INH is a normal serum component designed to curtail sporadic or excessive activation of C1s. All the other choices listed are cell surface regulators of complement at the level of C3b. Each is a member of the RCA group whose inheritance originates on human chromosome 1. All members of the RCA group have long amino acid consensus repeat sequences.

3. In the alternative pathway of complement activation
   A. Components C6, C7, C8, and C9 do not participate
   B. Both C3a and C5a are produced
   C. Immune complexes are required
   D. Properdin is actually the first, not the last, unique serum protein involved
   E. All of the above

Answer B

When C3b is produced by the C3bBb convertase, C3a is also produced. The alternative pathway of complement activation then uses all the subsequent components after C3. Immune complexes are not involved in the alternative pathway. The terms "properdin pathway" and "alternative pathway" were once interchangeable, but the former term is gradually falling into disuse. Properdin is the last unique protein of the alternative pathway but is followed by C5, C6, C7, C8, and C9.

4. Which of the following is the C3 convertase of the alternative activation pathway of complement?

   A. C1s
   B. C4b2a
   C. C3bBa
   D. C3bBbP
   E. Factor D

Answer D

The complex C3bBbP is the stable form of C3bBb, both of which are C3 convertases of the alternative pathway. C3bBa does not exist, Ba being shed into the blood after factor D attacks the C3bB pair. C4b2a and C1s participate in the active pathway.

5. C3 has been described as the most critical element of the complement system. This is because

   A. C3 is more abundant in blood than any other component
   B. C3 participates in both the classic and alternative activation pathways
   C. More biologic properties are associated with C3 (including C3a and C3b) than with any other protein in the complement system
   D. It is the first component of the alternative pathway
   E. All of the above

Answer E

All of the statements are true. The sum of these supports the claim that C3 is the most important molecule in the complement system.

Case Study: Diagnosis Unknown

Nina T., a 15-year-old high school freshman, was referred to the University Hospital by her local physician for diagnosis of a possible deficiency of C1 INH. Over the past year, Nina had been stricken by episodes of fainting, difficulty in breathing, and edema of the throat and face. The first incidents were much milder than the more recent attacks. Extensive and repeated physical and laboratory examinations were unable to detect a cause for her condition. Because it was believed the increasing severity of her laryngeal edema might eventually create a life-threatening situation, she was referred to UH for further work-up.

Questions

1. What immunologic events could lead to repeated sporadic attacks of edema, and how are they diagnosed?

2. What are the normal control mechanisms for edema of immune origin?

3. What are the therapeutic possibilities for this condition?

Discussion

Among the first diagnostic considerations in a case like this is hereditary angioneurotic edema (HANE). HANE is a genetic disease resulting from an inability to synthesize C1 INH or to synthesize an inactive form of C1 INH. As a result of this loss, the affected person is unable to control those spontaneous, ordinarily trivial activations of the complement cascade that are easily controlled when C1 INH levels are normal. The C2 kinins and possibly the anaphylatoxins are allowed to express their full activity and produce the symptoms that Nina displayed.

The diagnosis of HANE can be made by immunodiffusion tests for C1 INH in Nina's serum. The radial immunodiffusion test is used for this (see Chapter 14). It would also be possible to determine the amount of complement activity in Nina's serum by doing hemolytic tests. Persons unable to slow or regulate the complement cascade have lower complement levels than do healthy persons.

The natural control of edematous eruptions originating from the complement system is based primarily on the adequacy of C1 INH. Other inactivators or inhibitors at the C4, C3, and C5 levels of the complement system are also contributors. AnaINH would play a very important part in destroying the C4a, C3a, and C5a anaphylatoxins.

Treatment of HANE by transfusions with normal plasma to reconstitute the C1 INH level is one therapeutic mode. The esterase inhibitor ϵ-aminocaproic acid has also been used. The preferred therapy is to use androgens that release C1 INH from its cellular storehouse in the liver.

Actually, in Nina's case a diagnosis of HANE was not possible. Serologic tests proved her to have the normal serum C1 INH level of 180 μg/mL. Efforts to identify an allergic cause of her attacks are in progress.

GLOSSARY

activation unit of complement Complement proteins C4, C2, and C3.

alternative complement pathway A system for activating complement, beginning at C3 and not involving a serologic reaction.

AnaINH Anaphylatoxin inhibitor.

anaphylatoxins C3a, C4a, and C5a, all of which cause degranulation of mast cells.

anaphylatoxin inhibitor An enzyme that destroys the biologic activity of C3a, C4a, and C5a.

C1, C2, and so on Components of serum complement numbered sequentially from 1 through 9.

C1 INH The serum inhibitor of the activated first component of complement.

classic complement pathway A system for activating complement that is initiated by a reaction of antigen with IgG or IgM.

complement fixation A serologic test using complement, antigen, and antibody.

CR1, CR2, and CR3 Designations for complement receptors on cells.

HANE Hereditary angioneurotic edema.

hereditary angioneurotic edema An edematous condition resulting from a deficiency of C1s INH.

immune adherence The adhesive nature of antigen-antibody complexes to inert surfaces when C3b is bound.

kinins Peptides or polyamines released during anaphylaxis that possess vasodilating and muscle-contracting activity.

MAC The membrane attack complex.

membrane attack complex Complement components C5b, C6, C7, C8, and C9.

RCA Regulators of complement activity.

recognition unit of complement Complement molecule C1.

regulators of complement activity In a generic sense, any inhibitor of complement; in a specific sense, chemically related complement inhibitors arising from chromosome 1.

CHAPTER 7

◆

Immunity

Every living being must defend itself against infection. Some do this indirectly by developing an unusually high rate of reproduction to ensure the survival of at least a few from an enormous population. The human animal evolved to master a more aggressive strategy, a strategy that is divisible into two major compartments. One compartment is permanently in place. It is constituitive and is known as **natural resistance**, though several synonyms are also in use. The second compartment is adaptive, a part of our defense system that is acquired from our encounters with infectious challenges. This **acquired immunity**, unlike natural resistance, may be considered a more economic type of immunity because it focuses on a specific invader, rather than on the broader spectrum of infectious threats.

This chapter is divided into two sections—natural resistance and acquired immunity. In the former section, several tissues and organs are considered from the viewpoint of their self-protection. This is followed by a description of activities and agents, such as phagocytic cells and complement, that are more widely distributed.

The discussion of acquired immunity is described both from its humoral or antibody source and from its cellular sources. A major section is devoted to active immunization, first against bacterial and then against viral diseases. Many of these vaccines will be changed in the future as new products are developed through recombinant DNA technology, synthetic molecules, and the anti-idiotypic network as described in the last section of this chapter.

Natural Resistance

The term "natural resistance" is usually equated with inherited or innate immunity and has traditionally been defined as an individual's ability to resist infection through the normal body functions typical of the human species. These functions will vary with the age, sex, nutritional status, and other characteristics of the individual. Natural resistance does not include resistance developed because of a previous exposure to a pathogenic organism or its toxic products. Therefore, natural resistance relies upon the nonadaptive, normal structures and functions of the body. Natural resistance is traditionally divided into two subtopics — the **external defense system** and **internal defense system** mechanisms. Both are based on anatomic and structural barriers, antimicrobial molecules found in the blood and the tissue, direct antimicrobial tactics of cells such as those of the phagocytic cell system, mechanical events such as peristalsis, the flow of

secretions, and even the influence of nonpathogenic organisms on the ability of pathogenic organisms to colonize and invade the body.

EXTERNAL DEFENSE SYSTEM

Although some pathogenic microorganisms can cause disease by their ability to colonize our external body surfaces and the secretion of toxins that wound underlying cells, most pathogens must transgress this outer cell barrier in order to cause disease. In this regard, because no cell layer is passed when an organism takes residence in the alimentary tract, the genitourinary tract, respiratory tree, or other invaginations of the body, these are subject to control by our external defense system. This system is very versatile, including keratinized, relatively impermeable cell layers, antimicrobial chemicals and cells, and protective physiologic functions (Fig. 7–1).

The Skin — More Than an Anatomic Barrier

The first resistance system encountered by externally located microbes is the intact outer cell layer of the dermis or the mucous membranes. The keratinized outer layer of the **skin** represents a formidable **anatomic barrier** to most microorganisms. Only a few

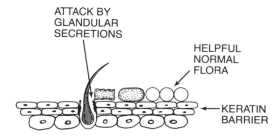

ATTACK BY
GLANDULAR
SECRETIONS

HELPFUL
NORMAL
FLORA

KERATIN
BARRIER

Figure 7–1. The bacterium next to the hair shaft is in a state of decay as it contacts secretions brought outward by the growing hair. The coccus-shaped bacteria represent normal flora that prevent occupation of that skin site by pathogens. The outer layer of the skin also represents a tough, resistant barrier to pathogens.

pathogens (including the spirochete causing syphilis, the bacterium causing tularemia, and the larvae of certain infectious worms) can penetrate intact, healthy skin, but in reality it is the activity of the glands underlying the skin that dominates immunity on these barriers. The skin is coated by *secretions from the sebaceous glands* that contain lactic acid and unsaturated fatty acids. These are both antibacterial and antifungal in nature. The skin is also coated by a large population of microorganisms that constitute the **normal flora**. These bacteria are ordinarily unable to cause disease, but they occupy an ecologic niche preferred by pathogenic organisms. In so doing, they exclude pathogens from a permanent residence upon the skin or mucous membranes. Potentially pathogenic organisms that do contact the skin may dry and thereby lose their vitality before reaching a population sufficient to cause disease. Certain organisms such as the gonococcus are especially vulnerable to drying.

Defense of the Mucous Membranes

The Respiratory System. Drying, of course, does not take place upon the mucous membranes, because the surface is continually moistened by additional heavy secretions. However, the mucosal surfaces often have additional protective devices. Upon the mucosal areas of the upper respiratory tract, a special kind of phagocytic cell, the **alveolar macrophage**, contributes significantly to natural resistance. These cells roam over the external surface of the lungs and through the mucus, and phagocytose inhaled objects, including microorganisms. **Mucus** is a mucilaginous substance upon which microorganisms impinge during deep inhalation and from which they cannot easily

escape. This mucous film is swept upward from the lungs and through the trachea at a rate of 1 or 2 inches per minute. It then passes the epiglottis and is swallowed.

The Genitourinary System. Mucous membranes of other surfaces have different protective functions. In males and females, the genitourinary system is *mechanically flushed with urine* that is slightly acidic and provides an unsuitable growth pH for microorganisms that are not mechanically removed by the flow of urine. The urine and mucosal surfaces of the eyes contain **lysozyme**, an enzyme that is actually able to dissolve the outer cell membrane of many gram-positive bacteria. Gram-negative bacteria are much more resistant to lysozyme, and it is interesting to observe that contagious pinkeye is caused by a gram-negative, lysozyme-resistant microorganism. Weeping tends to wash microorganisms from the eye.

The Digestive System. The digestive system, like the respiratory and genitourinary systems, is considered part of

---

MEMORY CHECK 7 – 1

The external natural defense system consists of

1. Skin as a physical barrier where drying takes place
2. Secretion of unsaturated fatty acids and lactic acid on the skin
3. Normal bacterial flora, especially in the bowel and female genitourinary system
4. Alveolar macrophages of the lung
5. Lysozyme in tears and urine
6. Peristalsis, the flow of urine and tears

the external system of the body. The **acidity of the stomach** may be as low as pH 1 and is destructive for many organisms that are fully exposed to it. However, certain microorganisms are aciduric and can escape the detrimental influence of this acid, especially when protected inside poorly masticated pieces of food. The population of normal flora bacteria in the bowel reaches 10^{15} per gram of feces. The residence of these organisms on the bowel surface and the antimicrobial compounds they secrete aid our resistance to gastrointestinal disease. Such immunity is not perfect, however. Invading microorganisms thus reach the small intestine, where they must overcome the natural flora before they can cause disease. The microbial flora of the small intestine serves an extremely important role in resisting invasion by potentially pathogenic organisms. Typhoid fever, cholera, and bacterial and amebic dysenteries are examples of diseases in which pathogens do supersede the normal flora (Table 7–1).

INTERNAL DEFENSE SYSTEM

After pathogens penetrate the external defense system and enter the true physiologic milieu of the host, they then encounter a large number of internal defense activities. Within the organs and tissues there are anatomic barriers that prevent direct extension of pathogens from one tissue to another. Organisms that are able to invade the blood stream or the lymphatic system avoid these barriers and are distributed through these systems to other tissues and organs where they may establish foci of infection.

Phagocytes

The most important activity in the internal defense system is phagocytosis. Although polymorphonuclear neutro-

Table 7–1
MECHANISMS OF
NATURAL RESISTANCE

Tissue Site	Active Agents
Skin	Keratinized anatomic barrier
	Lactic and unsaturated fatty acids
	Normal microbial flora
Respiratory system	Alveolar macrophages
	Mucous film
	Ciliary action
Genitourinary system	Mechanical washing by urine
	Acid pH of urine
	Lysozyme
	Mucus
	Normal microbial flora
Gastrointestinal system	Peristalsis
	Alkaline pH of small intestine
	Acid pH of stomach
	Normal microbial flora

philic leukocytes in the blood do contribute to phagocytosis, the most important of the phagocytic cells is the tissue macrophage. As described in Chapter 2, the monocytes leave the blood, enter tissues, and metamorphose into their more active phagocytic form, the macrophages. These cells are more motile, more adhesive to surfaces (phagocytosis is a surface phenomenon), more phagocytic, and far more cytocidal than monocytes. When the complement system of the blood is activated by the alternate pathway, chemotaxins are released that stimulate a directional motility of phagocytes. This is important in that it leads the phagocytes to the site and to the bacteria often involved in this type of complement activation. Enzymes released from tissues that have been damaged by the bacteria or their toxins may also activate the complement system. Macrophages stimulated by complement and the act of phagocytosis have been described as **activated, or armed, phagocytes** because they assume an even more aggressive attitude than the usual macrophage. These hyperactive macrophages are more destructive of invading organisms than the "standard" macrophage (Fig. 7–2).

The biochemical mechanism used by macrophages to destroy their phagocytosed foes relies heavily on their **oxidative metabolism**. The enzyme myeloperoxidase has been identified as a major contributor in this process with assistance from hydroxyl radicals, singlet oxygen, and other toxic varieties of oxygen.

Within the granules of human phagocytic cells, a battery of cationic proteins has been aptly named **defensins**. These are all low molecular weight peptides active against both gram-positive and gram-negative bacteria, fungi and even the enveloped viruses typified by herpes simplex virus. The concentration of these defensins in phagocytes exceeds that of myeloperoxidase or lysozyme by twofold (Fig. 7–3).

Large Granular Lymphocytes

A second cell type that is an important contributor to natural immunity is the **large granular lymphocyte** known simply as the **LGL** or **natural killer (NK)** cell. LGL or NK cells are large granular lymphoid cells that lack typical B-cell or T-cell markers; because of this they have been called null cells. Upon direct contact with a target cell, in the absence of any previous experience, the LGL cell is able to effect cytolysis of the target. The biochemical basis for this is only partially known — the LGL cells release **lymphotoxin (LT)**, also known as TNFβ, and **perforins** that may be their major weapons, as discussed in Chapter 4. Normally, tumor cells are the target for LGL cells; however, they may attack virus-infected cells or any cell with an extraneous antigen on its surface. LGL cells are considered part of the first line of defense against viruses, other intracellular pathogens, and tumor cells, and they may play an important role in graft rejection.

Complement

The **complement system** was described extensively in the preceding chapter. The participation of complement in immunity may originate either

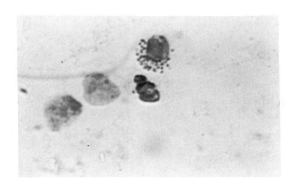

Figure 7–2. This phagocyte (upper center) has engulfed numerous bacteria. (See color figure after Table of Contents.)

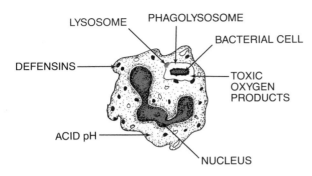

Figure 7-3. Three antimicrobial agents within neutrophil (shown here) and macrophages are the defensins, acid pH, and oxidative metabolism, the latter of which exists in multiple forms.

from the alternate, nonantibody-requiring pathway or the classic pathway. C3 and C5 contribute more to the immune functions of complement than the other components. **C3b** is a powerful **opsonin**. The presence of C3b receptors on monocytes, macrophages, neutrophils, and other granulocytes ensures that a C3b-coated organism will be engulfed. **Immune adherence** is another phagocytosis-promoting function of C3b. C5b is a powerful **chemotaxin** that draws phagocytes to antigen-antibody deposits. The clearance of C3b-bearing immune complexes from the blood is an important cleansing activity. The C3a, C4a, and C5a **anaphylatoxins** function in the inflammatory phase of host resistance by creating a local edema that dilutes toxic molecules deposited by infectious organisms. Of these, C4a originates solely from the classic system. Although lysis is not a major attribute of the alternate complement system, the inflammatory and phagocytosis-promoting activities of complement contribute significantly to the internal defense system.

Antimicrobial Chemicals

In addition to complement, other macromolecules in the blood may function importantly in natural resistance. For example, many viruses normally attach to glycoproteins on the external membranes of the host cells that they will invade. **Glycoproteins** found in the blood may coat the virus and function as false receptors, thereby preventing contact of the virus with its natural receptor on susceptible cells. **Iron-binding proteins** present in the blood and in secretions, when not saturated with iron, compete with bacteria for the iron present in the body fluids, iron that is needed for bacterial growth. Sequestration of iron by transferrin or lactoferrin can reduce or prevent bacterial growth. Other molecules such as polyamines, protamines, histones, spermine, and other **basic polypeptides**, because of their cationic nature, are able to attach to the surface of the negatively charged bacteria. In the neutral ionic state, the microorganisms are more easily approached and phagocytosed.

Regulation of Natural Resistance

It is clear that even young children, whose immunity is based largely upon natural resistance, differ from one another in the degree or extent of their resistance. In general, the very young and the elderly are the least resistant to infections, with the middle age groups being the most resistant. These differences are related to many factors such as sex, race, nutritional status, fatigue, and climate. Extensive **protein-**

calorie malnutrition increases the incidence of bacterial, fungal, and viral infection by interfering with many aspects of natural resistance. For example, when affected by malnutrition, phagocytic cells function at only 10% to 30% of their efficiency in normal individuals. Lysozyme levels are also depleted by malnutrition. In general, undernourished individuals not only suffer more frequent episodes of infectious disease; these episodes are more severe, and recovery is usually prolonged. **Hormonal modifications** also alter natural resistance. Individuals with diabetes are unquestionably more susceptible to staphylococcal, streptococcal, and certain yeast infections. Insulin deficiency has a direct effect upon the integrity of cell membranes, rendering cells more susceptible to invasion by pathogenic microbes. Hormonal changes that cause a thickening of the vaginal epithelium of adult women contribute to their resistance to infection. As the additional cells present in this thickened epithelium die and are shed, greater quantities of lactic acid are formed from the glyco-

gen stored in these cells in adult women than in prepubertal females. This acid, which is produced by the indigenous vaginal flora, deters infection by pathogenic organisms.

Acquired Immunity

Acquired immunity is dependent entirely upon new factors generated by the body as an adaptive response following a first contact with pathogenic organisms or their products. These acquired factors may act independently or cooperate with aspects of natural resistance. Acquired immunity is too often thought to rely entirely upon the activity of the antibody system. Although antibody-based acquired immunity is often the major source of protection against infectious diseases, there are important exceptions. Persons with genetic agammaglobulinemia contract the usual childhood viral diseases but recover from them normally, an expression of T-cell immunity. Phagocytosis, though improved by antibody, is still an important defense factor even in its absence.

ACTIVE IMMUNITY

Classification

Active immunity is **self-generated** by one's own tissues. Normally acquired immunity is highly effective because it uses both immunoglobulin and T-cell activities. It is also possible to have acquired immunity in advance of contact with an infectious agent, so that when contact does occur, the immune system fights with a small number rather than a large population of invaders. Active immunity requires an immunologic waiting period of 5 to 14 days to develop after the exposure to antigens

---

MEMORY CHECK 7–2

◆

The natural internal defense system consists of

1. Large granular lymphocytes, their perforins, and lymphotoxin

2. Phagocytosis and its oxygen-dependent and -independent microbicidal activities

3. Complement: its C3b opsonin, its C3a, C4a, and C5a anaphylatoxins, and the C5a chemotaxin

4. Cell-free basic peptides and amines, iron-binding proteins, and so forth.

of the pathogenic organisms before the immunoglobulin-producing B cells and the T cells are fully active. During this time, the invading organism could achieve very large numbers unless the individual was already immune. When a preceding infection stimulates the immunity, the condition is referred to as a **naturally acquired immunity**. This should not be confused with **natural resistance**. Immunity may arise from immunization with killed or attenuated vaccines, cellular subunits, purified products, or with detoxified products (toxoids) of microorganisms. If contrived immunizations are responsible for the immunity, it is described as an **artificially acquired immunity**. Here the use of **attenuated vaccines** rather than killed or subunit vaccines is preferred. Attenuated vaccines consist of weakened infectious agents that can grow in vivo and produce a mild infection that the host is able to control. This more nearly represents naturally acquired active immunity and is generally superior to the use of killed vaccines. The immunity developed as a result of immunization with toxoids is exceptionally strong and is preferred when the principal symptoms of a disease are related to an intoxication rather than an infection.

A major advantage of active immunity is that after proper booster doses, the decay of the serum antibody titer is prolonged because of isotype switching to the long-lived IgG. Consequently the immunity is of **long duration**. Moreover, the ability to repeat the booster injections of antigen on demand means that active immunity can be easily reactivated. **Booster injections** restimulate both antibody-mediated **(humoral) immunity** and T-cell **(cell-mediated) immunity** (Table 7–2).

MEMORY CHECK 7–3

◆

Acquired immunity is

1. Naturally acquired active immunity resulting from previous disease
2. Artificially acquired active immunity resulting from immunization
3. Of long duration
4. Easily reactivated by booster vaccinations
5. Based on antibody and T-cell immunity

Table 7–2

CHARACTERISTICS OF ACTIVE AND PASSIVE IMMUNITY

	Active Immunity	Passive Immunity
Origin	Self-generated	Received by injection
Mechanism	1. Immunization	1. Injection
	2. Disease	2. Maternal antibody passed across the placenta
Booster effect	1. Easily done	1. Easily done
	2. Little danger	2. Risk of anaphylaxis with animal sera
	3. Boosts both T and B cells	
Effectiveness	1. High	1. High, prophylactically
	2. Long duration	2. Low, therapeutically
		3. Short duration

Immunoglobulins

Immunity based on antibody formation is the most formidable type of immunity against bacterial toxins, against some but not all bacterial pathogens, and in some instances against viral pathogens, particularly those viruses that must pass through the blood to reach their target tissues. *The most effective of the immunoglobulins is IgG*, although IgM also plays a significant role in immunity. IgG is the antibody whose synthesis is often stimulated preferentially by protein antigens such as toxoids. The combination of the antitoxin with a toxin is very firm, with little opportunity for the toxin to dissociate and attack host cells. IgG also has a prolonged half-life of approximately 25 to 30 days. IgM synthesis is favored by exposure to polysaccharide antigens, such as those present on the surface of many infectious bacteria. Combination of **IgM** with these antigens **opsonizes** the bacteria, so that they become highly susceptible to phagocytosis. IgA of serum plays a questionable role in immunity despite the recognition of true antibody activity in this globulin. **Secretory IgA**, by virtue of its coating of mucosal membranes, may actually be more significant in immunity than serum IgA by preventing direct contact of the pathogen with host cells, thereby reducing the risk of an infection. These immunoglobulins mask the attachment site used by viruses to contact their receptor on host cells. Although it possesses certain antibody activities, IgD is of questionable value in immunity, partially because of its scarcity in serum. IgE may contribute to immunity, in part, by its generation of potent inflammatory responses. IgE bound to the surface of eosinophils arms these cells for a lethal attack on animal parasites and pathogenic bacteria.

Antibodies bound to antigen are able to activate the classic complement pathway, a system that generates several protective functions of complement as described earlier.

Antibody-Dependent Cell Cytotoxicity

Antibody-dependent cell cytotoxicity (ADCC) is a unique expression of target cell toxicity expressed by antibody acting in concert with cells. Cells of diverse origin — polymorphonuclear, monocytic, and lymphoid — are all known to cooperate with antibody in the destruction of tumor, transplant or viral-infected cell targets (Fig. 7–4). It is believed that these cells will attack and kill any host cell that has a foreign antigen on its surface. The method of cell killing differs for each of the cell types. Polymorphonuclear neutrophilic leukocytes and macrophages have surface **receptors for the Fc fragment** of IgG. When this antibody combines with its target antigen, phagocytosis is enhanced and the internalized target cell is killed by oxygen-dependent or oxygen-independent pathways available to the phagocyte. Eosinophils use IgE for this activity. Lymphoid cells are

---

MEMORY CHECK 7–4

Immunoglobulins function in acquired immunity by

1. Being opsonins and stimulating phagocytosis
2. Activating complement and generating its several immune functions
3. Arming cells for ADCC reactions
4. Neutralizing toxins
5. Coating viruses so they cannot combine with their receptor on target cells

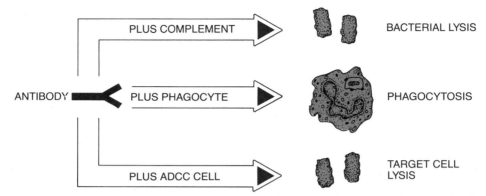

Figure 7–4. Immunoglobulins participate in target cell destruction by three different mechanisms: (1) directly with the assistance of complement, (2) indirectly by functioning as an opsonin, and (3) with ADCC active cells in target cell lysis.

not phagocytic. They destroy target cells by releasing perforins and lymphotoxin from their cytoplasmic granules.

Phagocytes

The role of phagocytes in acquired immunity is essentially the same as in natural resistance except that it is embellished by the opsonic and complement-activating properties of antibody.

T Lymphocytes

T cells are important in ADCC immunity. A small population of T cells, the Tγ cells, have Fc receptors for IgG. When this IgG is directed toward a "forbidden" antigen, this T cell, also known as a **killer (K) cell**, will attack and destroy the target. By means of the antibody specificity, normal host cells are spared. These T cells offer protection against viruses, other intracellular parasites, malignantly transformed host tumor cells, and transplanted cells. These Tγ cells secrete perforins that bore a hole in the cell membrane of the target cell. The cell cytoplasm leaks through this hole and the cell dies.

The cytotoxic **CD8+ T cell, or cytotoxic T lymphocyte (CTL)**, does not rely upon antibody as its binding agent for cells that it will ultimately destroy. The CTL uses its standard antigen receptor to combine with MHC class I proteins as anchoring sites for the target cell. CD8+ T cells destroy cellular targets by secreting perforins and lymphotoxin, as described in Chapter 4. Of course, the T helper cell is important in acquired immunity because of its positive influence on other T cells and the immunoglobulin-secreting B cells.

PASSIVE IMMUNITY

Passive immunity relies upon the acquisition of the immunity from some other animal — either another human or a lower animal. This may result from the transplacental transfer of maternal antibodies from the mother to the child **(natural passive immunity)** or may be conferred by injection of immunoglobulins from immune donors **(artificially acquired immunity)**. The effectiveness of passive immunity is often quite low but can be acceptable if proper quantities of antibody are used. This type of immunity is more effective if used prophylactically rather than therapeutically. Fortunately, passive immunity is provided immediately upon transfer of the immune substances to the recipient; unfortunately, however, passive immunity may have a very short life span — perhaps only a few days or weeks. In the case of human antibody transfers, the immunity may last several weeks, but when antibodies from lower animals are transferred the half-life of the immunoglobulins is rather low. This is due to the development of antibodies to the lower animal globulins that accelerates their removal from the host animal. The reinjection of animal sera into humans is potentially dangerous and can result in the production of serum sickness or life-threatening anaphylaxis (see Chapter 12).

Transfer of bone marrow or lymphocytes between individuals within the same species can be successful if proper transplantation matching has been done to ensure a long-term survival of the transferred cells. This is known as **adoptive immunity**. The availability of recombinant interferon, IL-1, IL-2, and other interleukins has

opened a new vista to prophylaxis and therapeusis of infectious disease. These immunostimulants are already in use against viral infections and cancer.

Immunization

Historically, the most important aspect of immunity has been the ability to develop immunizing schemes that confer protection against the more serious toxic and infectious diseases such as smallpox, tetanus, and poliomyelitis. Owing to the success of vaccinations, the World Health Organization has declared the world free of smallpox. The last natural case of smallpox was in 1977. Research is continuing with the goal to develop and improve vaccines against diseases such as typhoid fever, cholera, whooping cough, and chickenpox and to develop vaccines against diseases that are rare or unknown in the United States but that constitute major world health problems (malaria, schistosomiasis, and trypanosomiasis).

BACTERIAL DISEASES

Diphtheria, Pertussis, and Tetanus

Protection against diphtheria, pertussis (whooping cough), and tetanus by active immunization is recommended by the American Academy of Pediatrics. Immunization against these diseases is provided by the injection of a polyvalent vaccine. The diphtheria, pertussis, and tetanus (DPT) vaccine contains **diphtheria toxoid, killed cells of the whooping cough organism** (*Bordetella pertussis*), and **toxoid of the tetanus bacillus**. This is administered at 2, 4, and 6 months of age; at $1\frac{1}{2}$ years old; and at 4 to 7 years old or at preschool age (Table 7–3).

MEMORY CHECK 7–5
◆

Passive immunity is

1. Acquired naturally from maternal transplacental antibody
2. Acquired artificially from injections of antibody
3. Of shorter duration than active immunity
4. Potentially dangerous to reactivate
5. Created also by adoptive immunization with cells

Table 7-3
IMMUNIZATION AGAINST BACTERIAL DISEASES COMMONLY
PRACTICED IN THE UNITED STATES

Disease	Agent	Immunizing Product
Diphtheria	*Corynebacterium diphtheriae*	Diphtheria toxoid
Whooping cough (pertussis)	*Bordetella pertussis*	Whole, killed, bacterial cells
Tetanus	*Clostridium tetani*	Tetanus toxoid
Pneumonia	*Streptococcus pneumoniae*	Polyvalent capsular polysaccharide
Meningitis	*Haemophilus meningitidis*	Hib, group b capsular polysaccharide
Meningitis	*Neisseria meningitidis*	Quadrivalent capsular polysaccharide
Tuberculosis*	*Mycobacterium tuberculosis*	Bacille Calmette-Guérin, attenuated bovine strain of tubercle bacilli

*Not widely used except for special risk groups.

The serum level of diphtheria antitoxin achieved by immunization can be estimated by the **Schick test**. To conduct the Schick test, the skin is injected with dilute diphtheria toxin and observed for an appearance of an erythematous reaction. If the injected person has sufficient immunity, no reaction will be observed.

Unfortunately, in the case of tetanus, no simple skin test such as the Schick test is available, but it is known that the amount of toxoid present in the DPT vaccine is sufficient to confer protection against tetanus for 10 to 12 years when the recommended series of injections is completed.

The killed B. pertussis organisms in the DPT vaccine are of the phase 1 type, since this is the capsular type of the organism responsible for human disease. The killed B. pertussis cells contain several antigens associated with disease—the capsule, a toxin, a cytotoxin, a dermonecrotic toxin, and a few others. B. pertussis, in addition to functioning as an antigen per se, also has an adjuvant effect that improves the immune response to the tetanus and diphtheria toxoid present in the vaccine. Reports of neurotoxicity re-

sulting from the use of the pertussis vaccine prompted studies to develop a new product and to reevaluate the incidence of untoward reactions to the vaccine. Although serious side effects to whooping cough immunization have an incidence of less than 0.1%, new acellular vaccines containing the pertussis toxoid are destined to replace the whole-cell vaccine. A Japanese product in use since 1981 has proved effective as an acellular vaccine of low toxicity, and other new vaccines may be patterned after it.

Streptococcal Pneumonia

Pneumococcal pneumonia due to *Streptococcus pneumoniae* accounts for nearly 25% of all cases of pneumonia in the United States. The primary virulence factor of this bacterium is its outer capsule, an antiphagocytic polysaccharide that shields the organism from the immune system. Immunity to the capsule of one strain of the organism does not protect against streptococcal pneumonia because there are 83 different antigenic representatives of this capsule. Fortunately, from the viewpoint of vaccine development, 23 of these capsular types cause 88% of the pneumonias. A relatively new **polyvalent vaccine containing capsular material** from these 23 types is recommended for the elderly, who have a fatality rate of 25% with this disease, and for those with splenectomy or other predisposing conditions. The vaccine is not very effective in children less than 2 years of age, who typically do not muster a good antibody response to polysaccharide antigens.

Hemophilus Meningitis

Haemophilus influenzae is the etiologic agent of several childhood diseases, but not of influenza. The organism exists in six capsular serogroups, and group b is the dominant human pathogen causing meningitis, otitis media, pneumonia, and septicemia, among others. It has been suggested that a successful Hib (*H. influenzae* type b) vaccine could prevent 85% of hemophilus infections in children, the most susceptible age group. The **Hib vaccine** contains a complex **phosphosaccharide** as its major immunogen, and this antigen is a poor stimulant of the young child's immune system. New formulations of the Hib vaccine have recently been licensed for use in infants as young as 2 months of age. One is a conjugate of Hib with meningococcal protein, the other of Hib with diphtheria toxoid.

Neisserial Meningitis

A **quadrivalent vaccine** containing **polysaccharide** from the four serologic types of *Neisseria meningitidis* that cause virtually 100% of its infections is advised for young children, military groups, and others at risk. As with the Hib vaccine, the fault of this vaccine is the inadequacy of the polysaccharide vaccine in infants less than 6 months old, the age group with 85% of all childhood neisserial infections.

Tuberculosis

An attenuated strain of *Mycobacterium tuberculosis*, known as the **bacille of Calmette and Guérin (BCG) strain**, has been used since 1921 as a vaccine against tuberculosis. The history of this vaccine over the past 70 years has been checkered with reports of protection ranging from 0% to 80% in different trials. These results have been ascribed to improper preparation (freeze-drying), faulty storage (especially in tropical countries), and mutations of the parent vaccine strain. BCG vaccine is recommended in many countries, particularly those with a high incidence of tuberculosis and low living standards. It is not recommended in the United States, with rare exceptions (eg, children living in a home with adults who have active tuberculosis). The attenuated tubercle bacilli grow in the skin for a few weeks before the immune response eliminates them. This leaves

---

MEMORY CHECK 7-6

1. Toxoids are used for active immunization against tetanus and diphtheria (probably pertussis too).
2. Polysaccharide vaccines are used to combat streptococcal, hemophilus, and neisserial infections.
3. The BCG vaccine is the only attenuated bacterial vaccine.
4. Immunity to tuberculosis is T-cell–dependent, not antibody-dependent.

a small scar on the skin. The vaccine recipients are then old tuberculin (OT)–positive and this is taken as evidence of immunity. *Immunity to tuberculosis is one of the few instances in which an antibacterial immunity relies on T cells, not antibody.*

VIRAL DISEASES

Poliomyelitis

The first successful vaccine for immunization against poliomyelitis was the formaldehyde-inactivated or **killed poliomyelitis vaccine (KPV)** developed by Jonas Salk. In time, the Salk vaccine was replaced by the attenuated oral polio vaccine **(OPV) or Sabin vaccine,** which contains infective virus (Table 7–4). The infection caused by the attenuated strains (there are three antigenic types of polio virus) is restricted to an invasion of the intestinal mucosa. The attenuated virus cannot enter the central nervous system to produce

Table 7–4
IMMUNIZATION AGAINST VIRAL
DISEASES COMMONLY
PRACTICED IN THE UNITED STATES

Disease	Vaccine
Poliomyelitis	1. Killed, Salk vaccine
	2. Attenuated, Sabin vaccine
Measles (rubeola)	Attenuated, Moraten virus strain
Mumps	Attenuated strain
Rubella (German measles)	Attenuated strain
Hepatitis B*	Hepatitis surface antigen (HBsAg), natural or recombinant
Varicella (chickenpox)	Attenuated virus
Influenza	Inactive or "split" vaccine

*Used primarily for high-risk groups.

crippling poliomyelitis characteristic of fully virulent virus. Because the Sabin vaccine provides immunity at the level of the gastrointestinal tract, which is the natural entry port for the virus, it has been considered the superior of the two vaccines. In addition, those persons who receive the Sabin vaccine will shed virus and can serve as a source of immunization for their close associates. In contrast, recipients of the Salk vaccine do not develop intestinal immunity. Therefore, they are subject to an intestinal infection with wild virus that could serve as a source of wild-type infection for nonimmune persons.

Because the use of the Salk vaccine in Scandinavia and northern European countries has had a high rate of success, the present situation regarding poliomyelitis immunization has become somewhat confused. The Salk vaccine can never revert to a live virulent virus, as the Sabin vaccine has apparently done. As a consequence, there is a tendency to return to the Salk vaccine in many countries, including the United States. Regardless of which vaccine is used to prevent poliomyelitis, it is essential that immunity to all three antigenic types of the virus be developed. These three forms of the virus are included in a single injectable solution for the Salk KPV vaccine. The OPV vaccine is administered as a solution of the virus, sometimes offered on a sugar cube. Oral poliomyelitis immunizations should follow the same schedule as DPT vaccination.

Measles (Rubeola)

Protection against measles is now possible in virtually 100% of all 1-year-old children who receive this vaccine. The vaccine is a modified **attenuated** strain, the Moraten strain, which produces a much lower incidence of febrile episodes than the earlier vaccine. The measles vaccine should be given when the child is 12 to 15 months of age and can be incorporated with the mumps and rubella (German measles) vaccines in a single dose.

Mumps

The **attenuated mumps virus vaccine** may be incorporated into the measles-rubella preparation or given separately. It is an important aspect of the childhood immunization program because natural mumps infections cause orchitis in about 20% of postpubertal males. Mumps can also cause sterility. Unfortunately the general populace does not realize the seriousness of mumps infections and has apathy toward mumps vaccination. The attack rate of the mumps virus has remained steady at two to five persons per 100,000 population for several years.

Rubella (German Measles)

German measles pose the greatest threat to the unborn child. Maternal infections with the rubella virus regularly pass through the placenta and infect the fetus. Fetal infection in the first trimester of pregnancy usually culminates in one or more of the **congenital rubella syndrome**: microcephaly, micro-ophthalmia, retinitis, deafness, encephalitis, diabetes, or numerous other abnormalities. Fetal protection is afforded by vaccination of all women before childbearing age, which is estimated to spare $1 billion in medical costs annually in the United States. The importance of the rubella vaccine is not that it protects against a serious childhood infection but that it prevents fetal malformation by the rubella virus. It may also prevent abortion or stillbirth. To prevent such a risk, all children should be immunized prior to puberty. The vaccine consists of an attenuated virus usually given in a mixture with the attenuated mumps and measles viruses.

Hepatitis B

Hepatitis B virus (HBV) infection is indigenous to homosexuals and many people in Third World countries. It is known to be a predisposing factor for hepatoma. Virus carriers are the source of infection for nonimmune individuals, yet these carriers have also proven to be the source of protection against hepatitis. Persons with hepatitis B infections have whole virus (Dane particles) in their blood, but they also have a subfraction of the virus—the **hepatitis B surface antigen (HBsAg)**—an additional submicroscopic element of the virus circulating in the blood. HBsAg can be purified from the blood and used successfully as a vaccine. It is given in three doses and is claimed to be 100% effective. The AIDS virus, also occurring frequently among homosexuals, is not copurified with HBsAg. A recombinant HBsAg vaccine is also available.

Chickenpox (Varicella)

The mortality of chickenpox is admittedly only 2 per 100,000 cases but extensive morbidity exceeds 6.5 per 100,000 cases. Chickenpox has a mortality rate of 28% in leukemic children. The varicella virus is one of the most easily transmitted viruses. Consequently, these attack rates are expected to remain high unless the vaccine now completing a successful trial is licensed for general use. This attenuated virus vaccine has reduced the disease rate by 50% in children known to be exposed to chickenpox.

Influenza

The **A strain of the influenza virus** is the only one of the three strains that causes a significant incidence of human influenza ("flu"). One remarkable property of the virus that allows it to continue as an important human pathogen is known as **antigenic drift**. This refers to minor antigenic changes in the virus and must be distinguished from **antigenic shift**, a major change in antigenic properties. Antigenic drift occurs with sufficient frequency that a population immune to influenza as a result of immunization or disease last year can be susceptible to the "drifted" strain this year. For this reason influenza monitoring stations throughout the world analyze new viral isolates for antigenic drift. When identified and perceived as threatening to cause an influenza pandemic, the new strain is placed into an accelerated program of vaccine production. This is why we are advised to receive the Hong Kong vaccine one year, the London vaccine the next, and so on. In the 1989–1990 winter, the influenza threat came from the Shanghai H3N2 strain. This H3N2 designation refers to the antigenic type of hemagglutinin (type 3) and neuraminidase (type 2) in the Shanghai strain. These two antigens are critical in developing resistance to influenza. The current vaccines are whole virus or chemically disrupted "split" vaccines; the latter are somewhat less toxic than the former.

Although some local tenderness and fever are associated with the flu vaccine, it is highly recommended for elderly persons.

AIDS

Human immunodeficiency virus (HIV) type I is the causative agent of acquired immunodeficiency syndrome (AIDS). The *HIV agent uses the CD4 protein* on the surface of the helper T cell as its avenue of entrance into the cell. Once entry is accomplished, HIV commands the cell to synthesize virus. In so doing, the cell loses the ability to replace its own vital cell components. Eventually the CD4 cell fails in its role of a helper T cell and the entire immune defense system gradually erodes into total decay. The normal CD4:CD8 T-cell ratio of 1.6:1 reverses during HIV infection. Efforts to maintain the normal relationship of these lymphocytes by injections with interferon or interleukins, IL-1, IL-2, etc., has been unsuccessful. Antibody levels, now no longer replenished by new synthesis, fall below protective levels. A wide spectrum of infectious diseases, rarely seen in individuals who do not have AIDS, become life-threatening in the absence of any substantial immunity.

Unfortunately progress toward an HIV vaccine has been slow. An attenuated vaccine is considered impractical because the viral genome is RNA and because the virus contains reverse transcriptase, the enzyme that can synthesize the DNA from which more virus is generated. One of the most external proteins on the virus coat, glycoprotein 120, has been considered the best prospect for an effective vaccine. This protein is a good antigen and initiates a good antibody response in primates but has not protected them against infection. Other proteins have been suggested, the most unusual being CD4 itself. This would not stimulate antibody formation, as human beings are tolerant to this self-antigen, but it would bind and mask the virus so that it could not bind to CD4-positive T_H cells. Presumably this type of receptor treatment would require regular infusions of CD4, a practice that now seems impractical.

Rabies

On a worldwide basis, rabies is still responsible for several thousand deaths each year. Since Pasteur's development of the first rabies vaccine, numerous modifications in the choice of source material has reduced untoward reactions to the vaccine. The initial Pasteur vaccine caused allergic encephalomyelitis in 1 to 8 of every 10,000 vaccinees due to the myelin present in the central nervous tissue taken from rabid rabbits used in the vaccine. Duck embryo vaccines had the drawback of causing allergy to egg and was not totally protective. Poor protection was the complaint against mouse brain vaccines also. The current vaccine is taken from cell cultures and chemically inactivated. It provides good protection. Attenuated vaccines are under trial.

Because rabies often has a long incubation period, it is possible to wait and determine whether the biting animal actually had rabies before beginning the vaccination.

Smallpox

Jenner discovered, nearly 200 years ago, that smallpox did not develop in persons who had recovered from an infection with the closely related cowpox virus. Jenner then pursued a program of vaccination with cowpox virus to prevent smallpox. Despite errors and confusion about the true nature of the immunizing virus, jennerian vaccination proved to be tremendously successful in preventing the disfiguring and lethal smallpox. Vaccination according to the protocol of Jenner has now eliminated smallpox as a natural disease, **the last natural case occurring in 1977**. This success was the result of a massive immunization effort by the World Health Organization.

Elimination of poliomyelitis through the use of an intensive immunization program, similar to that used for smallpox, is a genuine prospect for the future. Whenever a disease is exclusively that of the human being, with no ani-

mal reservoir or other source of the disease, and when effective vaccines are available, the possibility to repeat the smallpox story exists.

MEMORY CHECK 7-7
◆

1. Attenuated viral vaccines include those for poliomyelitis, measles, mumps, rubella, chickenpox, and rabies.
2. Smallpox vaccination (another attenuated viral vaccine) is no longer practiced.
3. Killed viral vaccines include those for poliomyelitis, influenza, and hepatitis B.

Passive Immunization

Hyperimmune gamma globulin has been very effective in preventing hemolytic disease of the newborn (Chapter 13), and this reveals the primary utility of passive immunization as a prophylactic rather than a therapeutic device. **Passive immunization** of international travelers into zones where hepatitis is common will afford temporary immunity, as opposed to the more permanent protection of active immunity. Hyperimmune gamma globulin is used for this purpose. Victims of severe or multiple bites from rabid animals may also be given both antiserum and active immunization (Table 7-5).

Antisera are also administered to persons with botulism, gas gangrene, tetanus, or other exotoxin-caused disease, but the success rate is extremely variable. Passive immunization is required for certain examples of B-cell (immunoglobulin) immunodeficiency to provide the antibodies the person is unable to produce (Chapter 8).

Table 7-5
CONDITIONS FOR WHICH PASSIVE IMMUNIZATION IS PRACTICED

Disease	Comment
Hemolytic disease of the newborn	Anti-RhD within 72 hours of delivery by Rh⁻ mother of an Rh⁺ child
Hypogammaglobulinemia	Periodically with pooled human gamma globulin for immunodeficient patients
Tetanus	If not immune
Rubella	Children and women prior to exposure to rubella
Hepatitis A	Prior to or immediately upon exposure

Newer Approaches in Vaccine Technology

The statement attributed to Louis Pasteur that "it is in the power of man to make parasitic maladies disappear from the face of the globe" has been an enormous challenge to microbiologists, immunologists, physicians, and other biomedical scientists. For the first time a step toward this goal has been taken —the earth has been declared by the World Health Organization free of natural smallpox. Immunization against smallpox by a procedure first described in 1796 completed this task 180 years later. New techniques drawn from genetics and biochemistry may enable immunologists to accelerate this conquest via synthetic, recombinant, and anti-idiotypic vaccines.

SYNTHETIC VACCINES

Immunization with intact bacteria or viruses burdens the immune system with an unnecessary assortment of antigens because only one or two antigens of the infectious agent are usually identifiable as the virulence antigens. Even the use of just two or three antigens in a purified state is potentially an overly ambitious immunization because each antigen contains numerous epitopes. An immunity against any one of the epitopes will be expressed against the complete antigen. Based on this logic, the use of a restricted number of epitopes for immunization has proved successful. Poliomyelitis virus peptide of only nine amino acids contains its critical epitope. The dominant epitope in the malarial circumsporozoite is a tetramer of only four amino acids repeated many times. A small peptide from HBsAg is its protective epitope. In most instances the critical epitope is only 5 to 20 amino acids, ie, is haptenic in character. Therefore, it has been necessary to link these epitopes to existing antigens (tetanus toxoid is an example), for successful immunization. Because of the limited complexity of these epitopes, biochemists have prepared these small peptides as **synthetic vaccines** and this has eliminated the cumbersome fractionation and purification steps required to secure the important epitopes from the parent organism (Fig. 7-5).

RECOMBINANT VACCINES

Genetic techniques have proved very advantageous to immunologists needing a specific antigen from an organism that is difficult or even impossible to cultivate. Through **recombinant DNA technology** it is possible to isolate the

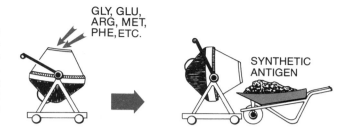

Figure 7–5. Synthetic antigens representing key epitopes of important pathogens can be prepared and used in vaccines. Because of their size, such peptides are often treated as haptens and must be coupled to an antigenic carrier.

GLY, GLU, ARG, MET, PHE, ETC.

SYNTHETIC ANTIGEN

genomic DNA corresponding to an important antigen and insert that DNA into a bacterial plasmid or bacteriophage. A plasmid is an infectious extra-chromosomal form of DNA found in many bacteria and a bacteriophage is a bacterial virus. Infection of the bacterial host by the plasmid vector or phage that contains the foreign gene is followed by an expression of this gene. The *bacterial host synthesizes* and excretes *the gene product*, a protein, into its growth medium, from which the protein is recovered and used as an antigen (Fig. 7–6). Variations of this technique permit the in-

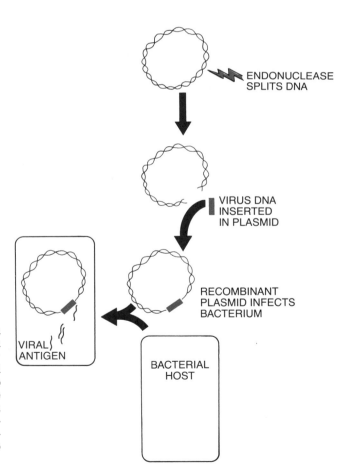

ENDONUCLEASE SPLITS DNA

VIRUS DNA INSERTED IN PLASMID

RECOMBINANT PLASMID INFECTS BACTERIUM

VIRAL ANTIGEN

BACTERIAL HOST

Figure 7–6. When plasmid DNA is "opened" by the action of an endonuclease, it can be "filled" with viral DNA. The resealed plasmid carries the new DNA to its bacterial host which makes the gene product of the DNA. Thus, a bacterial cell that is easily cultivated can be the source of antigens that are otherwise difficult to produce.

sertion of *foreign DNA fragments into viruses.* The smallpox vaccine virus, vaccinia, has been chosen as a vector because it is a large virus and has space for several additional genes. Implantation of several genes in vaccinia DNA would enable the familiar smallpox vaccine to immunize against several diseases at one time. Recombinant vaccines for rabies, herpes simplex, influenza, hepatitis B, malaria, and several other diseases have been tested and proved to raise high levels of antibody under experimental circumstances.

ANTI-IDIOTYPIC VACCINES

If an antibody contains the reverse image of an epitope in its HV regions, an anti-idiotypic antibody must carry the reverse image of the antibody's idiotope (Fig. 7–7). According to common logic, if two things bear an identi-

cal relationship to a third, then the two things are equal. With this logic in mind, **anti-idiotypic antibodies** were tested as antigen substitutes and found to be successful. Anti-idiotypic immunization has successfully developed high titers of antibody against schistosomiasis, pneumococcal pneumonia, hepatitis B, poliomyelitis, and several

---

MEMORY CHECK 7–8

◆

The three new vaccines are

1. Chemically synthesized peptides

2. Recombinant antigens

   a. Secreted by bacterial hosts

   b. Carried by a virus (vaccinia) in active immunization

3. Anti-idiotypic globulins

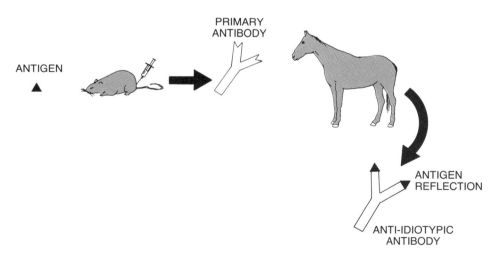

Figure 7–7. An antibody to an antibody (an anti-idiotypic antibody) reflects the structure of the original antigen because the antigen is also a reflection of the primary antibody. Trials with anti-idiotypic vaccines have shown that they can be successful.

other diseases of medical and economic importance. These anti-idiotypic vaccines carry no risk of causing disease as exists with attenuated vaccines. It is important to use a highly purified antigen for the immunization to produce the idiotypic antibody; otherwise, the anti-idiotypic antiserum will contain numerous antibodies, some of which would be nonessential to the immune state.

References

Arnon, R (ed): Synthetic Vaccines. CRC Press, Boca Raton, FL, 1987.

Atassi, MZ (ed): Immunobiology of Proteins and Peptides, Vol. V, Vaccines. Plenum Press, New York, 1989.

Germanier, R (ed): Bacterial Vaccines. Academic Press, Orlando, FL, 1985.

Hiernaux, JR: Idiotypic vaccines and infectious disease. Infect Immun 50:1407, 1988.

Plotkin, SA and Mortimer, EA, Jr (eds): Vaccines. WB Saunders, Philadelphia, 1988.

QUESTIONS AND ANSWERS

1. Which of the following contribute(s) to both natural resistance and actively acquired immunity?

    A. IgG

    B. Interferon

    C. Large granular lymphocytes

    D. Sebaceous skin secretion

    E. Defensins

Answer E

IgG and interferon are both part of the adaptive immune response and are thus a part of active immunity. Conversely, skin secretions are constituitive agents that are normally present as part of our natural resistance system. Synonymous with large granular lymphocytes are natural killer cells, which indicates their place in immunity. Defensins are present in granulocytes and macrophages. Because these cells participate in both antibody-dependent and antibody-independent phagocytosis, defensins contribute to both natural resistance and acquired immunity.

2. A person never before immunized against tetanus is exposed to this disease. A physician decides to administer passive immunization. This should consist of an injection of

    A. Tetanus toxoid

    B. Tetanus antitoxin

    C. Tetanus toxin

    D. Pooled human gamma globulin

    E. Blood

Answer B

Tetanus toxoid is used in active immunization to prompt antitoxin formation. Tetanus toxin is not used as a human injectable because of its extreme toxicity. Tetanus antitoxin should be given in this instance. Pooled human gamma globulin and blood may contain tetanus antitoxin, but the concentration would be unknown and would normally be lower than in an antitoxin preparation.

3. Resistance to infection upon recovery from that infection is known as

    A. Passive immunity

    B. Natural immunity

    C. Artificial active immunity

    D. Natural active immunity

    E. Natural passive immunity

Answer D

Active immunity implies immunity that is self-generated. If this immunity origi-nates from a natural infection, as the question indicates, the response is that of natural active immunity. Natural immunity, answer B, is sometimes used as a synonym for natural resistance.

4. An attenuated vaccine is used for immunization against
   A. Diphtheria and poliomyelitis
   B. Whooping cough and hepatitis B
   C. Tuberculosis and measles
   D. Tetanus and diphtheria
   E. Typhoid fever and rabies

Answer C

Attenuated vaccines are available for immunization against poliomyelitis, tuber-culosis, measles, and rabies; therefore, only answer C is correct. Toxoids are used to immunize against diphtheria and tetanus. Killed bacteria compose the vaccine for whooping cough and typhoid fever. Hepatitis B vaccines are either the natural or recombinant HBsAg antigen.

5. ADCC is a property of
   A. LGL cells
   B. Macrophages
   C. $T\gamma$ cells
   D. Eosinophils
   E. All of the above

Answer E

All the cell types listed have Fc receptors for immunoglobulins and can use cell-bound immunoglobulin in a cytolytic attack on target antigens. Macrophages complete their attack internally after phagocytosis. The other cells are not phago-cytic or, as in the case of eosinophils, are weakly phagocytic. LGL cells, $T\gamma$ cells and eosinophils contain toxic molecules that they release from their cytoplasmic granules. Eosinophils use IgE, not IgG, in their ADCC activity.

Case Study: Rabies Immunization

As Mildred, a 55-year-old housewife with a history of allergies, was placing her five-iron in her golf bag, an animal lunged from under her motorized golf cart and bit her on the ankle. The animal had brown fur and a smooth or nearly hairless tail, and moved rapidly. After biting her, the animal hid among some rocks that had been used to fill an abandoned well. A conservation agent was called to help retrieve and/or identify the animal but was unsuccessful. Mildred contacted her physician, who initiated the rabies immunization series.

Questions

1. What is the relative role of domestic and wild animals in the transmission of rabies?

2. How is the diagnosis of rabies determined in lower animals?

3. What is the currently preferred method of rabies prophylaxis?

4. In what way does an allergic predisposition influence the rabies immunization program for an individual?

5. Under what conditions is rabies antiserum administered?

Discussion

The incidence of human rabies has decreased in the United States to only one case per year. In domestic animals the incidence of rabies has also fallen sharply, but this has been accompanied by an increase of rabies in wild animals, especially skunks, foxes, and bats. Urban dwellers thus run little risk of exposure to rabies, but residents of rural areas and persons exposed to wild animals have a slightly higher risk. The animal involved in the case under discussion could have been a muskrat, weasel, opossum, or other animal.

Ideally lower animals suspected to have rabies should be impounded and observed for the development of the disease, which is believed to terminate invariably in death. Central nervous tissue can then be stained for Negri bodies or subjected to immunofluorescent examination. The latter method is also applied to the animal's brain when the animal has been killed and will identify rabies virus in putrefied or other damaged tissues that are unsuitable for the histologic identification of rabies virus inclusion bodies. The tissue preparation is flooded with rabies virus antiserum and then with a fluorescent antibody to the gamma globulin of the primary antiserum (Chapter 14). This indirect fluorescent antibody procedure is sensitive, rapid, and inexpensive. Its outcome can determine whether rabies prophylaxis need be initiated.

In those instances in which the suspected animal is not captured, and in which tissue examination is not possible, postexposure prophylaxis is recommended. This is especially the case with wild animal bites, bites of unvaccinated domestic animals, or severe bites from any animal displaying unusual behavior. Postexposure rabies prophylaxis was pioneered by Pasteur on the assumption that the long incubation time of rabies would permit a suitable immunity to be developed in the interlude between the bite and onset of the disease. This has been repeatedly confirmed.

The original Pasteur rabies vaccine consisted of an emulsion of dried spinal cord taken from rabid rabbits. Preparations used in the initial injections had been dried for several days and consisted of inactive virus. This allowed the individual to develop a level of immunity that would resist the later injections containing active virus. The original Pasteur vaccine and the Semple phenol-inactivated vaccine were given in 14 daily injections. The lengthy immunization schedule and the high content of rabbit brain and spinal cord antigens have been closely associated with neuroparalytic reactions occurring in about one out of every 8500 uses of these vaccines. This prompted the development of the Flury chick embryo or high egg passage (HEP) vaccine that avoided the problem of allergic encephalitis. Until recently, 90% of those receiving rabies prophylaxis in the United States were given the duck egg vaccine (DEV). Erythema, pain, tenderness, and pruritus at the inoculation sites are common with DEV. These may become more severe after 8 to 10 doses have been administered. Atopic individuals (those with allergies) should be observed carefully for systemic reactions and may require antihistamine and adrenergic drug support. The latest approved rabies vaccine is prepared in diploid tissue culture cells. New approaches to immunize against rabies have been tested in animals but are not yet approved for use in humans.

Rabies immune globulin (RIG) may also be advised concomitant with vaccination if the bite wounds are severe or near central nervous tissue, as on the head, face, and neck. In fact, there is good evidence that RIG in combination with vaccination is the best prophylactic course. Unfortunately, equine antirabies serum, which is the only preparation available in the United States, induces serum sickness in 20% of its recipients. Appropriate skin testing is necessary to reduce the risk of anaphylactic shock (Chapter 12).

GLOSSARY

---

acquired immunity   Immunity developed after birth, as opposed to inherited immunity.

ADCC   Antibody-dependent cell cytotoxicity.

antibody-dependent cell cytotoxicity   An ability of a cell to destroy a target cell with the aid of antibody by a complement-independent process.

anti-idiotypic vaccine   A vaccine consisting of an anti-idiotypic antibody that mimics the antigen that reacts with an idiotypic antibody.

attenuated vaccine   A vaccine consisting of an active (live) agent of weakened virulence.

defensins   A collection of broad-spectrum antimicrobial proteins isolated from the granules of neutrophils.

natural resistance   Inherited, not acquired, immunity.

passive immunity   Immunity contributed to one individual from another.

recombinant vaccine   A vaccine prepared by the use of recombinant DNA technology.

synthetic vaccine   A vaccine prepared by chemical synthesis.

vaccine   A suspension of living or dead organisms used as an antigen.

CHAPTER 8

◆

Immunodeficiency Disease

The immune defense system is based on the suitable functioning of three major cell systems: the phagocytic cells, the B lymphocytes, and the T lymphocytes. An array of other cells — those that synthesize components of the complement system, certain antimicrobial fatty acids, and other antimicrobial molecules — also contribute to immunity but are less vital than those of the major systems. In this chapter, deficiencies of the three major cell systems are considered in detail, with a briefer description of complement deficiencies (Fig. 8–1).

The phagocytic deficiencies are described first. In keeping with other sections of this chapter, this section begins with diagnosis and treatment of these deficiencies before describing the individual illnesses. The first group of deficiencies reflect abnormalities in oxygen metabolism. This is followed by a more heterogeneous set of phagocyte deficiencies.

The antibody deficiency states — Bruton's disease and selective IgA and IgG2 deficiencies — are described prior to a consideration of severe combined

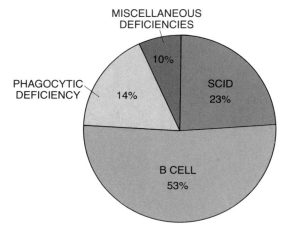

MISCELLANEOUS
DEFICIENCIES

10%

PHAGOCYTIC
DEFICIENCY   14%   SCID
                                 23%

B CELL
53%

Figure 8-1. Phagocytic cell deficiencies represented approximately 14% of all immunodeficiencies in the pre-AIDS era, B-cell deficiencies more than one half (53%), and severe combined immunodeficiencies 23%. Complement, complement receptor, and other deficiencies compose the remainder.

antibody and T-cell deficiency states; included here are the "name diseases" —Nezelof's syndrome, DiGeorge's syndrome, Wiskott-Aldrich syndrome —plus a few other diseases, including AIDS.

A brief section on complement deficiency diseases concludes the chapter.

CELL INTERACTIONS

It is important to recognize that phagocytic cells have an inherent phagocytic capacity that can be enhanced by products of the B and T lymphocytes. For optimal performance of these lymphocytes, an adaptive response triggered by an initial exposure to antigen or antigen fragments is essential. Normally, these changes in antigen structure rely on phagocytes in their function as antigen-processing and antigen-presenting cells. Because a bidirectional interaction of lymphocytes and phagocytic cells is essential to a perfect immunity, a loss or decrease in one arm of the immune system is destined to hamper other parts of the immune system. This is not limited to interactions between phagocytes and lymphocytes. Essential interactions between B and T lymphocytes are as necessary for good health as are interactions between lympho-

cytes and phagocytes. As a consequence of these interdependent relationships, a deficiency in one cell line often has ramifications elsewhere in the immune system.

ANTIGEN-SPECIFIC DEFICIENCY

Nevertheless, the antigen specificity of B and T lymphocyte responses makes it possible to have deficiency of a single cell line, which in normal health responds to an individual antigen. This would be expressed as a susceptibility to a single pathogen rather than as a general immunodeficiency disease. Pathogen-specific immunodeficiency is more prone to occur when a single cell line dominates immunity to that particular pathogen. Because phagocytic cells are not antigen specific, impairment of their function is expressed in a more general way.

Phagocytic Cell Deficiencies

DIAGNOSIS

Failure of the phagocytic cell system is normally expressed through an *increased incidence of bacterial infections*, with little or no change in the incidence or severity of viral or fungal diseases. Suggestions of a phagocytic defect from a medical history can be corroborated by determining the chemotactic, phagocytic, and cell-killing response of the patient's cells in vitro. At present, few clinical laboratories perform these studies, although the cytocidal activity of phagocytic cells may be examined indirectly through the **nitroblue tetrazolium (NBT) reductase test** (Table 8–1).

To perform the NBT test, phagocytes from the patient are exposed to an engulfable particle (latex spheres, killed yeast, or bacterial cells) in the presence of the dye nitroblue tetrazolium. This dye serves as a hydrogen acceptor, and if the phagocytic cells engage in the expected increased oxygen metabolism during phagocytosis, the dye becomes reduced. The reduced dye changes from colorless to dark blue and becomes insoluble. These dark blue granules within the phagocyte are accepted as evidence of its lethal potential.

TREATMENT

The treatment of phagocyte deficiencies is very difficult. Antibiotic therapy is important because phagocytic deficiencies are often reflected by an increased incidence of bacterial diseases. Granulocyte transfusions may be employed but are often unsuccessful owing to the short half-life of the cells. A greater potential for success may reside in treatments with the granulocyte-macrophage colony-stimulating factor (GM-CSF) or the granulocyte CSF (G-CSF). These proteins draw cells

---

Table 8–1
DIAGNOSIS AND TREATMENT OF IMMUNODEFICIENCY DISEASE

Immune system	Diagnosis	Treatment
Phagocytic cell	1. Clinical history of bacterial infections	1. Colony-stimulating factor
	2. Nitroblue tetrazolium reductase assay	2. γ interferon
B-cell deficiency	1. Clinical history of bacterial infections and vaccine response	1. Passive pooled plasma or gamma globulin
	2. Quantitative immunoglobulin analysis	
	3. B-cell enumeration	
	4. B-cell response to antigens or mitogens	
Combined T- and B-cell deficiency	1. Clinical history of viral and fungal infections	1. Thymus grafts
	2. Tests for delayed type hypersensitivity	2. Bone marrow grafts
	3. T-cell enumeration	
	4. Response to contact sensitizers	
	5. T-cell response to mitogens	
Complement	1. History of bacterial infections	1. Pooled plasma
	2. Complement titrations	

from the bone marrow and hasten their maturation. Partial success of this treatment was recorded after the 1986 incident at Chernobyl in Russia. Interferon γ may also be helpful.

CHRONIC GRANULOMATOUS DISEASE

Infectious Disease History

The first recognized phagocytic cell deficiency of genetic origin was **chronic granulomatous disease (CGD).** *CGD is a sex-linked recessive disease* that is recognized in the early months of life. Boys with this condition have a number of *infections with rather feeble pathogens* such as *Escherichia, Klebsiella, Proteus, Serratia,* and *Aerobacter,* as well as with the more virulent *Staphylococcus aureus.* Yeasts and fungi may also cause serious illnesses in affected children. It is interesting that these children may contract and recover from diseases caused by the most serious bacterial pathogens of childhood, bacteria in the genera *Neisseria, Haemophilus,* and *Streptococcus.*

Immunologic Status

As a result of these repeated infections, CGD patients usually have elevated immunoglobulin levels. The peripheral blood white cell count is either normal or elevated. In vitro studies indicate that neutrophils of these patients kill bacteria at a rate only about half that of the normal cells. However, tissue biopsies reveal extensive granuloma formation in which multinucleate giant or epithelioid cells representing fused white blood cells contain partially digested or undigested bacteria.

Biochemical Basis of CGD

The biochemical lesion in phagocytic cells of patients with CGD has been identified as an inability to produce hydrogen peroxide (H_2O_2) during phagocytosis. The critical lesion in phagocytes of CGD patients is *a loss of* **cytochrome b** in the electron transport chain. Cytochrome b is linked to NADPH oxidase, an essential enzyme in oxidase metabolism. As a consequence of this, the neutrophils are unable to function in normal aerobic metabolism, which is essential for the formation of the cytotoxic forms of oxygen. The inability to produce hydrogen peroxide is very clearly associated with the type of organism that causes disease in these patients. Those bacteria causing infections from which recovery is normal produce their own hydrogen peroxide inside the phagolysosome after they have been engulfed. This hydrogen peroxide is then converted by the phagocytes to other oxygen products — hypochlorite, hydroxyl radicals, and so on. Thus, *bacteria that produce H_2O_2 create a suicidal condition* within phagocytes and limit their own virulence. The more feeble pathogens (e.g., *Escherichia, Klebsiella,* and the like) are unable to produce hydrogen peroxide or, should they do so, also produce *catalases or peroxidases that detoxify the hydrogen peroxide* by converting it to oxygen and water. Consequently, these organisms never create the internal toxic environment that aborts their infection and are thus able to cause serious, even lethal, infections (Fig. 8–2).

MYELOPEROXIDASE DEFICIENCY

Enzyme studies of granulocytes of some patients with severe repeated bacterial infections have revealed that they have a myeloperoxidase deficiency. During phagocytosis, the normal phagocytic shift to aerobic metabolism takes place and normal amounts of hydrogen peroxide are produced;

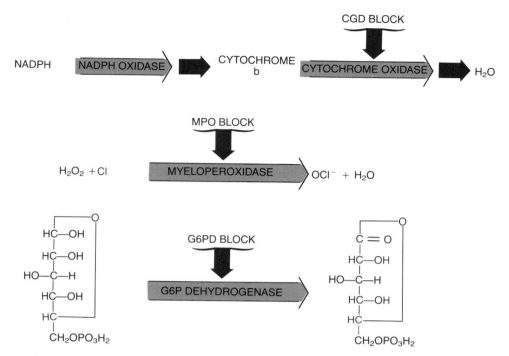

Figure 8-2. Three phagocytic cell deficiencies involving oxygen metabolism are illustrated. At the top, the loss of cytochrome b in CGD is presented. In the middle panel, the absence of myeloperoxidase prevents hypochlorite formation. The oxidative burst is prevented if phagocytes lack glucose-6-phosphate dehydrogenase, as shown in the bottom panel.

however, intracellular killing of microbes does not follow. The absence of myeloperoxidase *precludes the oxidative halogenation* of the engulfed organisms, thus sparing them. The relationship of patients with CGD to those with myeloperoxidase deficiency is apparent: the former produce no hydrogen peroxide but do have the myeloperoxidase enzyme; the latter lack myeloperoxidase but are able to produce hydrogen peroxide. Both systems are required for protection against many pathogenic bacteria.

GLUCOSE-6-PHOSPHATE DEHYDROGENASE DEFICIENCY

The enzyme that links the anaerobic glycolytic pathway to the aerobic pathway of carbohydrate metabolism is glucose-6-phosphate dehydrogenase (G6PD). Accordingly, the phagocytes of any individual who is devoid of this enzyme will be *unable to metabolize efficiently in the aerobic system.* Patients with G6PD deficiency produce only one-fourth the expected amount of hydrogen peroxide; consequently, they suffer numerous bacterial infections.

CHÉDIAK-HIGASHI DISEASE

Chédiak-Higashi disease (CHD) is characterized by albinism, extreme sensitivity to light, and frequent bacterial infections. The primary cellular defect observed in victims of CHD is the presence of *abnormally large granules* within their phagocytic cells and large granular lymphocytes. It is uncertain how this morphologic defect relates to their inability to handle infectious organisms. Studies indicate that the phagocytic capacity of neutrophils from these patients is normal but that their bactericidal activity is depressed. This retarded intraphagocytic killing is not the result of a failure to use oxygen but may relate to an *inability to degranulate and deliver myeloperoxidase* to the phagocytic vacuole.

LAZY LEUKOCYTE SYNDROMES

The failure of phagocytes to enter a nidus of infection may be due to a failure of the body to generate chemotaxins or of the cells to respond to chemotactic stimuli. The absence of this expected phagocyte response is referred to as the lazy leukocyte syndrome, three examples of which are presented here.

Hyperimmunoglobulinemia E

One phagocytic deficiency disease for which the underlying etiology is yet to be determined is hyperimmunoglobulinemia E, formerly known as **Job's syndrome**. Individuals with this disease are afflicted, as was Job in the biblical story, with boils, furuncles, skin abscesses and other skin infections caused by the usual skin pathogens — staphylococci, streptococci, and yeasts. Unfortunately there is a poor chemotactic response of white blood cells to these infections, which develop little if any inflammatory response. Failure to mount an inflammatory response is the basis of the description of these skin lesions as **cold abscesses**. Those phagocytes that do enter the infected regions have a weakened cytocidal power. Accordingly these skin infections are difficult to treat and are recurrent.

MEMORY CHECK 8–1

Phagocyte deficiencies

1. **Diagnosis:** History of repeated bacterial infections, and decreased NBT reductase assays

2. **Etiology:** Failure to form cytotoxic forms of oxygen, with the listed exceptions
   a. Chronic granulomatous disease — no H_2O_2 formed, cytochrome b loss, special bacteria involved
   b. Myeloperoxidase deficiency — no enzyme to combine H_2O_2 and Cl^- to form OCl^- and H_2O
   c. Glucose-6-phosphate dehydrogenase deficiency — inability to shift from anaerobic to aerobic metabolism
   d. Chédiak-Higashi disease — granule malfunction
   e. Lazy leukocyte syndrome — poor chemotaxis, associated with hyper-IgE, tuftsin deficiency, and actin dysfunction.

3. **Treatment:** No good immunologic therapy yet. Potentially interferon and colony-stimulating factors in the future.

Tuftsin Deficiency

Tuftsin, which is the natural tetrapeptide threonine-lysine-proline-arginine, is formed in the spleen by an enzymatic action upon a globulin substrate called leukokinin. **Tuftsin** *is a chemo-*

taxin and improves phagocytic motility, engulfment, and oxidative metabolism. A deficiency of tuftsin causes a loss of this activity and an increase in bacterial infections.

Actin Dysfunction

Actin is the protein that forms the microskeletal framework over which the cytoplasm of phagocytic cells flows during ameboid motion. Actin dysfunction, resulting from a *failure to form the filamentous actin network* from monomeric actin, retards the response of these cells to chemotactic stimulation and is a source of decreased phagocytosis and increased bacterial disease.

Immunodeficiencies Involving B Lymphocytes

The loss of functional B cells may be a genetically inherited condition or may be acquired. When only a single B-cell lineage is involved, only a single immunoglobulin isotype is affected. The extent of the immune penalty in these situations depends upon which immunoglobulin is missing. If it is a minor immunoglobulin (eg, IgD), the individual may note little if any increase in

bacterial disease. Such a person does not have an abnormal total globulin level. The opposite occurs in persons deficient in IgG. These individuals suffer an *increased frequency of bacterial diseases* and, because IgG represents 75% to 85% of our total globulins, have a lower gamma globulin level (Table 8–1).

Diagnosis

Assessment of past B-lymphocyte activities is determined by measuring the person's immunoglobulin levels. *The levels of the individual immunoglobulins must be measured.* This is an age-dependent variant, and standard tables should be consulted (Table 8–2). Reliance on the total serum globulin level is inadequate because a compensatory overproduction of one globulin may mask a loss of another globulin, especially when the missing globulin is normally in low concentration. Frequently, a history of successful immunizations with the usual childhood vaccines is used as an index of a satisfactory B-cell system earlier in life. Antibody titers, which will confirm the success of these immunizations, can be determined by specific serologic tests. Typical levels of the blood group antibodies also reflect a healthy B-cell sys-

Table 8–2
ONTOGENY OF THE IMMUNOGLOBULIN RESPONSE

Age	IgG	IgM	IgA
Newborn	1025* ± 200	10* ± 5	2* ± 3
6 months	425 ± 175	45 ± 15	30 ± 20
1 year	675 ± 200	55 ± 25	40 ± 20
10 years	1125 ± 225	80 ± 35	130 ± 60
Adult	1160 ± 300	100 ± 30	200 ± 60

*All values mg/dL.

tem. Assessment of concurrent B-cell function is accomplished by enumerating the B cells, by measuring an individual's *response to vaccines*, or by measuring the blastogenic *response of B cells to mitogens* (lectins), or antigens in culture.

TREATMENT

The treatment of B-cell deficiencies depends upon *infusions with pooled human plasma or gamma globulin*. Scheduled reinfusions or transfusions are required to maintain a protective level of antibody.

NEONATAL HYPOGAMMAGLOBULINEMIA

Transient hypogammaglobulinemia of newborn infants is a normal *regularly recognized phenomenon* present in all infants. The inability of the antigenically unstimulated unborn child to synthesize immunoglobulins, coupled with the sole transport of maternal IgG across the placental barrier, leaves the infant with approximately a 20% deficit of immunoglobulins—a deficit of all the immunoglobulins except IgG. Neonatal levels of IgM and IgA are usually 10% or less of the expected adult level. A significant concentration of IgM in neonates often reflects a maternal intrauterine infection.

Because of the gradual assumption of immunoglobulin synthesis by infants and the decay of maternal antibody in the infant's circulation, the neonate's antibody level dwindles over the first several months of life. Between 3 and 6 months of age the child's antibody titer is at its lowest level and it is at about this time that the child often experiences a rash of infectious diseases. These antigenic exposures stimulate the synthesis of immunoglobulins and their titers gradually ascend toward the norms of adulthood (Fig. 8–3). Neonatal hypogammaglobulinemia is *self-correcting*.

In instances of genetic hypogammaglobulinemia, the infant does not recover from its deficiency. Congenital hypogammaglobulinemia or agammaglobulinemia, of which there are several forms, were not recognized until antibiotics became available. Prior to the antibiotic era, these infants died of infectious diseases before a diagnosis of hypogammaglobulinemia could be made. Three examples—Bruton's agammaglobulinemia and two varieties of selective or common variable hypogammaglobulinemia—are described here.

BRUTON'S AGAMMAGLOBULINEMIA

Infantile sex-linked agammaglobulinemia is the official term for the disease

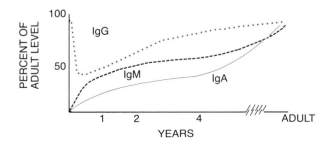

Figure 8–3. The normal increases in serum IgG, IgA, and IgM indicate the early loss of maternal IgG before the child begins to produce its own IgG.

commonly known as Bruton's agammaglobulinemia, Bruton's disease, or simply **sex-linked agammaglobulinemia**. This is a disease transmitted by a mother to only her male children. About the sixth month of the child's life, when the expected synthesis of antibodies does not develop and the child continues to suffer from repeated infections of childhood, a diagnosis of Bruton's disease may be contemplated. This is especially the case when these primary infections do not stimulate detectable antibody formation and recurrences of otitis media, sore throat, conjunctivitis, and more serious conditions such as septicemia develop. At this time, the gamma globulin level of these children may fall below 25 mg/dL which, though not being an absolute agammaglobulinemia, is clearly a significant hypogammaglobulinemia. It should be recalled that healthy adults have approximately 1250 mg/dL of IgG alone.

The immunologic lesion in Bruton's disease is a *break in the maturation of B cells*. Pre-B cells are present in the bone marrow of patients with this disease, but these cells do not progress through the normal stages of immature and mature B cells or to plasma cells. This may reflect a *fault in V-J-C and V-D-J gene rearrangement* or a more general failure to respond to growth stimuli.

COMMON VARIABLE HYPOGAMMAGLOBULINEMIA

A total loss of mature B lymphocytes reflected in Bruton-type agammaglobulinemia is a rare event. Instead, it is more likely that only one or two classes of immunoglobulins will be missing from the serum electrophoretic profile. These conditions have been described as dysgammaglobuline-

mias, referring to a disorder, a disease, or a disturbance in the balance of the gamma globulins. Individuals with **selective (or common variable) hypogammaglobulinemia** are the most difficult to diagnose on the basis of total globulin levels, since a decrease in one immunoglobulin is usually compensated for by a hypergammaglobulinemia of some other class of immunoglobulin.

Selective IgA Deficiency

Among the *most common of the variable hypogammaglobulinemias* is the loss of IgA. Different studies have suggested that the incidence of an IgA deficiency may range from 1 in 400 to 1 in 1000 persons. Both *serum and secretory IgA* are diminished or absent in these individuals despite the fact that the secretory component is produced. Individuals with the IgA form of common variable immunoglobulin deficiency have an increased incidence of sinopulmonary disease resulting from their loss of secretory IgA. The immunologic error is a *failure of the isotype switch* mechanism or an *excess of T_S cells*. These same mechanisms are postulated to account for other selective immunoglobulin deficiencies.

Selective IgG2 Deficiency

Persons with all possible combinations of dysgammaglobulinemia have been recognized and reported in the literature. These include single immunodeficiencies and all the expected pairs, all the expected triplets, and so on. Only those persons who have a loss of IgG, either singly or multiply with other immunoglobulins, suffer a significantly heightened incidence of infectious diseases. In children the loss of IgG2 has been associated with a variety of clinical manifestations. Nearly half of the children with an increased frequency of alimentary tract or upper respiratory tract infections were deficient in IgG2, either alone or combined with other IgG, losses. Deficiency of IgG1 and IgG3 in these children was represented in 13% and 16%, respectively. IgG2, with IgM, is a high responder to polysaccharide antigens, and the dominance of this chemical type of antigen on the surface of many infectious bacteria offers an explanation of the susceptibility of IgG2-deficient children to bacterial infections (Table 8–3).

Severe Combined B-Cell and T-Cell Immunodeficiencies

The loss of T-cell function without an accompanying loss of B-cell activities is extremely rare owing to the immunoregulatory role of T cells. Significant impairment of T-cell functions often present as a *viral or fungal infection* that fails to progress to its climax and recovery but continues to fulminate, eventually claiming the child's life. Children with T-cell defects are very prone to fatal disease from chickenpox, measles, rubella, and other common viral diseases of childhood. Other infections, including fungal disease and infections with *Pneumocystis carinii*, are also more common in these patients.

MEMORY CHECK 8–2

Neonatal hypogammaglobulinemia is

1. Normal; all infants have it
2. Due to
   a. Delayed maturity of immune system
   b. Inability of immunoglobulins except IgG to cross the placenta
   c. The minimal exposure to antigens in utero
3. Transient and self-correcting. If not self-correcting by 6 months to 1 year, suspect:

Bruton's agammaglobulinemia

1. Occurs in male children (alternate forms in females rarely occur)
2. No immunoglobulins detectable by quantitative immunoglobulin analysis
3. Treat with passive gamma globulin or plasma

Common variable hypogammaglobulinemia

1. Exists in all possible combinations
2. IgA deficiency is the most common type
3. IgG2 deficiency is an "emerging" syndrome

Table 8–3
IMMUNODEFICIENCY OF B LYMPHOCYTES

Condition	Etiology	Treatment
Neonatal hypogammaglobulinemia	Immaturity of cell systems	None, self-correcting
Bruton's agammaglobulinemia	Inherited failure of B cells to mature	Passive pooled plasma or gamma globulin
Selective IgA deficiency	Faulty isotype switch or excess T_S cells	None
Selective IgG2 deficiency	Uncertain	Pooled gamma globulin

DIAGNOSIS

The contemporary status of T-cell health can be determined by peripheral blood lymphocyte counts. A **lymphopenia** may signify a T-cell deficit, as 65% to 85% of peripheral blood lymphocytes are T cells. T-cell counts using the sheep erythrocyte rosette method is a more rapid and less expensive method than flow cytometry. It is also important to evaluate whether the cells are capable of the expected T-cell responses, and this can be done by stimulating the T cells in vitro with concanavalin A or other T-cell mitogens. Dermal sensitization of an individual with 30% dinitrochlorobenzene, which is successful in more than 95% of the healthy population, should also be used to evaluate the current status of the T-cell system.

TREATMENT

It is often necessary to effect a *transplant of thymus or bone marrow, or both*, to reconstitute a T-cell–deficient person (Table 8–4). Although bone marrow grafting alone will provide the T-cell precursors, a thymic environment that would permit their maturation may be absent. Likewise, the individual may have sufficient thymus but lack a source of pre-T cells. Some individuals appear to have the proper T-cell numbers, but these cells are metabolically arrested. Such cells can be stimulated into action by extracts of T cells from normal donors (transfer factor) and occasionally by T-cell–specific lectins.

AIDS

The discovery of human immunodeficiency virus (HIV) type 1 as the cause of acquired immunodeficiency syndrome (AIDS) once again focused attention on T lymphocytes as major contributors to immunity. HIV uses the **CD4 protein** on the surface of T_H cells for entry into these cells. Slowly the CD4 lymphocytes are killed and the normal human ratio of CD4:CD8 lymphocytes of 1.6:1 gradually reverses. During this time, a gradual erosion of

Table 8–4
SEVERE COMBINED B-CELL AND T-CELL IMMUNODEFICIENCIES

Condition	Etiology	Treatment
AIDS	Human immunodeficiency virus	Azidothymidine
Nezelof's syndrome	Genetic fault in thymus development	Thymus graft
DiGeorge's syndrome	Embryogenic error in thymus development	Thymus graft
Wiskott-Aldrich syndrome	Sex-linked inheritance	Bone marrow transplant
Ataxia telangiectasia	Failure of DNA repair enzymes	None successful
Purine enzyme deficiency	Loss of adenosine deaminase or purine nucleotide phosphorylase	Red cell transfusion, polyethylene glycol adenosine deaminase injection
Chronic mucocutaneous candidiasis	Isolated T-cell loss	Transfer factor therapy

CD4-dependent T-cell activities occurs. AIDS victims develop serious infections from endogenous herpes, cytomegaloviruses, and viruses from exogenous sources. Eruptions of Kaposi's sarcoma may also occur. These individuals also develop serious disease from other intracellular parasites such as *Mycobacterium tuberculosis* and *P. carinii*. A variety of fungi have emerged as life-threatening pathogens for AIDS patients, including *Cryptococcus neoformans*, *Coccidioides*, and others.

Because of a loss of immunoregulatory T cells, antibody levels also decay gradually. Entry of HIV into macrophages also affects the immune response. Neuropathologic sequelae of AIDS reflect the entry of the virus into CD4-positive cells of the central nervous system. All these factors have contributed to 160,000 cases of AIDS in the United States as of December 1990; the mortality exceeds 50%.

Transmission of the HIV agent is primarily through sexual contact and occurs particularly among homosexuals, although heterosexual transmission also exists. Intravenous drug users also represent a high-risk group to develop AIDS. AIDS can be diagnosed either by the presence of HIV antibodies, especially early in the disease, or by the presence of the virus determined by immunoblotting. Prevention and treatment of AIDS via vaccines is a logical hope, but experimental trials with simian AIDS have been disappointing. Treatment with antiviral drugs such as azidothymidine (AZT) has been useful, and other reagents also show promise. Immunotherapy with interleukins and interferons have been only partially successful to date. AIDS is considered a genuine threat to human survival because of its devastating effect on the immune system and its ease of transmission.

NEZELOF'S SYNDROME

Infants with Nezelof's syndrome are athymic by virtue of a *genetic recessive characteristic* that precludes normal lymphoid development in this gland. The thymus gland appears to have reasonably intact connective tissue and vascular and lymphatic supplies but is unable to fulfill itself as a lymphoid organ. Failure of the T-cell system in such instances is reflected early in one's lifetime by an increased susceptibility to numerous infections. Infections with *Candida albicans*, other yeasts, or fungi are usually severe and may be fatal. Childhood viral diseases such as chickenpox and measles, though mild in the normal healthy child, can prove fatal in one with Nezelof's syndrome. A high incidence of malignancy is also noted in these unfortunate children. The significance of the T-lymphocyte system in protecting against fungal and viral disease and malignancy is well documented by patients with Nezelof's syndrome.

DiGEORGE'S SYNDROME

DiGeorge's syndrome is the result of failure in the development of the third and fourth pharyngeal pouches during *embryogenesis* and the consequent inability to form a normal thymus gland. This is accompanied by inadequacies in the structure of the aortic arch, the mandible, the ear, and also the parathyroid gland. This gland is the regulatory organ for blood calcium. During fetal life, maternal parathyroid hormones control fetal as well as maternal blood calcium levels. After birth, the absence of the parathyroid gland allows a calcium deficiency to develop. *Low blood calcium* levels are expressed as an involuntary, rigid muscular contraction or tetanus. Consequently, tetany in newborn infants should suggest an examination for a thymus deficiency of the DiGeorge type. DiGeorge's syndrome is similar to Nezelof's syndrome but develops from an error in embryogenesis rather than from an inherited defect in thymus formation.

WISKOTT-ALDRICH SYNDROME

Victims of Wiskott-Aldrich syndrome, a sex-linked disease, suffer repeated bacterial, viral, fungal, and other infections characteristics of patients with *both B- and T-cell losses.* Eczema and thrombocytopenia are also typical of this disease. The T-cell loss in patients with Wiskott-Aldrich syndrome is seldom total. Moreover, sufferers may have elevated IgA and IgE levels, with normal or even elevated levels of IgG, the latter being a product of their repeated infections. The primary loss in the B-lymphocyte population is in *IgM-producing cells.* Blood group hemagglutinins are low or absent. Inadequacy of these cells results in poor production of IgM antibodies against polysaccharide antigens; consequently, these patients form poor agglutinating antibodies against gram-negative bacteria. Successful *bone marrow transplantation* has proved curative, but all other treatments (steroids, passive gamma globulin) have been inadequate.

ATAXIA TELANGIECTASIA

Ataxia telangiectasia is a disorder associated with losses of muscle coordination and the dilation of small blood vessels, most notably in the eye. This *autosomal recessive genetic disease* has an incidence of about 1 or 2 in every 100,000 persons. In terms of its cellular immune deficit, all patients have a hy-

poplastic thymus with an unfulfilled T-cell population. This is reflected clinically by repeated serious viral infections. These patients are also unable to develop a contact dermatitis to dinitrochlorobenzene. Malignancies develop in about 10% of these victims. IgG levels are often normal or may exceed normal as a result of repeated infections. IgE and IgM levels may be depressed, and IgA levels are depressed in approximately 40% of the cases. As might be expected, an increase in sinopulmonary infections is associated with the loss of IgA. An unexpected diagnostic aid for ataxia telangiectasia is the uniform high blood level of α-fetoprotein (AFP) in these patients. It is not yet possible to relate this to the T- and B-cell abnormalities in these patients. Data acquired in vitro indicate that patients with ataxia have a *reduced ability to repair breaks in DNA.* This prevents an expansion of the T-cell population after an antigenic stimulus and accounts for the high incidence of *malignancy and sensitivity to x-ray examination* expressed by these patients. Immunotherapy of patients with ataxia telangiectasia has encompassed injection of transfer factor, thymosin, and fetal thymic grafts, all with only partial success.

DEFICIENCY OF PURINE ENZYMES

Two enzymes in the **salvage pathway of purine metabolism** are essential for normal T-cell function. These enzymes—adenosine deaminase and purine nucleotide phosphorylase—assist in the recycling of purines, rather than in their de novo synthesis; hence the term "salvage pathway." Adenosine deaminase (ADA) converts the amino group of adenine in adenosine to a hydroxyl group, thereby creating inosine.

A phosphorolytic cleavage of inosine by purine nucleotide phosphorylase (PNP) produces hypoxanthine and ribose-1-phosphate. The end-products are slightly different if deoxyadenosine is the initial substrate.

Adenosine Deaminase Deficiency

T cells of ADA-deficient persons accumulate several forms of adenosine including adenosine triphosphate (ATP), deoxy ATP, deoxyadenosine, and S-adenosylhomocystine. The last of these molecules is considered a detoxification product of the four adenosine-containing molecules. These adenosyl derivatives *inhibit ribonucleotide reductase*, an essential enzyme in DNA synthesis. Adenosylhomocystine removes homocystine as a source of methyl groups that are required in the de novo pathway of purine synthesis. With both the salvage and de novo pathways of DNA synthesis blocked, the T cells are unable to enter the growth and differentiation phases essential to the antigen response. Curiously, B cells are not directly affected by ADA deficiency.

Transfusions from healthy persons of *whole blood* or *extracts of frozen erythrocytes* containing ADA are therapeutic, but the process must be repeated to replace ADA as it decays in the recipient. Recently a synthetic conjugate of ADA with polyethylene glycol has been used successfully to treat ADA deficiency.

Purine Nucleotide Phosphorylase (PNP) Deficiency

The biochemical basis of PNP deficiency is less clear than that of ADA deficiency. An accumulation of **deoxyguanosine derivatives** has been observed, but the metabolic influence of this is unclear. This accumulation does not occur in B cells that remain healthy but lack stimuli from T cells. Bone marrow transplantation has relieved both ADA and PNP deficiencies.

PARTIAL T-CELL DEFICIENCIES

Chronic Mucocutaneous Candidiasis

Partial losses of T cells have also been recognized, in which T cells specific for certain antigens are missing. One of these conditions is the serious disease of young children known as chronic mucocutaneous candidiasis, in which infants exposed to *Candida albicans* yeasts present in the mother's birth canal are unable to suppress the mild infection that many children develop shortly after birth. Consequently, the child is intensely colonized with the yeasts, particularly at the mucocutaneous borders. Erosion of the skin at these borders permits subsequent bacterial infections to develop. The normal features of the skin, particularly on the face, scalp, and arms, but also on other parts of the body, may be obscured by a crusty, serous exudate. It has been found that these children are able to respond immunologically to other yeasts and viruses controlled by the T-cell system. They have a *unique cellular defect* that does not allow a response to antigens of **Candida yeast**. Transfer factor injections are partially if not totally curative.

Leprosy

Leprosy is another disease in which a specific T-cell loss has been identified. Leprosy is separable into two forms:

lepromatous and tuberculoid leprosy. In the lepromatous form of the disease, the bacterial population is high and increases with further anesthesia and necrotic destruction of tissue. Tuberculoid leprosy, in which there is a lower load of bacteria and less tissue destruction, is associated with a better prognosis. Examination of the lymphocytes in these patients has revealed that those of the lepromatous person are not responsive to antigens of *Mycobacterium leprae*, whereas those from the tuberculoid patients are—a distinction that is believed to account for the major differences in the two forms of leprosy.

MEMORY CHECK 8–3
◆

Etiology of severe combined B- and T-cell immunodeficiencies

1. AIDS due to HIV infection
2. Nezelof's (genetic) and DiGeorge's syndromes (non-genetic)—failure to develop a lymphoid thymus
3. Wiskott-Aldrich syndrome—etiology uncertain
4. Enzyme-deficiency states
   a. Ataxia telangiectasia—DNA-repair enzymes missing
   b. Purine deficiency—Adenosine deaminase and purine nucleotide phosphorylase missing; decreased purine synthesis; toxic nucleotides accumulate
5. Chronic mucocutaneous candidiasis—isolated inability of T cells to respond to *Candida albicans* yeast

---

Deficiencies of the Complement System

DEFICIENCY OF COMPLEMENT COMPONENTS

Deficiencies of the complement system have been recognized at a steadily increasing pace since reagents have become more available to identify the individual complement molecules. Deficiency of the early-acting components C1, C2, and C4 is associated with immune complex diseases resembling lupus erythematosus and rheumatoid arthritis. Although one might anticipate that a deficiency of a complement component would be expressed by a heightened incidence of infectious disease, this is not always the case. **C3** is an extremely important component, and its loss has been associated with *repeated bacterial infections*. Depressed levels of the **late-acting components**—the membrane attack complex—are associated with an increase in *neisserial infections*. The cause of this specificity for only these bacteria is unknown (Table 8–1).

DEFICIENCY OF COMPLEMENT REGULATORS

Hereditary Angioneurotic Edema

One of the more interesting of the complement-related deficiencies is that of the C1 inhibitor (C1 INH). Deficiencies of this molecule can exist in either of two forms: a total or near total loss of the inhibitor molecule or the production of an ineffective molecule that is structurally similar to the normal inhibitor but lacks its biologic activity. Either of these situations permits incidental activations of complement component C1 to continue through the complement cascade. Normal C1 INH regulates the first step in this process. C1 INH also regulates the activity of activated Hageman factor and kininogenase, thus modulating the kinin-generating system. The *loss of C1 INH* allows the generation of *edema-producing molecules*, either from the complement component C2 or from the *kinin system*. This is expressed in the disease **hereditary angioneurotic edema (HANE)**, also known as giant edema. Severe gastrointestinal edema associated with the loss of C1 INH may cause severe pain, vomiting, and diarrhea, and respiratory involvement may result in laryngeal obstruction and asphyxia. Fortunately, the treatment is safe and effective, consisting of **transfusion with plasma** from healthy persons to supply the missing inhibitor or treatment with **androgens** to stimulate C1 INH synthesis (Table 8–5).

Paroxysmal Nocturnal Hemoglobinuria

For many years it has been known that the disease paroxysmal nocturnal hemoglobinuria (PNH) is related to an abnormality in erythrocytes, but only recently has the red cell lesion been identified. Patients with PNH *lack decay-accelerating factor (DAF)* on their erythrocytes. Consequently, C3b generated from either the classic or the alternate complement pathway accumulates on the CR1 molecule on the erythrocytes, serves as a binding site for the late-acting component, and allows lysis to occur. DAF normally destroys C3b and protects red blood cells from lysis.

MEMORY CHECK 8–4

Complement deficiencies are grouped as

1. Early-component deficiencies expressed as autoimmunelike diseases and, in the case of C3 loss, increased bacterial disease
2. Late-component deficiencies expressed as increased infections due to *Neisseria*

Complement regulator deficiencies are expressed as

1. Hereditary angioneurotic edema due to C1 INH deficiency
2. Paroxysmal nocturnal hemoglobinuria due to DAF deficiency

Table 8–5
DEFICIENCIES OF THE COMPLEMENT SYSTEM

Condition	Etiology	Treatment
Deficiency of complement components	Inherited	None
Hereditary angioneurotic edema	Loss or inactive C1 INH	Pooled plasma or androgen therapy
Paroxysmal nocturnal hemoglobinuria	Loss of DAF	None

References

Buckley, RH: Immunodeficiency diseases. JAMA 258:2841, 1987.

Davis, AE, III: C1 inhibitor and hereditary angioneurotic edema. Annu Rev Immunol 6:595, 1988.

Hassett, JM: Humoral immunodeficiency. Pediatr Ann 16:404, 1987.

Klein, E (ed): Acquired immunodeficiency syndrome. Prog Allergy 37:1, 1988.

Klempner, MS, Styrt, B, and Ho, Y (eds): Phagocytes and Disease. Kluwer Academic Publishers, Dordrecht, Netherlands, 1988.

Pachman, LM, et al: Primary immunodeficiencies in children: An update. Curr Probl Pediatr 19:9, 1989.

Stiehm, EE: Immunologic Disorders in Infants and Children. ed 3. WB Saunders, Philadelphia, 1989.

Webster, ADB: Immunodeficiency and Disease. Kluwer Academic Publishers, Dordrecht, Netherlands, 1988.

QUESTIONS AND ANSWERS

1. Which of the following is an enzyme-deficiency disease that does not involve T cells?

   A. Ataxia telangiectasia
   B. Adenosine deaminase (ADA) deficiency
   C. Purine nucleotide phosphorylase (PNP) deficiency
   D. Chronic granulomatous disease (CGD)
   E. None of the above

Answer D

All of the choices listed are enzyme-deficiency states. Ataxia telangiectasia results in part through a deficiency in DNA-repair enzymes and affects primarily T cells. Answers B and C also are deficiencies of T cells that involve two separate enzymes in the purine salvage pathway. Only CGD is a non–T-cell immunodeficiency. Its etiology is a loss of cytochrome b that then affects NADPH oxidase in phagocytic cells.

2. Which of the following is a good index of a B-cell immunodeficiency?

   A. Recurrent infections due to *Neisseria*
   B. Low peripheral blood lymphocyte counts
   C. Recurrent infections due to *Escherichia* and *Klebsiella*
   D. Very serious measles and chickenpox infections
   E. Recurrent infections due to *Streptococcus* and *Staphylococcus*

Answer E

Neisseria as the cause of repeated infections is indicative of a loss in the late-acting or membrane attack components (MAC) of the complement system. Low lymphocyte counts are more apt to reflect a T-cell rather than B-cell loss, as the majority of circulating lymphocytes are T cells. Chronic granulomatous disease is characterized by repeated infections of feeble pathogens represented by *Escherichia* and *Klebsiella*. T-cell deficiency states are characterized by an increased susceptibility to viral and fungal illnesses. Of the choices offered, repeated infections by streptococci and staphylococci are the most likely to result from an immunoglobulin deficiency.

3. If a thymic transplant does not cure DiGeorge's syndrome, it is possible that:

   A. Pre-T cells may not be produced by bone marrow of the patient with DiGeorge's syndrome
   B. DiGeorge's syndrome is primarily a B-cell deficiency disease
   C. T cells in the recipient have mounted a powerful host rejection of the thymus graft

D. The same autoimmune condition that destroyed the patient's own thymus has rejected the transplanted thymus

E. Suppressor T cells present in patients with DiGeorge's syndrome have minimized any T-cell help offered by the graft

Answer A

DiGeorge's syndrome is the result of pre-T cells failing to have a suitable environment (thymus) for their maturation upon release from the bone marrow; it is not a B-cell deficiency disease. If thymic grafting does not reverse this, then it is possible that a stem cell defect at the level of the bone marrow is the underlying cause of the condition. Individuals with DiGeorge's syndrome, by virtue of their T-cell insufficiency, do not have significant cytotoxic or suppressor T cells; therefore, answers D and E are incorrect.

4. The etiology of IgA deficiency is:
   A. A failure to synthesize secretory component (SC)
   B. A fault in H chain switch mechanism
   C. Excessive T_S cells
   D. None of the above
   E. Answers B and C only

Answer E

Failure to produce SC would prevent synthesis of secretory but not serum IgA. Two hypotheses have been forwarded to explain selective IgA deficiency: a faulty switch mechanism and undue restrictions of B cells by an overactive T_S population. Thus, only answer E is correct.

Case Study: Recurrent Bacterial Infections

Three-year-old Roger H. has suffered from recurrent infections for the past 2½ years. During this time, the child was hospitalized once for an undiagnosed meningitis that responded well to ampicillin. Numerous visits had been made to the clinic for other bacterial infections, including several episodes of sore throat and otitis media. These were treated successfully without hospitalization. Roger had not yet contracted any viral diseases.

Cultures taken at the present hospital admission for suspected pneumonia yielded group A β hemolytic streptococci. The antistreptolysin O (ASTO) test yielded negative results. Protein electrophoresis and quantitative immunoglobulin testing were requested.

Questions

1. What are the potential causes for recurrent bacterial infections?

2. How will the protein electrophoresis and quantitative immunoglobulin testing aid in establishing a diagnosis?

3. What are the normal values for serum proteins and globulins in a 3-year-old child?

4. What is the ASTO test?

Discussion

Recurrent bacterial infections could be related to defective phagocytosis or inadequate immunoglobulin synthesis. In the face of a negative ASTO titer, failure of immunoglobulin synthesis has to be the first consideration. Total protein in a child's serum should approach 8 g/dL and the gamma globulin level should be about 1150 ± 245 mg/dL. Of the latter, IgG, IgM, and IgA are, respectively, 1000 ± 250, 50 ± 20, and 100 ± 35 mg/dL. Roger had only 127 mg IgG, 5 mg IgM, and 7 mg IgA, as determined by quantitative immunoglobulin assays, and was considered to have Bruton-type, sex-linked agammaglobulinemia, pending further tests.

The ASTO test is a neutralization test used to measure antibodies to streptolysin O. Streptolysin O is an oxygen-labile hemolysin produced by group A β hemolytic streptococci. During infections, the streptococci secrete this hemolysin, which stimulates the formation of neutralizing antibodies. The titer of the antibodies is determined by the antistreptolysin O (ASTO) test. It is very unusual to have a negative test (no titer). In very young children or infants, a residue of maternal ASTO remains in their serum. If a child has had recurrent infections, some were almost certainly of streptococcal origin, and the ASTO titer should be elevated. Roger had no detectable ASTO, and this was considered to be further support for a diagnosis of Bruton's disease.

GLOSSARY

ADA   Adenosine deaminase.

ataxia telangiectasia   A disease characterized by a deficiency of T-cell function and IgA.

Bruton's agammaglobulinemia   A genetic (sex-linked) failure of B cells to mature and produce immunoglobulins.

CHD   Chédiak-Higashi disease.

Chédiak-Higashi disease   A phagocytic deficiency disease reflected by the presence of giant granules within white blood cells.

chronic granulomatous disease   A disease in which a deficiency of cytochrome b retards oxidative killing by phagocytes.

chronic mucocutaneous candidiasis   An isolated inability of T cells to defend against chronic infection by *Candida albicans*.

Common variable hypogammaglobulinemia   The loss of one or more immunoglobulin isotypes, most frequently IgA.

DiGeorge's syndrome.   Thymic aplasia of nongenetic origin.

HANE   Hereditary angioneurotic edema.

hereditary angioneurotic edema   A condition in which an inherited deficiency of C1s INH allows activation of complement and the production of extensive edema.

lazy leukocyte syndrome   Diminished response of leukocytes to chemotactic stimuli.

Nezelof's syndrome   Thymic aplasia of genetic origin.

nitroblue tetrazolium reductase test   An assay for the function of phagocytes by measuring their ability to reduce the dye nitroblue tetrazolium.

paroxysmal nocturnal hemoglobinuria   The sporadic loss of hemoglobin via the urine due to deficiency of decay-accelerating factor (DAF).

PNH   Paroxysmal nocturnal hemoglobinuria.

PNP   Purine nucleotide phosphorylase.

Wiskott-Aldrich syndrome   A genetic deficit in both T and B lymphocytes, with decreased IgM.

CHAPTER 9

$\blacklozenge$

Transplantation Immunology

Tissue transplantation and tumor immunology seem to be exact opposites, but it can be shown that they share many characteristics. The major problem confronting transplantation immunologists is that tissues with foreign surface antigens are often rejected when obviously the desire is to have them survive. In tumor immunology, neoplastic cells that have foreign antigens survive when the desire is to have them be rejected. Although transplanted cells and tumor cells are treated differently by the immune system, the two present essentially the same problem to that system.

In this chapter only transplantation immunology is discussed; tumor immunology is considered in the following chapter. The initial section in this chapter is devoted to allograft rejection—its terminology, its time frame, and its cellular and antibody basis. The transplantation antigens and techniques for their determination precede a description of graft survival strategies, including the dramatic improvement in graft "takes" when cyclosporin A and agent FK506 are used. Advances in bone marrow purging with immunotoxins are included here as well. The status of kidney, heart, liver, and bone marrow transplantation conclude the chapter.

Graft Rejection

The nomenclature used in transplantation immunology is a combination of immunologic and genetic definitions with a residue of surgical terms. Many earlier terms such as "homograft" and "isograft" have been discarded in an effort to arrive at a set of standard terms.

TISSUE TERMINOLOGY

An **autograft**, or a transplant involving autogenic tissue, is the correct term for situations in which the donor and the recipient are the same individual. The tissue is merely moved from one location to another. Such grafts are almost always successful if surgical and aseptic techniques have been adequate. This form of transplantation does not present an antigenic challenge to the individual. When tissue is transplanted from one person into a genetically identical individual, the tissue is described as **syngeneic**, or **congeneic**. (The prefix "syn-" means "together" or "common" and refers only to the antigens involved and not to other characteristics.) In humans this can occur only between identical twins or siblings with identical transplantation antigens. Again, this does not represent an antigenic challenge to the recipient, and the syngraft or congraft should be accepted. A graft that takes place between two nonidentical individuals within the same genus is an **allograft**, which involves allogeneic tissue. ("Allograft" replaces the earlier term "homograft," now obsolete.) Most grafts in humans are allografts. These grafts do represent an antigenic challenge to the recipient and are often rejected unless the recipient is immunoregulated to protect the graft. A **xenograft** involves xenogeneic tissues, tissues that are moved from one species to another. Although such grafts may have tempo-rary usefulness, they are rejected quickly. Rescue grafts are second grafts to replace an earlier and now failing graft.

When tissue is transferred from a donor to an unrelated recipient, rejection of the graft will follow one of three possible sequences. These are known as the hyperacute, first-set, and second-set rejection. Immunologic phenomena of different types and of varying degrees are involved in these three reactions.

HYPERACUTE REJECTION

In **hyperacute graft rejection** there is never a moment when the grafted tissue appears to be accepted by its new host. In these instances as soon as the vascular connection of a deep-seated organ is completed, it will become engorged with blood. The blood may quickly clot and block flood flow through the organ. This prevents the entry of oxygen into the tissue, which will assume a bluish-purple cast signifying that it is anoxic. Such tissue is clearly moribund, and the surgeon will remove the rejected organ during the same operation as the transplantation itself. In the hyperacute rejection of skin, the transferred tissue never becomes revascularized and remains a "white graft" that soon dries and is sloughed.

The hyperacute rejection sequence develops when the graft recipient has antibodies with a specificity for antigens in the donated tissue. *Grafts made across the ABO blood group barrier* into a recipient possessing the corresponding hemagglutinin(s) *are typically lost due to hyperacute rejection*. These antibodies arise naturally or may develop from previous blood transfusions. Matching of blood groups between the donor and recipient is clearly an essential first step in ensuring a successful transplant, but *blood group antigens are not* considered **transplantation (histocompatibility) antigens.**

FIRST-SET REJECTION

Even when cross-matching of the major and minor blood groups has proved satisfactory, the **first-set graft rejection** response may eliminate the transplanted tissue. In first-set rejec-tion, the initial events belie the fact that the graft will be rejected. Early on, the tissue becomes revascularized and assumes its normal hue, a feature eas-ily observed in skin grafts. In the case of organ transplants, the organ will quickly resume its physiologic func-tion—the excretion of urine by the kidney, the pumping of blood by the heart, the production of hormones by the pancreas, and so forth. Unfortu-nately, these events are destined to be short-lived. Within 5 to 10 days organ function will diminish in effectiveness. Skin grafts will acquire a deep purple hue that steadily progresses in the fol-lowing days to a blackened necrotic patch. The patient will usually develop malaise and fever if large areas of skin or a visceral organ are involved in the rejection. Depending upon the circum-stances, the first-step rejection se-quence will be complete between the 11th and 17th days, when the trans-plant no longer functions as a viable part of the recipient (Fig. 9–1).

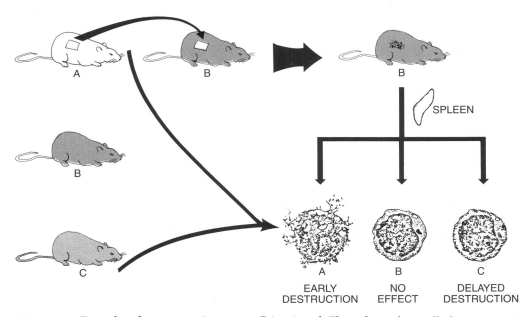

Figure 9–1. Transplant from mouse A to mouse B is rejected. Thereafter, spleen cells from mouse B quickly destroy A cells but not B cells in culture. B cells will attack other foreign cells (mouse C) but more slowly.

SECOND-SET REJECTION

If grafting again takes place between the recipient and the same donor, or a second donor antigenically related to the first, the graft again will be rejected. In this instance, skin is rejected within 3 to 4 days, and internal organs lose their function within a few days. The **second-set rejection** is an accelerated rejection sequence that reflects the sensitization of cells to the earlier exposure to antigen. As such, it is an anamnestic response. Second-set rejection must be anticipated in rescue grafts in which antigenically common donor tissues are used.

IMMUNOLOGIC MECHANISMS IN GRAFT REJECTION

Hyperacute graft rejection does not depend upon a response to histocompatibility antigens. As stated earlier, red blood cell antibodies in the recipient react with antigens on the donor tissue to deny transplant success. Despite this observation, successful grafting of A tissues into O recipients has been recorded, but this may involve circumstances in which the graft expressed only low levels of the A antigen or was such a large organ that the outermost cells in the graft sponged the anti-A antibody and permitted the internal cells to survive.

LGL Cells

The ability of LGL cells to lyse host cells bearing exogenous antigens is an important part of our early defense system against intracellular pathogens. These cells attack host cells when foreign antigens of the pathogen are expressed on the cell surface. LGL cells are also known to attack spontaneously arising tumor cells. The significance of LGL cells in transplant rejection is un-

certain. LGL cells have been identified in rejecting tissue, but there is no convincing evidence that they are active in the rejection process.

Cytotoxic T Cells

A histologic examination of tissues involved in first- or second-set graft rejection reveals that the tissue gradually becomes infiltrated with **macrophages, lymphocytes, and plasma cells**, which signifies that rejection is founded on immunologic grounds. Fibrin deposition and a loss of vascular patency are also seen. These features indicate that the grafted tissue is no longer able to receive a proper supply of nutrients, to effect proper gas exchange, or to dissipate its waste products, factors that ultimately terminate in cell death. The immunologic findings indicate that the T lymphocyte is primarily responsible for graft destruction. During the first few days after emplacement of the graft, T-cell sensitization develops. As the sensitized effector cells express their natural functions, graft rejection occurs.

The T lymphocyte is the cell primarily responsible for first-set allograft elimination. Of the several T-cell subtypes, the CD8$^+$ T cell (CTL), is believed to be the aggressor cell. This cell must rely on IL-2 from CD4$^+$ cells and this is compatible with the *mixed population of CD4$^+$ and CD8$^+$ cells in rejection sites.*

Cellular Interactions. Destruction of the allograft occurs through a two-stage process. The first stage is recognition. Antigen processing by macrophages is required to present antigen in the context of its MHC class II protein to the CD4$^+$ cells. CD4$^+$ cells then release IL-2, which magnifies the CD8$^+$ effector cell population. The awareness that allografts should be eliminated resides in the ability of CD8$^+$ cells to recognize antigen in the context of foreign histocompatibility antigens. This is presumed to be through a different mechanism than that by which this cell recognizes its own MHC and foreign viral antigens. It is possible that the $\alpha 1$ and $\alpha 2$ domains of foreign human leukocyte antigens (HLA) represent the epitope, as they differ from self-HLA, and that the $\alpha 3$ domain represents the agretope.

Biochemical Mechanisms. The second stage relies on the cytodestructive property of the CD8$^+$ cells. The dominant opinion is that the CTLs maintain a store of cytotoxins in their cytoplasmic granules, which they release upon contact with target cells. A major component of the granules is perforin, a pore-forming protein that is structurally and antigenically related to C9. **Perforin, also called cytolysin,** polymerizes in the presence of Ca^{2+} to form channels similar to those produced in the complement system. These channels through the cytoplasmic membrane allow the escape of the cytoplasmic contents and end the cell's life.

Alternative mechanisms include **granzymes**, a collection of proteases also released from CTL granules. There are seven of these enzymes—A through G—which contain an essential serine. Inactivation of these enzymes by serine-targeting chemicals spares the tissue graft.

TNFβ (LT) is another potential killer molecule. In one study, purified LT had the same target-cell spectrum as the intact killer cells. LT does not kill by creating pores and some studies have indicated that target-cell DNA fragmentation is the mechanism. TNFβ is described in Chapter 4.

Immunoglobulins

In second-set rejection, immunoglobulins and T cells combine to deny graft acceptance. This combinations hastens graft rejection compared with the first-set reaction. The antibodies involved are of two separate types. The first co-operates with cells, the second with complement. The first type of antibody participates in antibody-dependent cell cytotoxicity (ADCC). Several cells are active in ADCC. Each cell must have an Fc receptor for antibody and a mechanism to kill the target cell with which the antibody reacts. Macrophages, granulocytes, LGLs, and some T cells meet these criteria. Phagocytic cells kill after ingesting the target cell or by releasing toxic agents from their granules, or by both mechanisms. Released oxygen radicals may also kill extracellularly located targets. Nonphagocytic cells kill by means of perforins, granzymes, TNFβ, and possibly other agents. The ADCC reaction is a complement-independent method of cytolysis.

Dispersed cell grafts of bone marrow, circulating white and red blood cells present a unique situation in which the surface of every cell in the graft is exposed to antibody. Thus antibody and complement can lyse and totally destroy the cells in mismatched grafts of this type. This is a typical complement-dependent reaction, thereby differing from ADCC reactions (Fig. 9–2).

MEMORY CHECK 9–2

Graft rejection

1. By first-set rejection is due mainly to a cellular response

2. Of dispersed cell grafts depends heavily on antibody and complement

3. Sites are infiltrated by CD4$^+$ and CD8$^+$ lymphocytes

4. Is potentially dependent upon perforins and granzymes from lymphocytes

5. Is potentially associated with TNFβ from lymphocytes

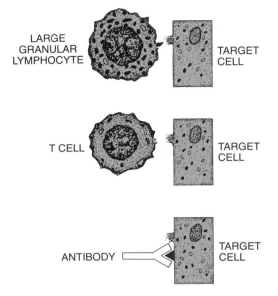

LARGE
GRANULAR
LYMPHOCYTE   TARGET
                                 CELL

T CELL   TARGET
                                 CELL

ANTIBODY   TARGET
                                 CELL

Figure 9-2. LGL, T cells, and antibody all participate in target cell destruction. The cells do so by releasing toxic agents from their granules. Antibody can cooperate either with the cells or with complement.

Transplantation Antigens

MHC REVISITED

The major histocompatibility complex is described in the introduction of this book. In those pages the importance of the MHC gene products as regulators of the immune response is emphasized. From a more cellular viewpoint this is restated in discussions of the antigen-presenting cells in Chapter 2 and of lymphocytes in Chapters 3 and 4. This early introduction to the MHC correctly emphasized the vital importance of this system to cellular interactions in immunity. Here the function of the MHC in graft rejections is presented. The magnitude of these two separate roles of the MHC is the basis for placing these contributions in separate sectors of the text.

The major human histocompatibility antigens originate from **chromosome 6**, the chromosome that *has genes for the class I, class II, and class III proteins.* The proteins of the class III genes are of no special concern in transplant immunology, except for dispersed cell grafts that are sensitive to lysis by antibody and complement. *The class II proteins are the immune-associated proteins controlled by the human DP, DQ, and DR genes* (see Figs. I-1 and I-2). These proteins on cells transplanted against unlike DP, DQ, or DR cells in the recipient do affect graft survival, but the *class I proteins are the major histocompatibility or transplantation proteins.* These major graft-regulating proteins were first recognized on leukocytes and are referred to as the **human leukocyte antigens (HLA).** Three separate gene loci—HLA-A, HLA-B, and HLA-C—determine these gene products (Fig. 9-3)

MHC CLASS I ANTIGENS

The HLA class I proteins are believed to be present on all nucleated cells except muscle and nerve cells. These proteins are glycosylated molecules of approximately 45,000 Mr. The structure of each HLA protein is divisible

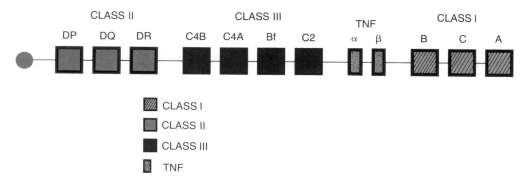

Figure 9-3. Human chromosome 6 contains the genes for the HLA-A, -B, and -C proteins to the right of the class III genes. The class II genes are to the left (see also Figures I–1 and I–2).

into discrete domains—three extracellular, a transmembrane, and a cytoplasmic domain. The transmembrane sector occupies 40 amino acids and the cytoplasmic tail consists of 30 amino acids (Fig. 9-4). The $\alpha 1$, $\alpha 2$, and $\alpha 3$ extracellular domains consist of about 90 amino acids each. The $\alpha 2$ and $\alpha 3$ domains have the expected disulfide bond characteristic of proteins in the **immunoglobulin supergene family**. The $\alpha 1$ domain lacks the cysteine-cysteine bond but is otherwise like the domains in the proteins of the supergene family. *The $\alpha 1$ and $\alpha 2$ domains harbor the alloantigenic determinants that give antigen specificity to each class I protein.*

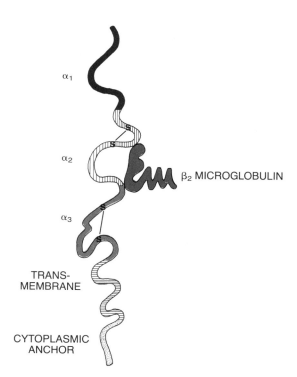

Figure 9-4. The MHC class I antigen has three domains that extend from the cell membrane, a transmembrane, and a cytoplasmic domain. The $\beta 2$ macroglobulin appears to be most closely associated with the $\alpha 2$ and $\alpha 3$ domains.

β2 MICROGLOBULIN

Constantly *associated with each HLA protein is the β2 microglobulin*, a protein of 12,500 Mr. With a single exception, all β2 microglobulins of human origin are identical; hence, this protein cannot function as a transplantation antigen. Through noncovalent forces, the β2 microglobulin is associated with the α2 and α3 domains of the HLA protein.

MEMORY CHECK 9-3

◆

The MHC class I

1. Proteins are noncovalently associated with the β2 micro-globulin
2. Proteins are members of the immunoglobulin supergene family
3. Protein domains of α1 and α2 probably represent their antigenically unique sections
4. Proteins are the major histocompatibility antigens

HLA GENETICS

Each of the HLA genes is allelic and highly polymorphic. Fifteen variations of the A gene are known and an additional nine antigens are believed to emerge from the A locus. HLA-B has 21 definitely established alleles and approximately 30 additional forms are believed under its control. The HLA-C antigen number is highly uncertain but is presumed to contain at least 11 variations. The accepted antigen specificities associated with a gene are numbered (eg, HLA-A1, HLA-A2, HLA-B7, HLA-B27). The numbering system is not completely sequential

because of the removal of specificities erroneously assigned to a gene locus. Table 9-1 lists some of the HLA antigens of known frequency.

The genes of presumed or indefinite assignments carry the suffix "w" (eg, Cw1, Bw70, Aw19) to indicate that the expert committee responsible for ordering these proteins has reserved the exact assignment until their annual workshop makes a definite determination.

The paired chromosome system of human genetics dictates that *each person will have two A proteins, two B proteins, and two C proteins*. The complete

Table 9-1
SELECTED HUMAN HLA-A AND HLA-B GENES AND THEIR FREQUENCY

Antigen	Frequency
HLA-A	
1	16
2	28
3	14
9	7
10	3
11	5
25	2
26	4
28	4
29	4
HLA-B	
5	6
7	10
8	10
12	14
13	3
14	5
15	6
17	5
18	3
27	6
37	2
40	10

genotype of a hypothetical individual could be HLA-A1,11; B12,14; Cw3,8, and since each of these antigens can be detected by serologic means, the person's genotype and phenotype are identical. *The term* **haplotype** *refers to the HLA proteins on a single chromosome.* Genetic studies are necessary to determine this. Thus, if the father of the individual just cited was HLA-A1,26; B14,40; Cw3,6, then it is clear that A1, B14, and Cw3 represent the paternal-derived haplotype. The maternal haplotype is thus HLA-A11, B12, and Cw8.

Information of this nature is extremely important in the *genetic determinations necessary to establish parenthood or individual identity.* In most instances, the genotype of the mother is easily determined. Thus, if the known mother of the hypothetical individual referred to above was HLA-A11, B12, Cw8, then the father must be HLA-A1, B14, Cw3. Because of the enormous number of HLA combinations possible, it can be calculated that, aside from identical twins, the chance for two persons to have identical HLA profiles is less than one in a billion. Thus, a putative father of a child who has a haplotype that agrees with that of a known mother is the true father (Table 9–2).

CLASS II GENES AND PROTEINS

The genes and proteins of the class II MHC are also important in graft rejection. It is well known that the class II proteins not matched with T cells are a potent stimulant of those T cells. The general acceptance of T_C cells as significant contributors to graft rejection emphasizes this interaction. Moreover, the destruction by radiation of so-called passenger cells in donor tissue —dendritic, Langerhans', and other class II–positive cells—prolongs graft survival. Whether this is directly due to stimulation of T cells or simply to their role as antigen-presenting cells is uncertain.

MHC AND AUTOIMMUNITY

Because the class II genes dictate the structure of the DP, DQ, and DR proteins and these proteins govern the interactions among macrophages, B cells, and T cells, it is not unexpected that errors in this interplay would allow a self-directed immune response. Several autoimmune diseases are associated with an inheritance of D region genes or, in instances wherein the D region gene product cannot be measured, with an HLA gene. An ex-

Table 9–2
HAPLOTYPE INHERITANCE OF HLA-A AND HLA-B ANTIGENS

Father	A1	A3	B7	B8
Mother	A2	A9	B5	B12
Children*				
First	A1	A2	B5	B8
Second	A1	A9	B8	B12

*The shaded antigens of the children represent the maternal haplotype, and the unshaded the paternal haplotype. Note that the two children represent a half-match (A1 and B8 being common).

MEMORY CHECK 9–4

◆

The HLA gene(s)

1. Are on human chromosome 6
2. Haplotype consists of one gene each of HLA-A, HLA-B, and HLA-C
3. Are related to autoimmunity (see Chapter 11)
4. Are more useful than blood grouping in establishing personal identity

panded discussion of this relationship is found in Chapter 11 on autoimmune disease.

Histocompatibility Testing

The assessment of graft success relies on a determination of the antigenic similarity between the donor and the recipient. This can be determined by analyzing tissues of each participant for the coincidence of the major histo-compatibility antigens by serologic methods or, alternatively, by the mixed lymphocyte technique. The mixed lymphocyte reaction (MLR) is an assay for an antagonistic reaction between tissues of the donor and those of the recipient. These tests are intended to determine the compatibility of donor and recipient tissues as they would be expressed in vivo.

MICROCYTOTOXICITY TESTING

The antigenic specificities in the α1 and α2 domains of the HLA antigens are recognized by antisera. The original source of these sera was persons who had received numerous blood transfusions or from multiply gravid women. Monoclonal antisera are available now for many antigens. These sera are used to identify the HLA class I and class II antigens on lymphocytes of potential transplant donors and recipients. Various serologic tests are appropriate for this, but the most common is the microcytotoxicity test.

In the **microcytotoxicity assay**, it is assumed that antibodies are available for each of the known HLA antigens. This may not be absolutely true and is a potential source of tissue-match uncertainty. Nevertheless, these antisera

are used to identify the antigenic mosaic of both donor and recipient cells as far as is possible. Lymphocytes of both donor and recipient are adjusted to 10^6 cells/mL for use in the microcytotoxicity test. A few microliters of these lymphocyte suspensions are added to separate samples of many HLA antisera in a paired test. This mixture is incubated, complement is added, and the test is incubated further. Thereafter, the cells are stained with trypan blue or eosin to determine if they are living or dead.

Living cells take up these dyes and reduce them to their colorless form. Dead cells become stained the color of the dye. By determining which histo-compatibility antisera were toxic for donor and recipient lymphocytes, the HLA formula for each can be determined.

MIXED LYMPHOCYTE REACTION

When lymphocytes from unrelated donors are placed in culture, lympho-cyte transformation, observed as a stim-ulation of DNA synthesis, enlargement of the cell nucleus, increase in mitotic figures, and cell enlargement and divi-sion, is observed (Fig. 9–5). These changes can be detected microscopically, but this is time-consuming and subject to interpretative error. To hasten the process and to increase the test's sensitivity, tritiated thymidine is added to the cultures. Incorporation of isotope is then used as an index of DNA synthesis and cell proliferation.

Mixed lymphocyte reactions appear to reflect disparities only in the major histocompatibility antigens, and differences in the minor antigens apparently go undetected. Because some grafts matched by cytotoxicity testing are rejected, the MLR may be measuring antigens that are highly critical to graft

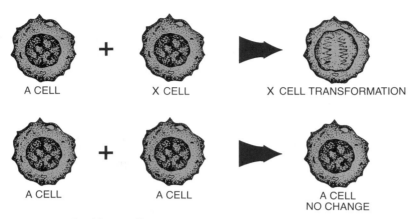

Figure 9-5. Mixture of unlike T cells, as in microcytotoxicity testing (*upper panel*), results in T-cell growth, represented here by mitotic division. Like cells do not stimulate each other (*lower panel*).

success. One of these antigens is an MHC class II protein on donor B cells that stimulates foreign T cells.

One obvious drawback to the MLR test is the potential for donor T cells to respond to class II proteins on recipient lymphocytes. This would be interpreted as a histocompatibility mismatch when in reality it is measuring cell incompatibility in the wrong direction. In the MLR test the only important determination is whether recipient T cells are reacting against donor cells. This can be determined if donor lymphocytes are poisoned with mitomycin C or killed by irradiation before being added to the culture. Mitomycin C blocks DNA metabolism. Lymphocyte transformation after either of these treatments is an index only of the recipient's response. This form of the test is known as the **one-way MLR** test.

PRIMED LYMPHOCYTE REACTION

The second disadvantage of MLR testing is the delay of several days before the results of the test are available. To compensate for this, a panel of lymphocytes that have been preexposed to specific histocompatibility determinants is maintained. Stocks of these cells can be preserved under liquid nitrogen and removed when needed. These presensitized cells transform rapidly upon reexposure and shorten the MLR test to a day or two.

Graft Survival Strategies

Transplant immunologists realize that some anatomic locations are immunologically privileged sites where transplants are accepted despite mismatching of class I proteins. Likewise, some tissues that are immunologically privileged can be moved across histocompatibility barriers. Very few tissues are in either of these categories; consequently, immunosuppression must be practiced for all except those rare, perfectly matched grafts. Pretransplantation blood transfusions is one means of enhancing graft survival, but a major emphasis has been placed on the evaluation of chemical immunosuppressants. The use of these compounds is invariably associated with a risk of infectious disease, and in some circumstances, of graft-versus-host disease.

PRIVILEGED SITES AND TISSUES

In the case of maternal-fetal relationships, the fetus contains antigens inherited from the father that are different from those of the mother. The fetus represents a transplant of foreign tissue that is not rejected: it is in a privileged site. This immunologic escape may be based on the trophoblastic layer of tissue that physically separates the uterine wall of the mother from the tissues of the fetus. Each cell in this trophoblastic layer surrounds itself with a mucoprotein shell, and it is believed that T lymphocytes are unable to migrate through this layer.

The cornea is one of the most generally accepted privileged tissues. Surgically successful corneal transplants in which vascular tissues are not ruptured are normally accepted. However, if the vascular bed is damaged during surgery, an immune reaction will develop, clouding the transplanted cornea and rendering it unusable. Likewise, if the cornea is not transplanted to the eye but is placed in some other region of the body, rejection takes place much as with any allograft. The success of corneal grafts into their natural location resides in the failure of recipient T cells to contact corneal antigens. Antigen release from the cornea is minimal under normal circumstances and is usually insufficient to stimulate an immune response. In unnatural locations, corneal antigen is released in adequate quantities to initiate rejection.

IMMUNE ENHANCEMENT

The phenomenon of immunologic enhancement was discovered as the result of exercises in tumor immunology in which it was expected that immunization with tumor antigens would pre-

vent subsequent tumor graft success. In these experiments, the tumor "take" was more successful in the immunized animals than in those exposed to the tissues for the first time. *Immunologic enhancement is based on the development of blocking antibodies*, which coat the transplanted tumor cells, thereby shielding them from sensitized lymphocytes or cytotoxic antibodies. These antibodies do not participate in ADCC or complement-dependent cytolysis.

Immune enhancement may have a role in graft prolongation by blood transfusion prior to tissue transplantation. This was first noticed in human kidney grafts. In 1972, when the kidney survival rate was only 29%, it was found that recipients receiving 1 to 10 units of blood had a kidney take at 43%. This rose to 66% success in patients receiving more than 10 units of blood. The basis for this is still not fully understood. Some evidence points to an increase of T_S cells responsive to HLA antigens present on the transfused white blood cells and on the kidney implanted later. This seems a more likely explanation than the promotion of anti-idiotypic antibodies directed against antigraft globulins or FcR blockade, as antibodies are not considered to have a major role in kidney rejection.

IMMUNOSUPPRESSION

Even though tissue antigens can be closely matched between donor and recipient, it is rare that the match can ever be perfect. For this reason, *it is necessary for the recipient to receive posttransplant immunosuppressant therapy.* The exact regimen will vary from one hospital or surgeon to another, as well as from one patient to another, but it usually involves chemical immunosuppression with azathio-prine, corticosteroids, and the antibi-otic cyclosporin A. A second antibiotic, FK506, appears to be as useful as cyclo-sporin A. In some instances antilym-phocyte globulin is also used.

MEMORY CHECK 9–5
◆

Graft survival may depend upon

1. Transplantation to a privi-leged site
2. Transplantation of a privi-leged tissue
3. A good antibody response to the graft (immune en-hancement)
4. Suitable immunosuppression

Antilymphocyte Globulin

Antilymphocyte serum (ALS) or anti-lymphocyte globulin (ALG) is nor-mally prepared by using human pe-ripheral lymphocytes (primarily T cells) as the antigen to immunize horses. If a purified preparation of T cells is used, the antiserum is desig-nated as ATS. The resulting antiserum, or more usually its globulin fraction, can be given by intravenous inocula-tion or by other routes to the transplant recipient. Despite the fact that ALG, ATS, or ATG (anti T cell globulin) is administered together with chemical immunosuppression, *hypersensitive re-actions typical of serum sickness*, or less often of an anaphylactic nature, often develop. Consequently, antilym-phocyte therapy is temporary and is usually withdrawn after about 1 month.

Azathioprine and Prednisolone

Purine and pyrimidine analogs may function at several levels to inhibit T-cell proliferation. **Azathioprine** is known to inhibit synthesis of the nor-mal purine bases. Incorporation of the purine base of azathioprine into mRNA results in the formation of defective proteins that stunt cell growth. Other analogs of nucleic acids are substituted for azathioprine in some protocols, but azathioprine is one of the most widely used in the triple regimen with pred-nisolone and cyclosporin A.

Prednisolone is but one example of a long list of corticosteroid drugs used to prolong the life of grafts. The steroid drugs inhibit protein synthesis, and this impact on IL-1 and IL-2 production impairs macrophage activation of T_H cells and of CTL. B-cell differentiation and proliferation is also inhibited be-cause of the unavailability of T-cell interleukins.

Cyclosporin A

Cyclosporin is an ineffective antimi-crobial antibiotic isolated from *Tolypo-cladium inflatum*. The structure of cy-closporin A is that of a cyclic peptide of 12 amino acids, some of which are rarely encountered in biologic sources. By 1976 this antibiotic was found to have potent immunoregulating char-acteristics.

The role of cyclosporin A in trans-plantation immunology is based on its ability to inhibit T-cell activation. Its primary site of action is the *inhibition of IL-2 synthesis*. This occurs at the level of gene transcription where mRNA transcription for IL-2 was in-hibited 100% by cyclosporin at a con-centration of 1000 μg/L. The activation of other T-cell genes is also blocked. Activation of IL-1 genes in monocytes is also impeded by this immunoregula-tory antibiotic.

Blockage of IL-2 formation blocks the autocrine induction of IL-2 receptors.

This prevents clonal expansion of cytotoxic T cells and protects the transplanted tissues. Proliferation of cells already exposed to IL-2 is not prevented by cyclosporin.

The success of cyclosporin as a specific T-cell suppressant has advanced the triple-drug regimen of azathioprine, prednisolone, and cyclosporin as the most effective combination of immunosuppressants.

FK506

A macrolide antibiotic isolated in Japan from *Streptomyces tsukubaensis*, **FK506** has had an impact on human transplant success that parallels that of cyclosporin A. This as yet unnamed drug has proved to be 10- to 100-fold greater in immunosuppressive activity than cyclosporin. It is also cheaper and less toxic. Its successful early use in liver transplants indicates FK506 may replace cyclosporin in the triple-drug regimen or may be added to it to create a quadruple combination.

FK506 prevents T-cell activation by either antigens or mitogens. Effector T cells cannot be generated, and the graft is protected against CTL. FK506 blocks early events in T-cell activation, probably at the early transcription level of activation genes, the same target hit by cyclosporin. Failure of T_H cells to produce IL-2 suspends all T-cell subsets in an inactive state and allows graft survival.

Infectious Disease Risks

Cytostatic and cytotoxic drugs that act upon lymphocytes and macrophages have been major contributors to the growing success of transplantation. The lack of target specificity for most compounds has hampered progress in improving graft success and has ren-

dered *transplant recipients sensitive to the emergence of infectious diseases*. These infections are often a reactivation of a latent infection. The herpes viruses, including herpes simplex, varicella virus, and cytomegalovirus, are most prominent in this category. A second group of agents best described as opportunistic pathogens includes agents such as *Candida albicans*, *Pneumocystis carinii*, *Cryptosporidum*, and others. It is important to monitor the peripheral blood granulocyte count of patients receiving immunosuppressant drugs so they do not become overly susceptible to pathogenic bacteria, viruses, and fungi.

GRAFT-VERSUS-HOST DISEASE

In transplantation immunology, the primary emphasis is on host-versus-graft reactions, which reflects the primary direction of rejection. This is the major cause of transplant failure. However, a graft-versus-host (GVH) reaction may develop when immunocompetent tissues are transferred to an immunologically handicapped host — one who has been heavily immunosuppressed. Graft-versus-host reactions are the result of an adaptive immunization in which T lymphocytes from the donor respond to and attack recipient tissues. In certain maternal-fetal relationships when maternal lymphoid tissues accidentally pass the placental barrier and enter the fetus, a GVH reaction may develop. When it was found that experimental GVH reactions were seldom fatal, transplantation of adult lymphoid tissues or bone marrow into T-cell–deficient children or children with other marrow deficiencies was initiated. Many of these children progress through a graft-versus-host reaction, but both donor and recipient tissues survive. Karyotyping of the newly generated cells reveals that both donor and recipient cells are present; that is, the marrow recipient is a true blood-cell chimera. For transplants of nonlymphoid tissue, it is possible to destroy the few resident T lymphocytes by irradiation or perfusion with immunosuppressant drugs so that GVH reactions are unlikely.

PURGING BONE MARROW

Purged bone marrow has been one avenue for the control of GVH disease. Purged marrow is depleted of T cells. Purging can be accomplished with monoclonal antibodies and complement or by immunotoxins. It has been demonstrated, however, that T cells may be helpful for sustained proliferation of engrafted cells.

Immunotoxins

Purging of bone marrow with immunotoxins has been useful both in transplantation and tumor immunology. Immunotoxins are a synthetic combination of an antibody with a toxin. The most used toxins are those like diphtheria toxin or ricin, which have a clear structural division of their toxic portion (A or active region) and cell-binding region (B region). A monoclonal antibody to T cells such as anti-CD3 will transport the toxin to T cells. When the toxin enters and kills these cells, the marrow, purged of all T cells, can be used with minimal risk of graft-versus-host reactions (see Fig. 10–5).

Antibody and Complement

Immunotoxin purging of bone marrow is a more technical approach to the procedure that can also be accomplished with antibody and complement. Both procedures have been used effectively.

MEMORY CHECK 9 – 6

Immunosuppression

1. With antilymphocyte globulins is usually terminated because of allergic reactions
2. Has the hazard of lowering immunity to infectious agents
3. At the level of IL-2 synthesis is a property of cyclosporin A and FK506
4. Usually requires multiple agents to be effective
5. Of the recipient may lead to graft-versus-host disease

Organ Transplantation

KIDNEY TRANSPLANTATION

The 1-year survival rate for kidney grafts is now nearly 90% when there is a double-haplotype match; this falls to 75% with a single-haplotype match, and to 50% if there is no match. This is the result of several factors, not the least of which is the success of the triple suppressive regimen of azathioprine, steroids, and cyclosporin. Even so, the earliest renal transplants in the United States were performed prior to knowledge of the MHC class I proteins. Transplants were unwittingly made across the MHC barrier and an unexpected percentage of them have survived. The basis for this is speculative.

HEART TRANSPLANTATION

The first human heart transplant was performed in 1967. The 5-year survival of transplanted hearts is still only 40%.

This has placed an inordinate amount of attention on the development of artificial hearts. Artificial hearts have a useful role as temporary organs, but blood clotting problems have been a persistent problem. Because of this it is anticipated that natural heart transplants will continue indefinitely as the best heart replacement procedure. Temporary grafting with hearts from lower animals has been a deplorable aspect of heart transplant history.

Heart tissue is less sensitive to rejection than skin in histoincompatible transfers. This does not mean that the risk for immune rejection is slight; it is customary to treat heart recipients with high-dose steroids, cyclosporin, and a purine or pyrimidine analog. When rejection develops, there is a pronounced infiltration of mononuclear cells into the myocardium. Both T_H and T_C cells enter the heart. LGL cells also enter heart tissue early in the rejection sequence, although there is little evidence that LGLs contribute to heart rejection. Immunoglobulin and complement also deposit in the tissues but are considered secondary agents in graft rejection. Immune complex deposits alter vascular permeability and contribute to fibrosis.

Arteriosclerosis is a chronic problem for heart transplant patients. Within 4 years after grafting 25% will have arteriosclerosis, and 11% of cardiac transplants deaths are due to this.

LIVER TRANSPLANTATION

One-year survival of liver transplants hovered near 30% until being doubled by the introduction of cyclosporin. Some centers are now reporting survival as high as 80%, a factor that has contributed to multiorgan transplant trials. A potential feature allowing this high rate of success is that hepatocytes are class II MHC negative, suggesting that they may be poor antigen presenters. Liver transplantation is considered appropriate for the repair of malignancy, several metabolic disorders, and liver cirrhosis. Donors should be ABO compatible and as closely HLA matched as possible. Surprisingly, 10 liver transplants from blood group A donors to O recipients have had a 70% 1-year survival. Grafting against the blood group barrier may be more possible for the liver than for other organs because of its large size and high population of phagocytic cells.

Immunosuppression with azathioprine, steroids, and cyclosporin is usually practiced. FK506 has been used extensively as a fourth suppressant or as a substitute for cyclosporin. This combination severely reduces IL-2 production and the expression of class II MHC proteins. Macrophage production of IL-1 is inhibited slightly. ALG and anti-CD8 monoclonal sera have been used occasionally, but these are complicated by allergic side effects. Rejection episodes are treated with bolus steroids, repeated as necessary.

BONE MARROW TRANSPLANTATION

Transplantation of bone marrow as a treatment for leukemias and aplastic anemia has been practiced for 30 years. This modality is also applied to repair severe combined immunodeficiencies and certain metabolic abnormalities such as thalassemia, Gaucher's disease, and Franconi's anemia. Bone marrow transplants between siblings matched at the HLA-A, HLA-B, and class II loci are obviously most apt to be successful. Partial matches are at risk for powerful GVH disease because marrow in the recipient is destroyed by total body irradiation, chemotherapy, or both. Purging of donor bone marrow with immunotoxins will minimize the potential for GVH disease.

Hematopoiesis in the recipient is usually seen within 2 to 3 weeks of engraftment. GM-CSF therapy may accelerate the recovery phase. In some patients, recipient cells that escaped destruction may regenerate and produce a mixed blood cell chimera. Ten-year survival is projected to approach 80% for grafted aplastic anemia patients. Graft resistance in haploidentical transfers has been attributed to LGL

cells. These cells appear to be more radioresistant than other lymphocytic cells.

MEMORY CHECK 9 – 7
◆
Transplantation

1. **Of kidney has the highest survival rate of organ transplants**
2. **Of bone marrow purged by an immunotoxin can minimize GVH disease**
3. **Is usually accompanied by immunosuppression with cyclosporin, azathioprine, and prednisolone**

References

Bach, FH and Sachs, DH: Transplantation immunology. N Engl J Med 317:489, 1987.

Catto, GRD (ed): Clinical Transplantation: Current practices and future prospects. MTP Press, Boston, 1987.

Cramer, DV: Cardiac transplantation: Immune mechanisms and alloantigens involved in graft rejection. CRC Crit Rev Immunol 7:1, 1987.

Martin, PJ, et al: Human marrow transplantation: An immunological perspective. Adv Immunol 40:379, 1987.

Meryman, HT: Transplantation: Approaches to graft rejection. Alan R Liss, New York, 1986.

Milford, EL (ed): Renal Transplantation. Churchill Livingstone, New York, 1989.

Roberts, JP, et al: Liver transplantation today. Annu Rev Med 40:287, 1989.

Shaw, LM: Advances in cyclosporine pharmacology, measurement, and therapeutic monitoring. Clin Chem 35:1299, 1989.

Thomson, AW (ed): Cyclosporin: Mode of action and clinical applications. Kluwer Academic Publishers, Dordrecht, Netherlands, 1988.

Wallwork, J (ed): Heart and Heart-Lung Transplantation. WB Saunders, Philadelphia, 1989.

Williams, JW (ed): Hepatic Transplantation. WB Saunders, Philadelphia, 1990.

QUESTIONS AND ANSWERS

1. A major consideration in bone marrow transplantation is
   A. Graft-versus-host disease
   B. Adequate purging of T cells from the donor marrow
   C. Failure of total body irradiation, thereby allowing graft rejection by recipient T or LGL cells
   D. Appearance of latent viral infections
   E. All of the above

Answer E

All of these are serious aspects of bone marrow transplantation. Since the lymphoid population of the recipient should be totally destroyed by total body irradiation or chemosuppressant therapy, or both, a potential for graft-versus-host disease always exists. GVH disease is especially likely if donor T cells have not been completely purged. If recipient cells have not been adequately destroyed, the opposite may occur and the graft rejected. In virtually all transplant situations, recurrence of latent herpes, cytomegalovirus, or other viral disease is a threat.

2. Which of the following immunosuppressant agents is most specific against nonsensitized CD4$^+$ T cells?
   A. Cyclophosphamide
   B. Cyclosporin A
   C. Corticosteroids
   D. Antilymphocyte globulin
   E. Azathioprine

Answer B

Most agents that are toxic for lymphocytes will show dual activity against both B and T cells, and this is true for the agents listed in the question. Cyclosporin A and FK506 are highly specific for unsensitized T cells that are unable to secrete IL-2. This arrests T_H cell development and blocks activation of other T-cell subsets, as well as hindering B-cell growth.

3. Which of the following is the father of a child with HLA-A2,9; B5,27; Cw1,3; DR3,- from a known mother of HLA-A2, B5, Cw1, DR3?
   A. HLA-A2,9; B5,27; Cw2,4; DR23-1
   B. HLA-A9,11; B5,17; Cw-,7; DR-,-
   C. HLA-A9,11; B5,27; Cw3,-; DR-,-
   D. HLA-A2,-; B5,-; Cw1,-; DR23,-
   E. HLA-A2,29; B5,27; Cw1,3; DR3,-

Answer C

The maternal haplotype is subtracted from the child's genotype in the following expression to determine the paternal haplotype.

Child	A2,9	B5,27	Cw1,3	DR3,-
Mother	A2	B5	Cw1	DR3
Father	A9	B27	Cw3	DR-

Only answer C has this as a potential haplotype.

4. Immunotoxins
   A. Have no influence on hyperacute graft rejection
   B. Are a conjugate of an antibody and lytic complement
   C. Used for bone marrow purging are usually specific for MHC class I proteins
   D. Used for bone marrow purging are usually specific for MHC class II proteins
   E. Are used with the intent to destroy all B cells in bone marrow

Answer A

Immunotoxins used in bone marrow purging are directed against T cells. Answers C, D, and E are inappropriate. These toxins are intended to replace antibody and complement. Because hyperacute graft rejection depends upon ABO incompatibility between donor and recipient, and immunotoxins are T-cell directed, answer A is the only correct response.

5. The genes of the major histocompatibility complex can be described as all of the following *except*
   A. Autosomal
   B. Located on human chromosome 6
   C. Polymorphic
   D. Sex-linked
   E. Codominant

Answer D

The human MHC genes, located on chromosome 6, are codominantly expressed, autosomal genes with many variations. Only answer D is wrong.

Case Study: Corneal Graft Rejection

In Hosptial X, 348 patients were given corneal grafts over a 5-year period ending in July 1989. During this period, follow-up examination was possible on 304 patients of which there were 26 graft failures. These graft failures were analyzed in order to answer the following questions.

Questions

1. Is ABO matching important in corneal grafting?

2. What is the importance of HLA matching?

3. In corneal rejection, is antibody or T-cell function the most important?

4. What is the effect of immunosuppression on corneal graft acceptance?

Discussion

In 1987 over 30,000 corneal transplants were made in the United States alone. The failure rate when all grafts are considered is below 10%. Graft failure is affected by numerous nonimmunologic factors including secondary diseases in the recipient and the use of unfit cornea with latent viral or other infectious agents. Nevertheless, evidence is increasing that cornea, though avascular and relatively inert, can succumb to graft rejection.

ABO blood group antigens are present in the cornea, yet ABO incompatibility does not adversely affect graft survival. Both class I and class II antigen are found in the cornea, the latter on dendritic cells. Particularly in patients with a prior history of graft rejection or corneal vascularization, HLA matching may be beneficial. Retrospective studies confirm a partial immunologic privilege for cornea but good class I matching lowers graft rejection. It is assumed that class II matching will further corneal graft success.

Maintenance of corneal grafts amid GVH disease has centered on blocking the T-cell component of the immune response. Topical cyclosporin has proved very helpful. Locally injected anti-CD3 induces remission of rejection symptoms even when used alone. Irradiation of the corneal endothelium prior to grafting has also been practiced successfully in some centers. The newer FK506 has proved useful in animal models and is under test in humans.

GLOSSARY

allogeneic   Of a different genetic structure than another individual in the same species

allograft   A grafted tissue that contains antigens not present in a recipient of the same species.

autograft   A graft of tissue from one location to another in the same individual.

congeneic   Genetically identical to another individual except at one allele.

cyclosporin A   An immunosuppressant antibiotic that blocks IL-2 synthesis by T_H cells.

first-set rejection   The rejection of an allograft after its first transplantation.

graft-versus-host (GVH) disease   The attack of immunocompetent tissues in a graft placed in an immunocompromised host.

haplotype   The genes present on one of the two chromosomes.

histocompatibility antigen   An antigen on the surface of a cell that induces the response leading to graft rejection; synonymous with transplantation antigen.

human leukocyte antigen (HLA)   Antigens on leukocytes and other cells derived from the class I MHC genes.

hyperacute rejection   An accelerated rejection of a graft owing to the presence of preformed antibodies.

immune enhancement   Improved survival of a transplant in hosts possessing antibodies against antigens in the transplanted tissue.

immunotoxin   A conjugate of an antibody and a toxin.

microcytotoxicity test   A test to determine histocompatibility by measuring antigens on donor and recipient lymphocytes.

mixed lymphocyte reaction   A test to determine histocompatibility by cocultivation of donor and recipient lymphocytes.

rescue graft   A second graft used to replace an earlier failing graft.

second-set rejection   An accelerated form of first-set rejection.

transplantation antigen   Histocompatibility antigen.

CHAPTER 10

◆

Tumor Immunology

In the preceding chapter, the ideologic conflict of tumor immunology and transplantation immunology was used as the introduction. That introduction is equally appropriate here. To repeat briefly, self-generated tumor cells, though expressing new antigens, are too often capable of escaping the immune surveillance system — a system that can attack and destroy transplanted tissues through immune mechanisms directed against newly presented antigens. In this chapter, the antigens unique to malignantly transformed cells are described and the means by which these cells escape the immune system considered. Immunologic approaches to the diagnosis and treatment of cancer are also described.

Specific topics discussed include the T-cell leukemia viruses, and Burkitt's lymphoma in the portion devoted to the viral etiology of human cancer. Hairy-cell leukemia, Hodgkin's disease, multiple myeloma, and Waldenström's macroglobulinemia are all considered, in each instance with a specific description of the marker for that particular tumor. Immunotherapy with lymphocytes, immunotoxins, interleukins, and bacille Calmette-Guérin (BCG) vaccination are discussed in the final pages of the chapter.

Tumor-Specific Transplantation Antigens

When a neoplastic cell develops, it expresses a large set of new properties not possessed by the surrounding cells; among these is the formation of new antigens. Some of these antigens are restricted to the intracellular portion of the tumor, but others are located on the cell surface. The former are anatomically protected from the defense system of the host, whereas those on the cell surface, like the histocompatibility antigens of any foreign cell, are situated in a vulnerable position where they are exposed to the host's immune system. Despite this, these cells avoid an immune-mediated demise, and proliferate. This interrupts the physiologic and structural pattern of surrounding tissues, and may cause the eventual death of the host.

Nevertheless, it is possible to demonstrate protection by the immune system against tumors. If a small number of tumor cells is transferred between otherwise identical animals, the recipient's immune response against the exposed antigens of the tumor is able to destroy it. This response is parallel to the immune rejection of allogeneic cells between genetically unlike recipients; **tumor-specific transplantation antigens (TSTAs)** are the novel antigens on the surface of the tumor cell. TSTAs are not always able to engender a protective immune response. When a large number of tumor cells are transferred to a new host, the host's response is inadequate to provide protection.

CHEMICALLY INDUCED ANTIGENS

Public health officials have identified an increasing number of carcinogenic chemicals in tobacco smoke, pesticides, herbicides, etc. Application of many of these compounds to the skin of an animal will induce a local tumor. *Tumors provoked experimentally in animals by carcinogenic chemicals are, with few exceptions, antigenically unrelated*, even when multiple tumors are induced in different locations on the same animal. This suggests that the carcinogenic chemical has affected the genetic apparatus of sensitive cells at different sites, and each tumor cell has made its own adjustment in protein synthesis. The conclusion from this is that one cannot develop a simple serologic system for identifying all tumors because of the antigenic variety that they represent. Neither is it possible to develop an anticancer vaccine against these chemically induced tumors. The situation with virus-induced tumors is slightly different.

VIRUS-INDUCED ANTIGENS

When oncogenic viruses transform a cell to a neoplastic state, they also induce the synthesis of new proteins; however, these *are antigenically constant from tumor to tumor* or from animal to animal. A number of oncogenic RNA viruses such as those in the leukemia-sarcoma group, mouse mammary tumor virus, and the oncogenic DNA viruses in the herpesvirus, adenovirus, and papillomavirus groups are known to induce tumor-specific antigens characteristic for that virus (Table 10–1).

The fact that these viruses induce TSTA suggests the possibility that an immune response directed only against the TSTA antigens would destroy the tumor with no effect on other host cells. It is also apparent that detection of the TSTA antigen would assist in the diagnosis of cancer, and the quantitation of TSTA levels in blood or other

Table 10–1
VIRUSES IMPLICATED IN HUMAN CANCER

Agent	Cancer
Human T lymphotrophic viruses	
HTLV-I	T-cell lymphoma
HTLV-II	T-cell leukemia
Epstein-Barr virus (EBV)	Burkitt's lymphoma
	Nasopharyngeal carcinoma
	Other lymphoproliferative diseases
Hepatitis B	Hepatocarcinoma
Human papilloma viruses (HPV)	
HPV-1	Plantar warts
HPV-2	Common hand warts
HPV-6	Genital condyloma
HPV-11	Laryngeal papilloma
HPV-16	Cervical cancer
HPV-18	Cervical cancer

tissues of a patient would serve as a prognosticator of therapeutic efficacy.

MEMORY CHECK 10–1

Tumor antigens

1. Behave like transplantation antigens when transferred between congeneic hosts
2. Induced by viruses are antigenically constant
3. Induced by chemicals are antigenically inconstant

T-Cell Leukemia Viruses

In 1980, the first confirmed isolation of a virus from a human cancer led to the later acceptance of that virus as the cause of the cancer. The disease was T-cell lymphoma, a malignant proliferation of T cells. The virus was a retrovirus, an RNA virus later termed **human T-cell lymphotropic virus I (HTLV I)**. In 1982, a second virus isolated from patients with T-cell leuke-mia was identified as a retrovirus and named **HTLV II**. These were forerunners of the feared **HTLV III** virus of AIDS, discovered in 1984 and now re-named **human immunodeficiency virus (HIV)**. It too is a retrovirus. HTLVs I and II are transforming viruses causing T cells to reproduce in an uncontrolled fashion. Thus, HTLVs I and II are conclusively proven human oncogenic viruses. HIV infection of T cells is lethal to the cells.

Burkitt's Lymphoma

Prior to the association of the HTLV agents with leukemia, Burkitt in 1958 suggested that the lymphoma he first noted in children living in the mosquito belt of central Africa might have a viral etiology. This intuitive opinion was based on the restricted geographic distribution of the lymphoma known at that time. Since then, **Burkitt's lymphoma** has been recognized worldwide, though not with the incidence noted in Africa.

Support for the viral etiology of Bur-

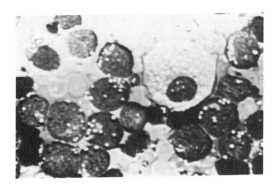

Figure 10-1. The smaller, dark-staining cells are typical of Burkitt's lymphoma and are of B-cell lineage. (See color figure after Table of Contents.)

kitt's lymphoma came forward in 1964 with the visualization of typical C-shaped structures characteristic of a herpesvirus in Burkitt's cells. The affected cells are early B cells, though not all at the same stage of development (Fig. 10-1). Nearly 95% of these cells will have surface IgM, and many express CD21, the complement receptor 2 protein that is the receptor for Epstein-Barr virus (EBV). Some cells will have FcγR. Patients with Burkitt's lymphoma have antibodies to one or more antigens of the **Epstein-Barr virus**, *a herpesvirus also associated with the nonmalignant disease infectious mononucleosis and with the malignancy* **nasopharyngeal carcinoma**. Intact Epstein-Barr virus, a DNA virus, is rarely found in cells, but the C-shaped structures and the strong immunologic association of EBV antibodies with Burkitt's lymphoma has convinced many that this cancer has a viral etiology.

Aside from its viral relationship, Burkitt's lymphoma has an interesting connection to immunoglobulin genetics. Human chromosome 14 is the location of the structural genes of immunoglobulin heavy (H) chains. Approximately 75% of the patients with Burkitt's lymphoma *exchange a piece of DNA between chromosome 14 and chromosome 8.* Chromosome 8 has a

sequence related to the avian myelomatosis oncogene. It is believed this translocation places the oncogene under the control of the H gene promoter. Activation and expression of the oncogene results in Burkitt's lymphoma. Most of the remaining Burkitt's patients have *translocations between chromosome 8 and 2 or between 8 and 22.* It should be remembered that chromosomes 2 and 22 house the genes for the human immunoglobulin light (L) chains.

Nasopharyngeal Carcinoma

EBV DNA has also been associated with nasopharyngeal carcinoma. This disease is more common in Southeast Asia than elsewhere, and is particularly common in the Chinese population. Patients with nasopharyngeal carcinoma are more likely to have elevated anti-EBV titers than patients with Burkitt's lymphoma. C-shaped structures have been seen in the tumor cells. Here again, the evidence is highly in favor of a herpesvirus as the etiologic agent of a human cancer.

Other Potentially Oncogenic Viruses

A few additional viruses have been incriminated in cancer, but the evidence is not always complete. **Hepatitis B virus** infection is a known risk factor for developing hepatoma. This hepatoma may develop as a result of constant replacement of cells lost by the virus infection, and the eventual appearance of a neoplastic cell. Cervical cancers may be related to recurrent **papillomavirus number 16** infection in the same way. **Penile warts (condyloma accuminata)** and warts on other parts of the body have a known viral

etiology, but because of their benign character these have not engendered much interest among tumor immunologists. At present, many cancers are being analyzed to determine if they produce unique antigens that would be useful in diagnosis or as therapeutic targets.

CARCINOFETAL ANTIGENS

Carcinofetal proteins, also called oncofetal proteins, represent a second class of antigens found on tumors. These are best characterized as *tumor-associated* rather than tumor-specific antigens, as cancers from diverse tissues may express the same antigen. The synthesis of these proteins is clearly unrelated to viral oncogenesis. The distribution of the carcinofetal antigens is restricted to fetal tissues and to cancers of the same tissues in the adult (Fig. 10–2). As the tissue degenerates from its normal adult state to the neoplastic condition, it regresses biochemically to the point at which proteins that were synthesized in fetal life are again produced. The antigen is detectable in tissue, and traces are shed

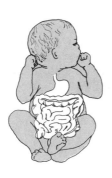
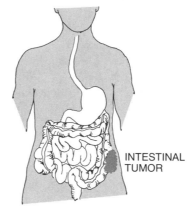

INTESTINAL TUMOR

Figure 10–2. Carcinofetal antigens are produced at a high rate in fetal tissues and in tumors of those tissues in adults; shown here is the situation with carcinoembryonic antigen.

into the blood where it can be detected serologically.

Carcinoembryonic Antigen

The first of the oncofetal antigens to be studied was **carcinoembryonic antigen (CEA)**. In 1965 this unique protein was first discovered to be present in embryonic gut and human colon cancers, but it is also seen in other *cancers of the digestive tract*—stomach, small intestine, rectum—and in associated tissues such as the pancreas and liver. Enzyme-linked immunosorbent assay (ELISA) and radioimmunoassay (RIA) have revealed that *cancers in many other organs also produce CEA*.

These facts led to the early assumption that the identification of CEA in blood would be a superb diagnostic test for cancer. Compatible with this idea was the apparent disappearance of CEA from the blood at birth. Progress in serology complicated the situation. The advent of enzyme-linked immunosorbent assay (ELISA) and radioimmunoassay (RIA) revealed low levels of CEA in the blood of healthy persons. It then became clear that CEA synthesis does not cease at birth; it does diminish sharply, however. Very shortly CEA was found in nonmalignant inflammatory states, including alcoholic cirrhosis of the liver, chronic obstructive pulmonary disease, ulcerative colitis, pancreatitis, and other conditions.

The *presence of CEA in the blood of adults, therefore, is not itself diagnostic of cancer*. The quantity of CEA may be diagnostic, or at least highly suggestive. This requires titration of the CEA blood level. The normal adult blood level ranges between 2 and 3 ng/mL, and elevations a fewfold above this suggest a neoplasm.

CEA titrations are *probably most useful as an index of the success of cancer therapy*. If posttherapeutic CEA levels do not fall much below pretreatment levels, then the treatment can be considered inadequate. CEA levels that fall but then gradually rise again indicate tumor regrowth, a sign that the treatment was only partially successful. If the CEA level remains low, the prognosis is more hopeful. Periodic CEA titrations are advised after surgery for many cancers as an index of successful treatment.

CEA is a β-glycoprotein of 200,000 Mr. All CEA molecules are not antigenically identical but are closely related and cross-reactive. Because of this fact, monoclonal anti-CEA is not necessarily superior to polyvalent sera if the epitope that reacts with the monoclonal antibody is not widely distributed among all CEAs.

Alpha-Fetoprotein

Alpha-fetoprotein (AFP) is a carcinofetal protein of 70,000 Mr found in the α1-globulin fraction of human serum. Hepatomas secrete this protein, as does fetal liver. *Many parallels exist between AFP and CEA*. Initially the mere presence of the protein in blood of adults was considered diagnostic of a liver cancer. Then it was found that individuals with noncancerous liver disease had low levels of circulating AFP. Subsequently the development of sensitive serologic methods identified AFP at levels below 25 ng/mL in sera of healthy adults. Now it is recognized, as with CEA, that AFP quantitation is helpful in diagnosis but is probably more useful in evaluating prognosis after cancer treatment.

An unexpected role of AFP in the diagnosis of neural tube defects comes from the analysis of this protein in amniotic fluid. *Failure of the neural tube to close during embryogenesis (spina* bifida) results in the escape of AFP into the amniotic fluid. Excess APF determined upon amniocentesis may influence decisions about abortion because serious neural tube defects, including anencephaly, may be indicated.

Other Cancer Markers

The α2-hepatic protein (AHP), a globulin of 600,000 Mr having a high iron content, is another oncofetal protein present in hepatomas. AHP is found in low levels in healthy adults, in high levels in fetal liver and hepatomas, and at various levels in persons with nonmalignant liver disease.

Several enzymes described as carcinoplacental enzymes have been associated primarily with a broad range of cancers. Among these are the isozymes of alkaline phosphatase, particularly the **Regan isozyme**. This enzyme is present in the sera of persons with various forms of cancer and is not restricted to those with placental or trophoblastic tissue tumors. Other enzymes associated primarily with hepatomas include aldolase, glycogen phosphorylase, glucosamine-6-phosphate synthetase, and amino acid transaminase.

MEMORY CHECK 10-3
◆

Tumor-associated antigens

1. Differ from TSTA because they are not associated with a single form of cancer
2. Such as CEA and AFP are very useful in evaluating therapy
3. Are produced by fetal tissues and cancers in adults
4. Can be useful in cancer diagnosis if quantitated carefully

---

Immune Surveillance

The immune defense system is versatile and normally provides resistance to any intruder that has a foreign antigenic marker. The part of our armament that is most useful in controlling tumor growth is the lymphocyte population. The two most important segments of this group are the LGL and the T cells. Under certain conditions these cells are assisted by antibody and their participation in antibody-dependent cell cytotoxicity (ADCC) reactions. Antibody plus complement can also be effective against dispersed cell tumors. Because these same activities participate in transplant rejection and are discussed in Chapter 9, they are not described here.

It has been demonstrated both in human subjects and in experimental animals that the immune response may actually favor the survival of cancers. This occurs when noncytocidal tumor cell antibodies coat the tumor cell and protect its surface from contact with LGLs, T cells, and cytotoxic antibodies. These blocking antibodies are responsible for the phenomenon of immune enhancement that follows immunization with tumor antigens.

Immunoproliferative Disease

A neoplastic state of either B or T lymphocytes presents serious problems to tumor immunologists, oncologists, and other health scientists. Excesses in nonfunctional or only partially functional cells can erode the immune defense system. Excesses of B- and T-cell products can disturb the physiologic balance, causing an array of detrimental side effects. Burkitt's lymphoma has already been mentioned as an immunoproliferative disease of the B-cell line, though no mention was made of its disfiguring side effects, which fortunately are resolvable by treatment. Multiple myeloma, mentioned briefly in Chapter 5, is described further here, along with Waldenström's macroglobulinemia and B- and T-cell leukemias.

THE LEUKEMIAS

The leukemias represent a heterogeneous collection of malignancies involving any of the white blood cell lines. Attention here will be directed to the lymphocytic leukemias with but a brief reference to Hodgkin's disease. Aberrations in lymphocyte maturation have been useful in establishing the ontogenetic development of these cells. It is important to identify the lymphocyte involved because this markedly affects therapy and prognosis. Surface markers on malignant lymphocytes suggest whether the leukemia is a B-cell or T-cell leukemia (Fig. 10–3).

Non-T Acute Lymphoblastic Leukemia

The **non-T acute lymphoblastic leukemias (non-T–ALL) are equivalent to B ALL and pre-B–ALL** used in some classification schemes. The progression of the B cell through its maturation stages is used to grade the leukemia. In the earliest stages, the cell is class II MHC and Tdt positive. Soon the **B4 antigen (CD19 protein)** is found on the cell surface and shortly thereafter the **common acute lymphocytic leukemia antigen (CALLA)** as the cell matures. By this time μ chain rearrangement is detectable. Later κ and/or λ chain rearrangement follows, IgM synthesis is completed, and this immunoglobulin appears on the cell surface. Chronic lymphocytic leukemia cells lose

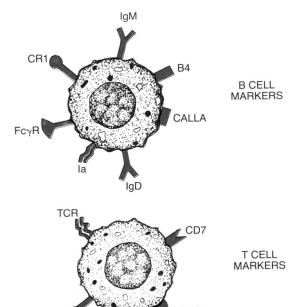

Figure 10–3. Characteristic surface markers used to classify malignant lymphocytes as a B-cell (*upper*) or T-cell (*lower*) lineage.

Table 10-2
DISCRIMINATION OF THE LEUKEMIAS

Leukemia	Key Characteristics
Non-T acute lymphoblastic leukemia (non-T-ALL)	Essentially equivalent to B-ALL, has Ig gene rearrangements, CALLA and B4 antigens
Hairy-cell leukemia	Mature B-cell leukemia, secretes immunoglobulin
T acute lymphoblastic leukemia (T-ALL)	A T-cell leukemia, TCR genes may be rearranged
Chronic lymphocytic leukemia (CLL)	A suppressor T-cell leukemia
Cutaneous T-cell leukemia	Synonym of Sézary-cell leukemia, a helper T-cell leukemia

CALLA, have all of the other markers, and may be at a slightly more advanced stage because they have IgD, FcγR, and CR1 on their surface (Table 10-2).

With the exception of B4 and CALLA, most of these surface markers have been described earlier. The B4 protein found on 95% of non-T-ALL cells behaves as a 40,000-Mr to 80,000-Mr protein in a potential monomer-dimer relationship. Recognition of B4 is important in identifying the leukemia as a B-cell leukemia because H chain rearrangements have been noted in a few instances of what otherwise were T-cell leukemias. The CALLA protein is a 100,000-Mr glycoprotein. The DNA for CALLA indicates it contains 750 amino acids with hydrophobic and hydrophilic tail sequences of only 24 amino acids. It appears relatively early in B-cell development but is lost, again emphasizing the need to identify B4 for the diagnosis of a non-T-cell leukemia. MHC class II proteins, FcγR, CR1, CR2, and several other surface markers are not specific for B cells.

Hairy-Cell Leukemia

The next maturation step leads to **hairy-cell leukemia**, a malignancy of mature B cells at a stage near that of the plasmacytoid B cell observed in Waldenström's macroglobulinemia (Fig. 10-4). This cell may secrete IgM

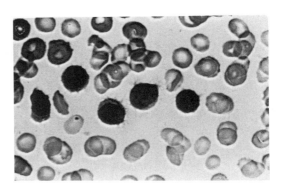

Figure 10-4. Hairy-cell leukemia was so named because the malignant B cells had fine hairlike protrusions, which are barely visible in this photograph. (See color figure after Table of Contents.)

and have one or more other immuno-globulins on its surface. One study of 64 cases revealed that 57% had switched to IgG synthesis and 25% expressed both IgG and IgA. After differentiation, multiple myeloma cells appear that secrete a single immuno-globulin and/or light chains.

T-Cell Acute Lymphoblastic Leukemia

Between 15% and 25% of all cases of ALL are related to a malignancy of T cells. In **T-cell acute lymphoblastic leukemia (T-ALL)** the earliest cell is Tdt and CD7 positive. The Tdt enzyme is only transiently present and is quickly lost. CD7, a 40,000-Mr protein, persists through all later levels of development. The TCR β chain may also be rearranged in these early cells. As the malignant T cell is seen at later stages, it will have lost Tdt and acquired CD3 and CD4 and/or CD8. The cells of T-cell **chronic lymphocytic leukemia (CLL)** appear to be derived from **suppressor cells**. *Cells of several other categories—adult T-cell leukemia, cutaneous T-cell leukemia (Sézary cells)—reflect characteristics of helper cells, ie, are CD4 positive.*

Non-B, non-T Acute Lymphoblastic Leukemia

Null cell leukemia is descriptive of those leukemic cells devoid of either T- or B-cell markers. This group is of interest because of the good prognosis during therapy.

HODGKIN'S DISEASE

Hodgkin's disease involves solid lymphoid tissues and circulating cells. The pleomorphism of the circulating cells and the variable expression of cell surface markers have made it difficult to determine the cellular origin of this disease. Binucleate Reed-Sternberg cells are usually observed in lymph node or bone marrow biopsy. This is an important criterion in the diagnosis, as are the pleomorphisms of the involved cells, which include plasma cells, eosinophils, and others, in addition to the Reed-Sternberg cells. The latter may be of T-cell lineage. This is compatible with the loss of delayed type hypersensitivity reactions in Hodgkin's patients. Complete remission of Hodgkin's disease is made possible by early treatment with the regimen of mechlorethamine, vincristine (oncovin), procarbazine, and prednisone (MOPP).

See also, the case study on page 232.

WALDENSTRÖM'S MACROGLOBULINEMIA

It should be noted that *immunoproliferative disease involving IgM is generally described as* **Waldenström's macroglobulinemia**. Waldenström's macroglobulinemia is distinguishable from multiple myeloma in that the proliferative cell appears more lymphocytic than plasmacytic and the punched-out bone lesions are more rare. Because of the hyperviscosity of blood in Waldenström's macroglobulinemia, vascular disease is more prominent than in the other myelomas. Of the myelomas, 60% are of the IgG class, 16% of the IgA class, and less than 1% each of the IgD and IgE classes. Waldenström's macroglobulinemia represents about 14% of the total. In about 10% of all myelomas, the only aberrant protein detectable is the Bence Jones protein, and none of the complete immunoglobulins can be found.

MULTIPLE MYELOMA

Multiple myeloma is the result of the neoplastic growth of plasma cells and is thus a **plasmacytoma**. This dyscrasia of plasma cells may encompass several histologic forms, but multiple myeloma is often noted as a proliferation of plasma cells in bone marrow with a concomitant erosion of the surrounding bone. Bone destruction is observable on x-ray examination as discrete holes in the osseous tissue and can be so extensive as to cause the fracture of long bones under moderate weight stress. Bone marrow aspirates may reveal that 10% to 20% of the cells are plasma cells, compared with about 3% or less of these cells in normal marrow (Fig. 10–5). These plasma cells will differ slightly in morphology from one case to another but are often classified as one of two types. The most easily recognized is the classic pyroninophilic plasma cell with a spokelike arrangement of its nuclear chromatin. The other cell will contain numerous acidophilic structures, disklike or globular in appearance, that are known as Russell's bodies. Russell's bodies are intracellular concretions of immunoglobulin. Because multiple myeloma is a malignant plasmacytoma, the cells and sera of these patients have unusually high concentrations of immuno-

globulins and/or light chains in their tissues, blood, and urine. Multiple myeloma is often diagnosed by recognizing these excessive gamma globulins in the blood. Alternatively, the diagnosis may be based on the recognition of the Bence Jones light chains in urine or blood.

Ordinary serum electrophoresis on paper or cellulose is helpful in establishing the diagnosis of multiple myeloma, which characteristically produces a sharp, abnormal peak in the tracing of the gamma-globulin portion of the serum profile. This peak, which appears in about 75% of sera from myeloma patients, represents the excess immunoglobulin produced by the neoplastic cells. This supplementary protein is known as the **myeloma (M) protein, or M component**. A single, sharp peak represents an electrophoretically homogeneous protein and indicates that a single clone of aberrant plasma cells has developed (Fig. 10–6). The protein is described as a **monoclonal** M component. Less frequent is the appearance of several new proteins, which represents a neoplastic development of several clones of plasma cells, or a **polyclonal gammopathy**. The electrophoretic positioning of the M component may indicate that the immunoglobulin is of the IgG, IgA, or other immunoglobulin class. Espe-

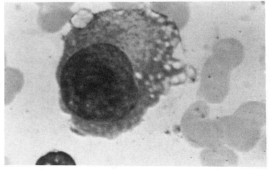

Figure 10–5. This abnormal B cell (plasma cell) was seen in a blood smear of a patient with malignant myeloma. (See color figure after Table of Contents.)

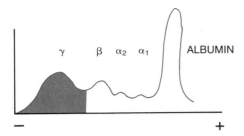

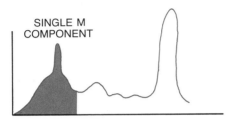

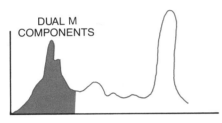

Figure 10–6. The upper electropherogram is of normal serum, the middle panel shows the same but with a single M component, and the lower shows a polyclonal gammapathy.

MEMORY CHECK 10–4
◆

Immunoproliferative disease(s)

1. Of B cells is responsible for multiple myeloma, Waldenström's macroglobulinemia, and numerous non-T lymphocyte leukemias

2. Can involve undifferentiated CD4-positive or CD8-positive T cells

3. Have been useful in following the ontogeny of B and T cells

4. Cannot be differentiated as B- or T-cell diseases by CALLA, as this is the common leukemia antigen

---

cially if the M component has a slow gamma mobility, myeloma of the IgG class can be anticipated. However, identification and quantitation of the M protein class is best confirmed by the use of specific antisera for IgG, IgA, and so forth, in radial immunodiffusion and nephelometric tests.

Immunotherapy of Cancer

The opinion that a failure in the immune surveillance system permits emerging cancer cells to perpetuate themselves is the basis of efforts to strengthen the immune system as the most logical therapy. An antigen-specific approach to this problem has been hampered by a general inability to recognize a unique antigen specific for a certain neoplasm. Furthermore, experiments that led to the discovery of immune enhancement discouraged early efforts to develop antigen-specific resistance through immunization. The prospect to identify specific tumor antigens has steadily improved and an antigen-specific approach to cancer therapy based on a cell-mediated response may yet prove feasible in the future (Table 10–3).

TUMOR-INFILTRATING LYMPHOCYTES

For the present, the nearest to an antigen-specific approach is the use of **tumor-infiltrating lymphocytes (TIL)**. The entire lymphocyte population present within tumors may not be activated by antigen, but their presence within the tumor suggests this. Elution of these TILs from a surgically removed tumor is followed by culture of these cells in *IL-2 to expand their numbers*. Reintroduction of these cells into the patient exposes the tumor to an enlarged population of cells. Therapeutic successes with TILS have been difficult to assess because of differences in the nature of the tumor, secondary health problems of the patients, variation in the number of cells reintroduced, further in vivo stimulation of these cells with IL-2, and other variables. Success has been observed but not with sufficient consistency to claim TILs as a cancer cure.

IMMUNOTOXIN

Immunotoxin therapy has been used on some patients with leukemia. The procedure begins with a harvest of the patient's bone marrow that is purged with an immunotoxin specific for cells carrying the leukemia antigen. The immunotoxin is usually a ricin or diphtheria-antibody conjugate (Fig. 10–7). The patient is then given intensive cytotoxic drug therapy and total body irradiation to destroy bone marrow totally. The purged bone marrow is returned to the patient. GM-CSF therapy may be added to accelerate the maturation of stem cells. Maturing cells then replenish the patient's circu-

Table 10–3
IMMUNOLOGIC APPROACHES TO CANCER THERAPY

Agent	Source and Use
Tumor-infiltrating lymphocytes (TILs)	Harvested from tumor, expanded in culture, and reinfused
Immunotoxin	Conjugate of a tumor-directed antibody and toxin, antibody targets the toxin on the tumor
Drug precursor	Drug precursor activated by enzyme—antibody conjugate at the tumor site
Lymphokine-activated killer cells (LAKs)	Peripheral blood lymphocytes are expanded in culture and reinfused with interleukins
BCG	Used as a vaccine and nonspecific stimulant of macrophages
Interferons	From T cells used as cell growth inhibitors

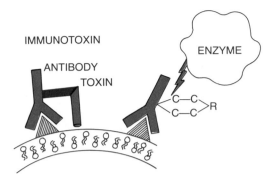

Figure 10-7. Antibodies to tumor-specific transplantation antigen (TSTA) may assist in tumor destruction by focusing a toxin or cytotoxic chemical on the tumor cell.

lating blood cells. Patients with T-cell leukemia and B-cell non-Hodgkin's lymphoma have been treated successfully in this way. Autografting with purged marrow avoids potential graft-versus-host (GVH) disease that may emerge after allografting.

DRUG PRECURSOR

A novel antibody conjugate that is a prospective immunotherapeutic agent for cancer carries an enzyme that activates a drug precursor. The prodrug is a phosphate derivative of a cytotoxic agent such as mitomycin phosphate or etoposide phosphate. The phosphate derivatives encounter an anticancer–alkaline phosphatase conjugate on the cancer cell surface and are hydrolyzed to the active form of the drug. Close contact of the cytotoxin with the tumor cell is expected to be more useful than systemic administration of mitomycin or etoposide in their non-phosphorylated form. Studies with laboratory models of cancer have given partial success with this technique.

LYMPHOKINE-ACTIVATED KILLER CELLS

Purification of lymphocytes from peripheral blood of a cancer patient is the first step in preparing **lymphokine-activated killer (LAK) cells**. These cells are incubated in culture with IL-1 alone or in combination with IL-2 and interferon (IFN). Again, IL-2 is used to expand the lymphocyte population. This expanded LAK cell population is reinfused into the patient who donated the cells. LAK cells have effected some cures but may be more useful in preventing metastases. Combined LAK plus IL-2 therapy achieved partial or complete remission in 5 of 32 renal carcinomas, 6 of 32 melanomas, and 2 of 17 colon cancers. Significant side effects include fever, rash, arrhythmia, and excessive weight gain due to massive fluid retention. LAK cells are of two types: typical T cells and asialo-GM1$^+$, NK1$^+$, NK cells (see also Chapter 4).

BCG VACCINATION

An earlier method designed to enhance natural resistance as a means of tumor therapy relied on the use of the **BCG vaccine against tuberculosis**. This attenuated culture of *Mycobacterium tuberculosis* variety *bovis* is used as an intradermal vaccine. Placement of the vaccine near nevi or melanomas sometimes unexpectedly cleared the skin of these growths. This occurs through the activation of macrophages by lymphokines elaborated by the T_{DTH} cells. The *antigen-nonspecific destruction of tumor cells* in the path of these macrophages is typical of their *indiscriminate attack on foreign substances*.

The molecular basis of the ability of macrophages to eliminate tumor cells apparently resides in their ability to secrete tumor necrosis factor α, described in Chapter 2. Intravesicle instillation of BCG weekly for 6 weeks has a 70% to 90% effectiveness on bladder carcinoma if no metastases have occurred, if the tumor burden is low, and if direct contact between vaccine and tumor is possible. BCG has not been nearly this successful in treating melanoma. Other nonspecific biologic response modulators— *Nocardia, Propionibacterium*, and extracts of these organisms—have also been used.

INTERFERONS

IFNα has proved successful in the treatment of chronic myelogenous leukemia (CML) and hairy-cell leukemia. In the CML group, 60% to 83% of the patients had complete remission depending upon the initial state of the disease; this included 36 remissions of 51 cases. Another study of CLL at the National Cancer Institute was less successful with only a 11% remission rate, but cutaneous T-cell lymphoma and B-cell non-Hodgkin's lymphomas had positive responses of approximately 50% of each group. These studies used recombinant IFNα but a second CML study of 74 patients treated with IFNβ had a 68% improvement. *IFNα is recommended for treatment of hairy-cell leukemia, CML, and Sézary syndrome.* Melanomas and lung, breast, and colon cancers are not responsive to the interferons.

MEMORY CHECK 10–5

Cancer immunotherapy

1. With BCG, LAK, and IFN are not antigen-specific methods

2. With immunotoxins, prodrug-immunoenzymes, and TIL are antigen-specific methods

3. Is directed at the cell-mediated, rather than the humoral, immune response

4. With TIL or LAK relies on IL-2 as a cell growth factor to expand the cell population

5. Has been very successful in hairy-cell leukemia but only partially successful in most other cancers

---

References

Ablashi, DV, et al (eds): Epstein-Barr Virus and Human Disease—1988. Humana Press, Clifton, NJ, 1989.

Balkwill, FR: Cytokines in Cancer Therapy. Oxford University Press, Oxford, 1989.

Beutler, B: The tumor necrosis factors: Cachectin and lymphotoxin. Hosp Pract 25:45, 1990.

Byers, VS and Baldwin, RW (eds): Immunology of Malignant Diseases. MTP Press, Boston, 1987.

Heppner, GH and Fulton, AM (eds): Macrophages and cancer, Boca Raton, CRC Press, 1988.

Kupchik, HZ (ed): Cancer diagnosis in vitro using monoclonal antibodies. Marcel Dekker, New York, 1988.

Lotzova, E and Herberman, RB (eds): Interleukin-2 and killer cells in cancer. CRC Press, Boca Raton, FL, 1989.

Maurer, AM (ed): The Biology of Human Leukemia. Johns Hopkins University Press, Baltimore, 1990.

Osborn, M (ed): Antibodies in cancer diagnosis and therapy. Seminars Cancer Biology 1:1, 1990.

Reisfeld, RA and Cheresh, DA: Human tumor antigens. Adv Immunol 40:323, 1987.

Revel, M (eds): Clinical Aspects of Interferon. Kluwer Academic Publishers, Hingham, MA, 1988.

Truitt, RL, Gale, RP, and Bortin, MM (eds): Cellular Immunotherapy of Cancer. Alan R Liss, New York, 1987.

QUESTIONS AND ANSWERS

1. The future role for carcinofetal antigens is probably
   A. As prognostic indicators of therapy
   B. As diagnostic antigens
   C. To induce enhancing antibody
   D. To induce blocking antibody
   E. More than one of the above

Answer E

Patient sera are often assayed for carcinofetal antigen concentration to determine if therapy has been successful. Answer A is correct. Answer B is also correct because precise measurement of CEA, AFP, and so on, by ELISA or RIA is useful with other data in the diagnosis of cancer. Answers C and D are incorrect. The answer to the question is E.

2. Immunologic therapy for tumors includes
   A. Passive immunization with tumor-specific antibody
   B. Active immunization with CEA
   C. Blockade of suppressor cells
   D. In vitro stimulation of lymphocytes
   E. Thymus grafting

Answer D

Passive immunization with tumor-specific antibody is more likely to result in tumor enhancement than in tumor destruction because these antibodies can function as blocking antibodies. Active immunization with tumor antigens also produces immune enhancement. Currently it is uncertain whether overactive T_S cells allow the emergence of tumors. Even if this were true, it would be difficult to control these cells without influencing other T-cell subsets. In vitro activation of lymphocytes—LAK and TIL—is a current modality showing promise in tumor control. Thymus grafting is not a therapeutic possibility.

3. Which of the following human cancers has a viral etiology?
   A. Burkitt's lymphoma
   B. T-cell lymphoma
   C. Adult T-cell leukemia
   D. Nasopharyngeal carcinoma
   E. All of the above

Answer E

T-cell lymphoma and T-cell leukemia are caused by infections of human T-cell lymphotrophic viruses I and II, respectively. Burkitt's lymphoma and nasopharyngeal carcinoma are accepted as Epstein-Barr virus infections.

4. Chromosomal translocations in human malignancy seem to involve _____ at a high level of frequency.
   A. H chain chromosome 14
   B. MHC chromosome 6
   C. κ chain chromosome 2
   D. λ chain chromosome 22
   E. MHC class III genes on chromosome 6

Answer A

Burkitt's lymphoma, both chronic T- and chronic B-cell leukemias, and follicular B-cell lymphoma are all associated with translocation or inversion of chromosome 14. Less than 20% of the reciprocal translocations in Burkitt's lymphoma involve immunoglobulin L chain genes alone. MHC genes are not associated with malignant transformation.

5. A TSTA is
   A. An antigen controlled by HLA-A, HLA-B, or HLA-C transplantation genes
   B. Specific for a certain tumor
   C. Synonymous with tumor-associated antigen
   D. A good antigen to use in immunization against cancer
   E. Exemplified by either CEA or AFP

Answer B

A is incorrect; TSTA is so named because it behaves like a transplantation antigen upon transfer of the tumor. B is correct. C and E are both incorrect. CEA and AFP are associated with many different cancers and are not specific. Immunization with tumor antigens has a high risk of creating blocking antibodies and is not practiced.

Case Study: Hodgkin's Disease

Joe, a 47-year-old postal carrier, was first seen in February 1982 for evaluation of a fever of undetermined origin. At that time he had no cough or sign of upper respiratory tract disease, although his tuberculin skin test result was positive. He weighed 178 pounds. The fever subsided spontaneously and no diagnosis was established. All cultures were negative for tubercle bacilli. In September 1982, the patient returned with complaints of lymph node swelling in his neck, fever, night sweats, and occasional chills. His weight at this time was 164 pounds; he appeared pale and acutely ill. His blood pressure was 112/88, and his temperature 103.2°F (39.6°C); the white blood cell differential count showed 67 polymorphonuclear leukocytes, 19 lymphocytes, and 14 monocytes, and the total white blood cell count was 4740 per mm³. A lymph node biopsy, sternal bone marrow aspiration, and serum protein electrophoresis were ordered. An immunologic assessment of the patient was indicated, and he was skin tested with tuberculin as the first step in that direction.

Questions

1. What cells of the immune system are involved in Hodgkin's disease?

2. What further immunologic tests are suggested to assist in the diagnosis of Hodgkin's disease?

3. In what way is the chemotherapy of Hodgkin's disease related to its immunocytology?

Discussion

Lymph node biopsy and bone marrow aspirations are recommended aids to the diagnosis of most immunoproliferative diseases. Peripheral white blood cell counts and differential counts are also useful. Hodgkin's disease is separable from the other lymphoproliferative diseases on the basis of two cytopathologic criteria: (1) the relative pleomorphism of the cellular constituents involved and (2) the near-constant appearance of Reed-Sternberg cells. In Hodgkin's granuloma, neoplastic elements are variable in appearance. A mixture of plasma cells, eosinophils, Reed-Sternberg cells, and fibrous elements is detectable. Variable foci of necrosis appear in the lymph nodes. Reed-Sternberg cells range from 12 to 40 μ in diameter, have a prominent lobulated nucleus, and may contain a pair of nuclei. The cytoplasm does not stain intensely and may be either acidophilic or basophilic. The presence of this type of cell establishes the diagnosis.

The position of the Reed-Sternberg cell in the lymphocytic system is uncertain but probably arises from a primitive, relatively undifferentiated cell. Hodgkin's disease appears to be a form of T-cell lymphoma, but the cellular defect escapes unequivocal positioning.

Serum protein electrophoresis and tuberculin testing were included as part of the immunologic evaluation of this patient. Changes in the immunoglobulin pattern of patients with Hodgkin's disease are variable, and either hypergammaglobulinemia or hypogammaglobulinemia may be noted. B-lymphocyte functions are not directly disturbed in this disease but are influenced by the progressive decay in T-cell function. The knowledge that this patient recently had a positive tuberculin skin test result is helpful in assessing his immunologic status. Other tests should include mumps virus and *Candida* skin testing, plus sensitization to dinitrochlorobenzene (DNCB) to determine the reactivity of the T-cell system. The incidence of delayed-type skin reactions to these tests in healthy adults and patients with Hodgkin's disease is tabulated as follows:

	Control Subjects (%)	Patients with Hodgkin's Disease (%)
Tuberculin	24	14
Mumps	88	63
Candida	52	36
DNCB	95	70

Retesting of the patient revealed a loss of his tuberculin sensitivity. No tests for B-cell functioning were deemed necessary.

Combined radiotherapy and chemotherapy are suggested for Hodgkin's disease; both are indicated for their destructive effect on lymphoid tissue. A nitrogen mustard such as mechlorethamine and an alkylating agent such as procarbazine are used, along with vincristine and prednisone. All of these agents are used with the recognition of their toxicity for T cells and the possible increase in viral and fungal disease that often follows. Chemotherapy alone can effect a cure of Hodgkin's disease.

GLOSSARY

adjuvant therapy   The nonspecific stimulation of macrophages as an avenue for immunotherapy of cancer.

alpha-fetoprotein   A tumor-associated antigen predominant in fetal liver and in patients with hepatoma.

Burkitt's lymphoma   A B-cell tumor associated with an infection caused by Epstein-Barr virus.

CALLA   Common acute lymphocytic leukemia antigen.

carcinoembryonic antigen (CEA)   A tumor-associated antigen secreted by fetal and cancerous adult intestinal and other tissue.

carcinofetal antigen   A generic term for an antigen found in fetal and cancerous adult tissues.

EBV   Epstein-Barr virus.

immunotoxin   A covalent combination of a toxin with an immunoglobulin.

LAK   Lymphokine-activated killer cell.

leukemia   A malignancy of any white blood cell line.

M protein   The immunoglobulin overproduced in multiple myeloma.

multiple myeloma   A neoplasm of plasma cells.

oncofetal antigen   Synonym for carcinofetal antigen.

TIL   Tumor-infiltrating lymphocyte.

TSTA   Tumor-specific transplantation antigen.

tumor necrosis factor α A protein from macrophages that is toxic to tumor cells.

tumor-specific transplantation antigen   A surface antigen specific for a tumor cell that behaves as a transplantation antigen.

Waldenström's macroglobulinemia   A neoplasm of IgM-producing lymphoblastoid cells.

CHAPTER 11

◆

Autoimmune Disease

The subject of this chapter is how and why an individual's immune system turns upon itself. Six different mechanisms are considered by which "self" can be treated or converted to "foreign," thereby initiating an immune response. These include not only factors related to the antigen but also alterations in T-cell control of the immune response and the potential role of excess class II major histocompatibility complex (MHC) proteins in exaggerating antigen presentation. This is followed by a discussion of the genetic control of autoimmunity.

Several autoimmune diseases are then described, including the relative role of immunoglobulin versus cell-mediated activities, the nature of the antigen, and the immunologic alterations noted in each disease. These autoimmune diseases span those involving haptens, enzymes, receptors, cross-reactive antigens, and several conditions of uncertain origin or immune relationships.

The demonstration that immunoglobulins may react with self-proteins or polysaccharides is no longer a startling event in clinical laboratories. Although technically more difficult to demonstrate, it can also be shown that T cells are stimulated by self-antigens. These events are not necessarily evidence that these immunoglobulins or reactive T cells are the cause of an autoimmune disease. These self-directed activities may only represent part of the normal checks and balances built into the immune system.

Autoantigens

SELF-TOLERANCE

Most body proteins, polysaccharides, and "would-be" antigens are synthesized previous to the maturation of the immune system. These molecules abort subsequent immune recognition by B and T cells by two different mechanisms. *The CD4$^+$/8$^+$ T cell encounters self-antigens in the thymus and is clonally deleted.* These cells actually die at a different rate than CD4$^+$/8$^-$ cells, for example. Because most antigens are TD antigens, the unavailability of helper T (T$_H$) cells to assist B cells is a major avenue toward self-tolerance. *As B cells encounter self-antigens, they simply become anergic* and fail to respond as they do to extraneous antigens. Consequently, the emergence of a self-directed immune response is explainable by assuming that a new generation of T cells has escaped deletion in the thymus, T$_H$ cells have arisen to assist B cells, new B cells have avoided anergy in some manner, or that an imbalance in T$_H$:T$_S$ ratios has permitted a forbidden response. *The number of T$_S$ cells diminishes in certain human autoimmune ailments.*

NEOANTIGEN

A "would-be" antigen may suffer alteration by the attachment of haptenic groups or partial physical distortion by heat, ultraviolet light, cold, or pressure to *create or expose new antigenic determinants.* If the immune response so generated is expressed against antigenic determinants that were present in the original molecule, then immunodestructive events can follow. If only the newly created epitopes are involved, then the autoimmune disease can be prevented or alleviated by avoiding exposure to the incitant chemical or physical agent. Some authorities prefer to consider a neoantigen etiology of autoimmune disease, as is discussed in the chapters on cytotoxic or immune complex allergy.

MATURATION ANTIGEN

If a protein, polysaccharide, or other molecule fulfilling the criteria of an antigen is synthesized after the immune response has matured, then the immune system may respond to it as it does upon first exposure to any protein or polysaccharide. This would be interpreted as an autoimmune response. For example, infertility related to aspermatogenesis could reside in an exposure of sperm antigens to the immune system after puberty. Well before puberty there is a plentiful supply of CD4$^+$ T$_H$ cells to foster an immune response.

CROSS-REACTIVE ANTIGEN

Another mechanism for an autoimmune response may be the close chemical *similarities between foreign antigens and autologous molecules.* Cross-reacting antigens need not be identical. The space-filling model of T-cell receptor (TCR)–class II MHC antigen interaction does not require this.

SEQUESTERED ANTIGEN

Many of the maturation antigens may also be considered as sequestered antigens. For example, lens proteins are biochemically inert with very little turnover and can be transplanted across the MHC barrier, yet exposure of lens proteins or uveal tissue of the eye to the immune system after ocular trauma may trigger an autoimmune ailment in the other eye. *Release of antigen from these hidden sites* into a mature immune environment enables an autoimmune disease to develop.

ANTIGEN-PRESENTING CELLS

The inflammatory cell infiltrates into tissues damaged by an autoimmune response are traditionally dominated by

---

MEMORY CHECK 11–1

Potential evasion of self-tolerance may develop from

1. Neoantigen formation upon contact with haptens
2. Release of antigens after the immune system has matured
3. Cross-reactive antigens shared by a microbe and its human host
4. Sequestered antigens released into the immune environment
5. Loss of immunoregulation by T cells — especially T_s cells
6. Excessive antigen-presenting cells

---

mononuclear cells. These include both monocytes and lymphocytes. Often both CD4$^+$ and CD8$^+$ lymphocytes are noted, frequently with B cells and plasma cells. More recently it has been recognized that an excessive number of MHC class II-positive cells, or an excessive density of these proteins, exists on cells in autoimmune lesions. This has advanced the prospect that antigen degradation—purposely by macrophages and accidentally by granulocytes—has been supplemented by intensive antigen presentation. This has forced neighboring B and T cells into activities they would otherwise be able to resist.

The MHC and Autoimmune Disease

The human histocompatibility antigens are cellular antigens that should be closely matched between donor and recipient to ensure the successful transplantation of tissue, as described in Chapter 9. The genes that regulate the synthesis of these class I transplantation antigens (HLAs) are located on human chromosome 6, the location of the genes for the class II immune response and class III complement proteins. Consequently, the *genes that dictate immune responsiveness and MHC antigens are transferred together.* If a disease has a genuine autoimmune etiology, then it may be possible to associate the disease with a specific class II gene.

HLA AND D REGION GENES

The three class II genes are the DP, DQ, and DR genes with numerous alleles at each locus. Because of the availability of antisera that recognize the products of some of these alleles, it is possible to associate specific DP, DQ, or DR genes with a specific autoimmune disease. When this cannot be done, it may be possible to associate the disease with a neighboring human leukocyte antigen (HLA) gene. The most proximal of the HLA genes to the class II genes is HLA-B, and this gene has been chosen in comparisons of autoimmune phenomena and MHC relationships because of the small chance of chromosome crossing over between them.

HLA-B15 antigen is four times more common in patients with systemic lupus erythematosus than in the rest of the population. Compared with healthy control subjects, HLA-B8 is twice as common in patients with myasthenia gravis, and HLA-B27 is about 12 times more common in patients with ankylosing spondylitis than in control subjects. In the latter disease, the presence of the HLA-B27 antigen is a cardinal diagnostic key if harmonious with physical data used to establish the diagnosis. Other examples of HLA associations with autoimmune disease are described subsequently.

RELATIVE RISK

Nearly 50 years ago, it was revealed that certain diseases, later found to display autoimmune phenomena, were more frequent in certain families (Table 11–1). The inheritance of this autoimmune tendency could not be related to other markers until the discovery of the HLA proteins. Unfortunately, the low incidence of any single HLA antigen precluded the use of ordinary statistics to affirm an HLA–autoimmune disease relationship. The formula designed to express the relative risk (RR) of autoimmune disease occurring in individuals with a specific HLA antigen is as follows:

$$\text{Relative risk} = \frac{\substack{\text{\% of patients with the} \\ \text{HLA antigen}} \times \substack{\text{\% of controls lacking} \\ \text{the HLA antigen}}}{\substack{\text{\% of controls with the} \\ \text{HLA antigen}} \times \substack{\text{\% of patients lacking} \\ \text{the HLA antigen}}}$$

Table 11–1
SELECTED DISEASES AND THEIR ASSOCIATION WITH SPECIFIC HLAs

Antigen	Disease	FREQUENCY (%)*		Relative Risk†
		Patient Number	Control Subjects	
B27	Ankylosing spondylitis	71–100	3–12	90.1
	Reiter's syndrome	65–100	4–14	36.0
	Anterior uveitis	37–58	7–10	9.4
	Salmonella arthritis	60–69	8–10	18.0
	Psoriasis	29	8	4.6
B8	Myasthenia gravis	38–65	18–31	4.4
	Juvenile diabetes	19–55	2–29	2.4
	Celiac disease	78	24	11.2
	Chronic hepatitis	68	18	9.7

*Number range refers to different studies.

†Relative risk = $\dfrac{\text{Frequency in patients with that HLA} \times \text{Frequency in controls lacking that HLA}}{\text{Frequency in patients lacking that HLA} \times \text{Frequency in controls with that HLA}}$

RR values greater than 10 are considered highly significant and values much lower (2 or 4) express a serious risk for autoimmune tendencies. Most of the RR numbers have been calculated for HLA, but now antisera are available for several human DP, DQ, and DR proteins. RR calculations for the DP, DQ, and DR proteins should yield slightly greater precision in identifying autoimmune genetic relationships.

IMMUNOLOGIC DIAGNOSIS OF AUTOIMMUNE DISEASE

Assessment of relative risk should be supplemented by immunologic findings to ensure a correct diagnosis of an autoimmune disease. The immunologic features of a disease will vary relative to the dominance of T cells or B cells in the disease. Obviously the total T-lymphocyte count may not be as useful as enumeration of the CD4$^+$: CD8$^+$ ratio. Loss of the suppressor cell population is often reflected in hypergammaglobulinemia. Excessive IgG and IgM levels may in turn be reflected by hypocomplementemia. Determination of C3 and C4 levels will indicate whether the complement loss is immune dependent or from some other cause.

Analysis of tissue biopsies to determine the type of cellular changes occurring in the diseased tissues may also aid diagnosis of autoimmune disease. Typically macrophages, B cells, and T cells are seen on occasion with cells expressing an excess of the class II MHC proteins. The success of certain immunotherapeutic agents is also supportive of a correct diagnosis of these diseases.

Immunoglobulin-Associated Diseases

A clear separation of autoimmune diseases into those that are immunoglobulin (B-cell) related and those that are T-cell–related is not possible. Indeed, the response of B cells to most antigens relies on their cooperative association with T cells, and stimulation by the T-cell interleukins. The classification of the autoimmune diseases listed hereafter as immunoglobulin or T-cell–related is meant to reflect the ease by which one or the other of these immune responses can be demonstrated, not that it is the sole cause of the condition (Table 11–2).

THROMBOCYTOPENIC PURPURA — A HAPTEN-RELATED CONDITION

Thrombocytopenic purpura (a platelet count of 20,000 to 100,000/μL of blood, associated with petechiae) may present as an idiopathic condition with an unknown etiology or may be drug associated. Some evidence exists that the idiopathic form, particularly when diagnosed in childhood, follows viral infections. The loss of platelets is reflected in a loss of control over the blood-clotting system that causes hemorrhagic petechiae to appear in the skin. Patients with thrombocytopenic purpura have antibodies that stimulate the platelet-release reaction expressed as an aggregation and degranulation of the platelets. In the presence of complement and antibody, the platelets are lysed.

Thrombocytopenic purpura is often an iatrogenic disease fostered by long-term therapy with drugs—antimalarials, antiarrhythmic drugs, antibiotics, aspirin, tranquilizers, sulfonamides, and so on. The thrombocytopenia invariably emerges during the course of the drug treatment and subsides when the drug is withdrawn. Reinitiation of the drug therapy causes an exacerbation of the disease. These features signal that a hapten-antigen complex, in which the dominant region of the antigenic determinant is as-

Table 11-2
CHARACTERISTICS OF SOME AUTOIMMUNE DISEASES

Disease	Antigen or Hapten	Immunoglobulin or T-Cell Dominance
Thrombocytopenic purpura	Hapten-platelet complex or hapten-protein complex absorbed onto platelets	IgG and IgM
Rheumatic fever	Streptococcal M protein	IgG and IgM
Glomerulonephritis	Streptococcal membrane lipoprotein	IgG and IgM
Rheumatoid arthritis	IgG	IgM
Systemic lupus erythematosus	DNA, RNA, many others	IgG
Myasthenia gravis	Acetylcholine receptor	IgG
Bullous pemphigoid	Skin basement membrane	All five immunoglobulins
Dermatitis herpetiformis	Dermal protein	IgA and IgG
Pernicious anemia	Intrinsic factor	Secretory IgA, IgG
Hashimoto's thyroiditis	Thyroglobulin	IgG and T cells
Postvaccinal encephalomyelitis	Myelin basic protein	T cells
Postinfectious encephalomyelitis	Myelin basic protein	T cells
Multiple sclerosis	Myelin basic protein	T cells
Sympathetic ophthalmia	Uveal protein	T cells

sociated with the hapten, is the incitant. One theory suggests that the hapten-antigen conjugate involves some protein or polysaccharide of the platelet itself, whereas an alternative suggestion is that a serum protein binds to the hapten and the platelet adsorbs to this complex (Fig. 11-1). In the latter instance, the platelet is lysed as a bystander cell by the antigen-antibody-complement complex and is not in reality a part of the antigen. This immunologic distinction does not alter the end result of thrombocytopenia. The dominance of the hapten is illustrated by the fact that passive immunization conveys the disease to a healthy individual only if the offending drug is also administered. In vitro mixtures of patient sera with platelets are inert until the drug is added, and then lysis occurs (when complement is also present).

GRAVES' DISEASE — AN ANTIRECEPTOR DISEASE

Patients with Graves' disease are in a state of hyperthyroidism because of their synthesis of long-acting thyroid stimulator (LATS). LATS is an antibody to the receptor for the thyrotropin-stimulating hormone. Unlike many antireceptor antibodies, *LATS stimulates rather than inhibits the receptor*, causing a continual release of the hormone. LATS, present in more than 75% of patients with Graves' disease, was *the first antireceptor antibody associated with an immune disease.*

In the thyroid gland, the antireceptor is easily detected by fluorescent antibody tests. CD8+ helper T cells are also present. An excessive density of HLA-DR on thyrocytes suggests that these cells have served as superfluous antigen presenters and are responsible for

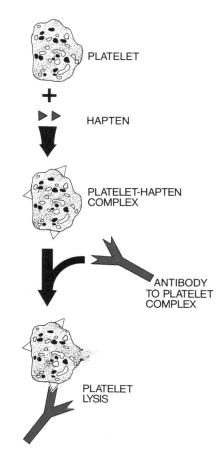

PLATELET

+

HAPTEN

PLATELET-HAPTEN
COMPLEX

ANTIBODY
TO PLATELET
COMPLEX

PLATELET
LYSIS

Figure 11-1. One potential mechanism for thrombocytopenic purpura is the creation of new haptenic determinants on the platelet surface by complex formation with a drug. Thereafter, antibody and complement lyse the platelet.

initiating the disease. Graves' disease has a relative risk of 2.6 associated with HLA-B8.

MYASTHENIA GRAVIS — ANOTHER ANTIRECEPTOR DISEASE

Extreme weakness of the muscles, even to the extent that chewing food is laborious, is a characteristic of myasthenia gravis (MG). Many of these patients have a thymoma or other thymic disease. The exact relationship of this to MG is uncertain because these patients may also have symptoms of other autoimmune diseases such as SLE or rheumatoid arthritis.

Antibodies to muscle proteins may be found in sera of patients with MG, but the most important finding is that of *antibodies to the acetylcholine receptor* (Fig. 11-2). Moreover, the severity of MG correlates well with the antibody titer to this receptor. Antibodies to the receptor interfere with neuromuscular transmission across the synaptic cleft because acetylcholine is blocked from combination with the postsynaptic receptor. This prevents depolarization and causes muscle exhaustion. Autoimmune myasthenia gravis can be produced experimentally

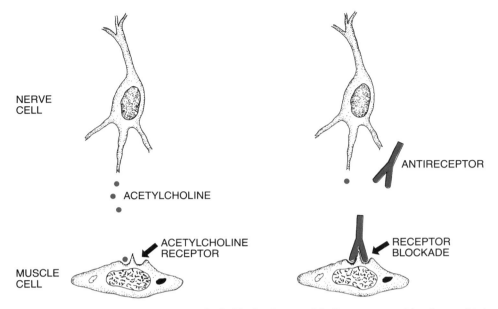

NERVE
CELL

ACETYLCHOLINE

ANTIRECEPTOR

ACETYLCHOLINE
RECEPTOR

RECEPTOR
BLOCKADE

MUSCLE
CELL

Figure 11–2. In myasthenia gravis, an antibody blocks the acetylcholine receptor either by combining directly with it, as shown here, or by steric hindrance resulting from attachment of the antibody near the receptor.

by immunization with the receptor protein. The common structure of the receptor in several animal species accelerated the discovery that MG patients have antibodies to epitopes in the α peptide of that protein.

PERNICIOUS ANEMIA — ANTI-B_{12}

Failure of intrinsic factor, secreted from parietal cells of the stomach, to bind properly with vitamin B_{12} is associated with a failure to absorb this vitamin and, consequently, with the disease pernicious anemia. Vitamin B_{12} is essential for hematopoiesis; failure to form red blood cells results in anemia.

Two different types of antibody that react with intrinsic factor have been described. One apparently *binds at or near the site of B_{12} binding and thus prevents B_{12} from occupying its proper site on intrinsic factor. This binding blocks both the transport and absorption of B_{12}. The other antibody binds to intrinsic factor after its union with B_{12}.*

This antibody impedes only the absorption of the intrinsic factor–B_{12} complex.

INSULIN-DEPENDENT DIABETES MELLITUS

Insulin-dependent diabetes mellitus (IDDM), or type I diabetes, is characterized by a decreased production of insulin. Type II diabetes is characterized by the lack of a response to insulin. *In IDDM, the islets of Langerhans, especially the beta cells, are in a state of decay and contain both IgG and complement.* The mononuclear cell infiltrate in the pancreas is of a mixed cell population and includes $CD4^+$, $CD8^+$, and LGL cells.

Numerous antibody activities are present in sera of patients with IDDM. These antibodies potentially arise because of a loss of T_S cells. An islet cell–specific antibody is found in the majority of these patients. A complement-fixing subclass of this antibody is found in approximately 50% of the sera. These two antibodies are especially suspect in the etiology of IDDM because of their potential to damage or lyse islet cells. The anti-insulin antibody found in approximately 30% of IDDM patients probably has a greater role in type II diabetes because it would neutralize insulin. Type II diabetes is also known as insulin resistance.

In both human and animal studies, there is a hereditary influence on the development of IDDM. In humans, DR3 and DR4 relate to susceptibility and DR2, DR5, and DR7 to resistance.

MEMORY CHECK 11–2

◆

Autoimmune diseases involving hormones and vitamins

1. May be antireceptor specific — Graves' disease and myasthenia gravis
2. May be related to an attack on their cell source — type I diabetes
3. May be stimulatory — Graves' disease
4. May be inhibitory — pernicious anemia, myasthenia gravis, and diabetes mellitus

---

POSTSTREPTOCOCCAL DISEASES — CROSS-REACTIVE ANTIGENS

Two important ailments traditionally may follow infections by group A β-hemolytic streptococci, both associated with an immune response directed toward streptococcal antigens and with the presence in human tissues of cross-reactive antigens. These diseases are rheumatic fever and glomerulonephritis.

Rheumatic Fever

Inflammation of the heart muscle, when associated with polyarthritis, subcutaneous nodules, fever, and, most importantly, with an earlier group A streptococcal illness suggests rheumatic fever. *Rheumatic fever is more likely than glomerulonephritis to follow a streptococcal infection; more than 50 types of group A streptococci have been associated with the former.* The accepted etiology for rheumatic fever is the presence of cross-reactive antigens in the bacteria and in human heart tissue. *The important microbial antigen is the M protein.* The M protein is unusual for two reasons: first, its size varies significantly from one strain of streptococcus to another, and second, each M protein contains a seven-amino acid sequence that is repeated numerous times. This *consensus repeat sequence is also present in myosin.* Cross-reaction of antibodies to the M protein with heart muscle myosin accounts for the cardiac symptoms in rheumatic fever (Fig. 11–3).

Patients who muster the most vigorous immune response to the streptococci, as witnessed by high antistreptolysin O titers, are the ones most likely to progress to rheumatic fever. It is for this reason that streptococcal diseases are treated with large doses of antibiotics — to eliminate the organisms as quickly as possible and to minimize the specific antibody response. These antibodies, usually IgG but also involving other immunoglobulin classes, deposit with complement throughout the myocardium. Fluorescent antibody staining with antihuman IgG, antihuman IgM, or anti-C3 has demonstrated these proteins in the tissues.

Glomerulonephritis

Group A streptococcal infection with one of the following serologic types —

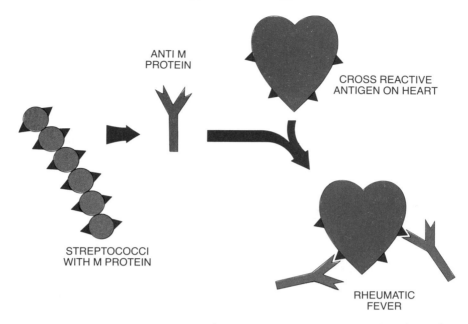

ANTI M
PROTEIN

CROSS REACTIVE
ANTIGEN ON HEART

STREPTOCOCCI
WITH M PROTEIN

RHEUMATIC
FEVER

Figure 11–3. In poststreptococcal rheumatic fever, antigens on group A streptococci stimulate antibodies that react with a cross-reactive antigen on human heart muscle.

4, 5, 12, 18, 25, 49, 52, and 55 — *may precede glomerulonephritis.* As with rheumatic fever, infections with these strains occur 10 to 15 days prior to the autoimmune sequelae. Just when it is clear that the streptococcal infection is being effectively combatted, signs of kidney disease appear. Fluorescent antibody tests demonstrate IgG and complement along the glomerular base-ment membrane of the kidney. These deposits are granular and unevenly distributed, unlike that seen in other forms of kidney disease. These deposits interfere with the normal filtration process of the kidney, a feature that is further complicated by the influx of polymorphonuclear cells that accompanies complement activation (Fig. 11–4).

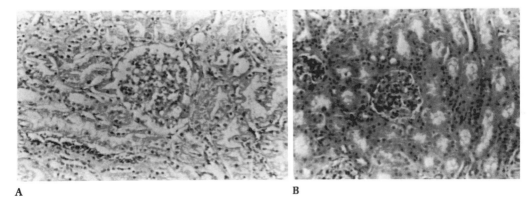

A   B

Figure 11–4. A normal kidney is seen in (A), and the congested kidney of a patient with poststreptococcal glomerulonephritis in (B). (See color figure after Table of Contents.)

The immunoglobulin deposits in the kidney are the result of an *immune response to a lipoprotein found in the cytoplasmic membrane of a restricted number of streptococcal types.* The antibody forms circulating complexes with the lipoprotein as it is released from the bacteria. These soluble immune complexes are removed from the blood by the kidney. When the deposits reach a sufficient size, or when a sufficient number of neutrophils have transgressed the glomerular basement membrane, the filtering efficiency of the kidney is lowered and kidney failure begins. Evidence is also accumulating that antibody to the bacterial lipoprotein is reacting directly with a similar protein in kidney.

RHEUMATOID ARTHRITIS — UNUSUAL SPECIFICITY OF RF

Entirely distinct from rheumatic fever is rheumatoid arthritis, a chronic disease in which swollen, deformed joints, particularly of the hands and feet, are the best known symptoms. Additional symptoms may include subcutaneous nodules, muscle atrophy, fever, and malaise. The paramount immunologic feature of the disease is the high incidence (75%) of rheumatoid factor (RF) in the sera of these patients. *RF is frequently an IgM* of normal size but may be a 7S IgM or even an IgG. *RF is unique in that the antigen with which it reacts is human IgG.* The specific antigenic determinants in IgG are the Gm markers located in the constant domains of the γ chain (see Chapter 5). RF-positive sera have been used to determine the distribution of the Gm allotypes in the four IgG subclasses.

The etiology of rheumatoid arthritis is unknown, and several theories have been espoused. One theory is that Epstein-Barr virus, a polyclonal B-cell ac-

tivator, activates numerous B-cell clones including those that are patterned to synthesize the anti-IgG rheumatoid factor. The subsequent serologic reaction of RF and IgG in the confinement of the joint space activates the complement system. Within the joint capsule, the attendant inflammatory consequences initiated by complement — chemotactic infiltration of neutrophils, lysosomal enzyme release, histamine release from neighboring cells — aggravate the original inflammatory response and convert it to a chronic condition. A slightly different scenario hypothesizes that antibody to a viral pathogen in the joint space encounters and activates complement. Neutrophils responding to the C5a chemotaxin release enzymes that partially denature IgG. This exposes Gm determinants and enables the formation of anti-Gm RF globulins.

An unusual development in rheumatoid arthritis research has been the discovery that the RF globulins are easily subdivided into only a few groups on the basis of small differences in their light chains. Most RF light chains are κ type. *Sixty percent of these RF have the same hypervariable region 2 sequence, the same J region sequence, and, based on total light chain amino acid sequence, are placed in κ chain subgroup IIIb.* Equally curious is the finding that an additional 20% of RFs all fit into a second subgroup. Why RFs are restricted to only a few light chain variants is puzzling.

ANKYLOSING SPONDYLITIS — THE HIGHEST RR

The autoimmune disease with the highest relative risk, a value of 90, is ankylosing spondylitis. This is an HLA-B27–associated disease occurring in Caucasians but not in Orientals, an observation that indicates other genetic traits are associated with susceptibility to this crippling disease. Although the etiology of this disease is unknown, one suggestion is that *Klebsiella* organisms may contain an antigen that cross-reacts with HLA-B27.

SYSTEMIC LUPUS ERYTHEMATOSUS — A RIBOZYME-RELATED DISEASE

Systemic lupus erythematosus (SLE) is a complex disease whose pathology is expressed through one or more of the following: an erythematous butterfly rash over the nose and cheeks, purpura, arthritis, nephritis, myocarditis, ocular lesions, and other organ involvements. DR2, DR3, and HLA-B8 are genetic associates of SLE. The immunologic phenomena displayed in SLE include the historically important lupus erythematosus (LE) cell, antinuclear antibody, and antibodies to other nucleoproteins. *The LE cell is a neutrophil that has phagocytosed the nucleus of another of its kind* (Fig. 11–5). The ingested nucleus is swollen, amorphous, and lighter staining than the multilobed nucleus of the active cell. Positive LE cells are demonstrable in the sera of about three fourths of SLE patients but can also be seen in persons with other autoimmune diseases such as rheumatoid arthritis. The LE cell de-

velops when antibodies to nuclear antigens enter into susceptible white cells, combine with their antigen, and with the aid of complement rupture the nuclear membrane. After this the viable neutrophil ingests the nucleus to form the LE cell.

Several kinds of *SLE antibodies can be demonstrated by fluorescent antinuclear antibody (FANA) tests.* Globulins from patient sera are allowed to react in vitro with nucleated cells and are then stained with fluorescent anti-human globulin. Several different staining patterns are possible, homogeneous, nucleolar, speckled, and nuclear membrane staining patterns being clinically the most important. The homogeneous and nuclear membrane staining patterns are closely associated with active SLE. The speckled and nucleolar patterns are also typical of SLE but are seen also in other connective tissue diseases, such as scleroderma or rheumatoid arthritis, and are accordingly less diagnostic. These antibodies may be directed to DNA, RNA, or proteins associated with DNA or RNA. Of these, *antibodies to double-stranded DNA are the most diagnostic of SLE.* Because these antibodies consume complement by the classic pathway, both C3 and C4 levels are lowered.

Interest in the speckled pattern of FANA staining by SLE sera has led to

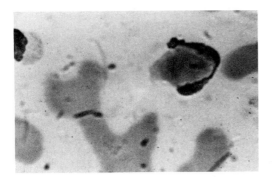

Figure 11–5. This photograph shows an LE cell, a phagocytic cell that has ingested the damaged nucleus of another cell. (See color figure after Table of Contents.)

the discovery that the antigen is actually a mixture of *small nuclear ribonucleoproteins (snRNPs)*. All of these contain a protein designated Sm and a uridine-rich ribonucleic acid (U-RNA). The U1, U2, and other U-RNAs are among the newest group of enzymes to be discovered. They have been called *ribozymes* by virtue of their nucleic acid composition. These unusual forms of RNA are able to cleave and to ligate RNA, thereby having an essential role in RNA processing. How this fits into the immunopathology of SLE is not yet known but is still a surprising new development in the study of this disease.

Polymyositis is another disease in which antibodies are reactive with self-nucleic acid complexes. In this instance, the antibodies are directed against the tRNA synthetases that add specific amino acids to the growing peptide chain on the ribosome.

BULLOUS SKIN DISEASES

Antibodies of all five immunoglobulin classes and components of both the classic and alternate complement pathways have been identified on the *underside of the epidermis in patients with* **bullous pemphigoid**. Below these deposits, blisters (bullae) separate the dermis from the epidermis. *Antibodies to proteins of the skin basement membrane* have been identified in the majority of these patients. The identity of the antigen is not yet known. Complement components have also been identified in the bullae—even in instances when only non-complement-fixing antibodies are deposited. It is presumed that this originates from the alternative pathway. The exact relationship of these phenomena to disease is uncertain; however, immunosuppressive therapy is the preferred treatment

and supports the idea that this is an immunologic disorder.

Deposits of IgA and C3 in the upper dermis are characteristic of **dermatitis herpetiformis**. Other immunoglobulins may also be present. This disease, which is also characterized as a bullous disease, involves vast areas of the skin—the back and shoulders, the inner surfaces of the arms, the neck, and the buttocks. A correlation of this disease with HLA-B8 and DR3 has been reported.

MEMORY CHECK 11–3

◆

Additional facts of importance

1. Multiple types of group A streptoccal infections precede rheumatic fever
2. Relatively few types of group A streptococcal infections precede glomerulonephritis
3. RFs are selected from a very limited array of HV2 and J genes
4. Ankylosing spondylitis has the highest relative risk of any autoimmune disease
5. Ribozymes are snRNPs and antigens of SLE

T-Cell–Associated Diseases

HASHIMOTO'S THYROIDITIS — A HORMONE-RELATED DISEASE

Pathologically, Hashimoto's disease is characterized by a loss of colloid from the thyroid gland, accompanied by an infiltration of lymphocytes and plasma cells (Fig. 11–6). Loss of the thyroid colloid creates a thyroid hormone insufficiency because thyroglobulin in

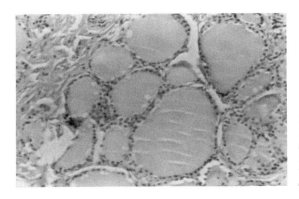

Figure 11–6. Normal thyroid as shown here has stored protein (colloid) in the acellular space. In thyroiditis the quantity of colloid is decreased and mononuclear cells infiltrate the area. (See color figure after Table of Contents.)

the colloid is a carrier for thyroid hormones. The thyroid gland enlarges slightly in an effort to compensate for this loss of hormone. *An antithyroglobulin can be detected in sera of Hashimoto patients* by a variety of serologic tests—immunodiffusion, passive agglutination, complement fixation, radioimmunoassay, enzyme immunoassay, and so on. Depending upon the titer of the antibody, and the sensitivity of the test, one or more of these tests may be negative even when disease is present. This has been proved by studies on experimental animal models of thyroiditis. The disease is more easily transferred with lymphocytes than with serum, and it is still somewhat uncertain which plays the greater role in pathogenesis.

POSTVACCINAL AND POSTINFECTIOUS ENCEPHALOMYELITIS

Encephalomyelitis following the use of vaccines that include neural tissues from lower animals, such as the rabbit spinal cord vaccine used in the early rabies vaccines, can now be explained on a rational basis. *The encephalitogenic protein is* **myelin basic protein (MBP),** a protein that is also involved in infectious encephalomyelitis and multiple sclerosis.

MBP is high in lysine and arginine and these contribute to its basic character. MBP represents more than 25% of the protein in myelin. MBP is only 18,500 Mr, yet several epitopes have been identified in this peptide. The epitopes critical to the individual demyelinating autoimmune diseases have been difficult to determine.

After either natural infections or immunization with active virus, viral replication may occur in nerve tissue. When viral antigens are expressed on the surface of these cells, cytotoxic T cells attack the cell in order to halt further virus replication. An associated result of this is postinfectious or postvaccinal encephalomyelitis. Viral infections of several types can be associated with this form of encephalitis—measles, mumps, chickenpox, herpes, and so on. An important feature of vaccination against the often mild viral diseases of childhood is to prevent the permanent sequelae of postinfectious encephalomyelitis.

MULTIPLE SCLEROSIS — ATTACK ON MYELIN

Multiple sclerosis (MS) is a neurologic disease of the central nervous system embodying various manifestations — muscle weakness, seizures, vision problems, ataxia, and so on — similar to the encephalitides just described. MS is closely associated with HLA-Dw2, HLA-A3, and HLA-B7. The involved areas of the central nervous system reveal demyelination and plaquelike regions where immunoglobulins are deposited. The free gamma globulin content of the cerebrospinal fluid is also increased. *Both anti-MBP and sensitized T cells seem to be involved.* One hypothesis for the disease is that the initial insult may be due to a neurotropic virus with ensuing CTL activation as seen in postinfectious and postvaccinal encephalomyelitis. Alternatively, myelin removal may be an activity of unchecked macrophages or other phagocytes. Antigen processing and presentation of myelin peptides to B and T cells would account for the anti-MBP globulins.

SYMPATHETIC OPHTHALMIA

Two weeks or more after a puncture wound or other damage to the uvea of one eye, the second eye may develop uveitis. This is expressed by the inability of the eye to accommodate light, by photophobia, and in more severe cases, by pain. More commonly, the inflammation is painless. The etiology of this disease in the sympathetic eye is related to the liberation of uveal antigens, perhaps altered by trauma, from the injured eye. Activation of T lymphocytes occurs, and sensitized lymphocytes in company with giant cells infiltrate the uvea of the second eye, causing disease. Patients with sympa-thetic ophthalmia exhibit delayed skin test reactions to uveal antigens. Topical or systemic corticosteroids are used in the treatment of what appears to be primarily a T-cell–mediated condition.

Treatment of Autoimmune Disease

If the autoimmune diseases reflect the abnormal behavior of components of the immune system, and if these specific components can be identified, then specific therapeutic interventions become possible. In the immunoglobulin-associated diseases, evidence of a B-cell attack on self-antigens is reflected in hypergammaglobulinemia, soluble immune complexes in the vascular system, deposits of immunoglobulins in or on tissues, and a participation of complement. A direct therapeutic attack on B cells by the use of **chemical or physical immunosuppressants, antilymphocyte serum**, and the like, though an obvious approach, is fraught with complications by the *generalized toxicity of these agents*, not only for all B cells but also for T cells and macrophages. Partial cell specificity of certain drugs such as cyclophosphamide for B cells or **cyclosporin for T cells** reduces the severity of this problem to some extent. Frequently the only recourse is to apply high-dose therapy with **anti-inflammatory steroids** despite its serious side effects. **Plasmapheresis**, recently applied in the treatment of immunoglobulin-associated diseases, involves periodic and repeated removal of serum proteins and spares the patient's red blood cells for reinjection. This procedure has provided relief for patients with SLE and other antibody-related connective tissue diseases.

References

Cohen, IR: Perspectives on Autoimmunity. CRC Press, Boca Raton, FL, 1987.

Cruse, JM, and Lewis, RE, Jr (eds): Cellular aspects of autoimmunity. Concepts in Immunology 6:1, 1988.

Cruse, JM, and Lewis, RE, Jr (eds): Genetic basis of autoimmune disease. Concept Immunol 5:1, 1988.

Mackworth-Young, C and Schwartz, RS: Autoantibodies to DNA. CRC Crit Rev Immunol 8:147, 1988.

Rose, NR: Current concepts of autoimmune disease. Transplant Proc (Suppl 4)20:3. 1988.

Samter, M (ed): Immunologic diseases, ed 3. Little, Brown, Boston, 1989.

Tan, EM: Antinuclear antibodies: diagnostic markers for autoimmune diseases and probes for cell biology. Adv Immunol 44:93, 1989.

QUESTIONS AND ANSWERS

1. In rheumatoid arthritis, RF is:
   A. Normally an IgM that reacts with the infectious agent that initiates the disease
   B. Usually an IgM that uses IgG as its antigen
   C. The cause of rheumatoid arthritis
   D. Totally unlike the RF recognized in systemic lupus erythematosus
   E. A Gm determinant

Answer B

All isotypes of RF have been identified but most are IgM antibodies that react with IgG as the antigen. Answer A is wrong; answer B is correct. Blood transfusion studies indicate that RF does not cause rheumatoid arthritis. SLE and other autoimmune diseases may present with positive RF test results; RF is not specific for rheumatoid arthritis. The antigenic determinant with which RF reacts is a Gm determinant. Gm determinants are *not* RFs.

2. In which of the following does an autoantibody stimulate rather than inhibit a cellular response?
   A. Hashimoto's thyroiditis
   B. Insulin-dependent diabetes mellitus (IDDM)
   C. Myasthenia gravis
   D. Graves' disease
   E. Pernicious anemia

Answer D

The long-acting thyroid stimulating (LATS) antibody of Graves' disease behaves as its name indicates, regardless of the fact that other autoantibodies may be present in this disease. In Hashimoto's disease, the major antibody reacts with and neutralizes thyroglobulin. In IDDM many antibodies have been recognized versus the beta cell and insulin but none are stimulatory. In myasthenia gravis, the responsible antibody is an antiacetylcholinesterase, an inhibitory antibody. In pernicious anemia, neutralizing antibodies interfere with the transport and absorption of vitamin B_{12}.

3. Which of the following is related to hypoactivity of T_s lymphocytes?
   A. Allergic encephalomyelitis
   B. Systemic lupus erythematosus
   C. Poststreptococcal glomerulonephritis
   D. Rheumatic fever
   E. Rheumatoid arthritis

Answer B

T cells participate in all immune responses, and even T_S cells regulate T-cell–independent antigens. In a few instances an imbalance of immunomodulating T cells is associated with an autoimmune disease and in systemic lupus erythematosus a loss of T_S cells is considered a key in the etiology of the disease.

4. Rheumatic fever is an autoimmune disease related to:
    A. A shared antigen
    B. A drug-altered antigen
    C. Excessive T_H cell activity
    D. Mutation of antibody-forming cells
    E. Biochemically altered antigens

Answer A

Current evidence indicates an antigen common to the M protein of certain group A streptococci and human heart tissue is responsible for poststreptococcal rheumatic fever. There is no evidence for any of the other mechanisms suggested. Poststreptococcal glomerulonephritis has an etiology similar to rheumatic fever but involves a different antigen.

Case Study: Drug-Related Systemic Lupus Erythematosus

Carol C., a heavy smoker, was first seen for hypertension 5 years prior to her present hospital admission. In the interim, she was treated with various combinations of diuretics, beta-blockers, and adrenergic neuron-blocking drugs. Episodes of allergic dermatitis were associated with some of the drugs, necessitating their withdrawal. Approximately a half year after the initiation of labetalol therapy, Carol developed polyarthralgia and myalgia and was given a thorough examination in the clinic. Stiffness in the shoulders, upper arms, and hands, and pain in the wrist and elbow were the major physical findings. Laboratory tests supported the possibility that the patient had a lupuslike syndrome.

Questions

1. What are the immunologic findings which support the diagnosis of drug-induced systemic lupus erythematosus (SLE)?

2. What drugs appear to be most frequently associated with iatrogenic lupus?

3. What are the recommended immunologic interventions suggested for the treatment of this condition?

Discussion

Primary serologic evidence leading to the diagnosis of drug-induced lupus can be determined by several procedures. Because lupus is an immune complex disease, it is common for the hemolytic complement level to be diminished, especially during the acute stage and when nephritis is present. The nephritis is the result of immune complex deposition in the kidney attended by complement activation and neutrophil infiltration.

Certain immunoglobulins formed in patients with SLE and lupuslike syndromes are antinuclear globulins. These are usually identified by the indirect FANA procedure. The homogeneous and nuclear membrane staining patterns are closely correlated with active disease. Anti-DNA globulins, which react with the natural double-stranded DNA, single-stranded DNA, or both, may be present. Of these, the anti-double-stranded DNA is the most important because antibodies to single-stranded DNA are present in several other conditions such as rheumatoid arthritis and liver disease. Anti-RNA globulins are less often indicative of SLE than anti-DNA globulins but are present in a majority of cases. Among these are the anti-snRNP globulins mentioned in the text.

A wide variety of drugs have been associated with the lupuslike syndrome. Several antibiotics (penicillin, streptomycin, tetracyclines, griseofulvin), the sulfonamides, isoniazid, hypertensive drugs, anti-inflammatory drugs, oral contraceptives, antimalarials, tranquilizers, and so on, are all represented in this list.

Treatment of SLE may involve the use of anti-inflammatory drugs (steroids, aspirin) and, in more serious cases, cytotoxic drug therapy. Recently, plasmapheresis has proved beneficial. In drug-associated SLE, removal of the drug from the therapeutic regimen is usually successful in halting the disease.

GLOSSARY

FANA   Fluorescent antinuclear antibody.

LATS   Long-acting thyroid stimulator, an autoantibody found in those with Graves' disease.

MBP   Myelin basic protein.

MG   Myasthenia gravis.

MS   Multiple sclerosis.

Multiple sclerosis   A demyelinating autoimmune disease.

Myasthenia gravis   An autoimmune disease related to antiacetylcholine receptors.

Myelin basic protein   Target antigen of the central nervous system in multiple sclerosis.

Relative risk   A mathematical expression that relates autoimmune diseases to MHC genes.

RF   Rheumatoid factor.

Rheumatoid factor   An antibody directed toward Gm determinants in IgG.

SLE   Systemic lupus erythematosus.

Systemic lupus erythematosus   An autoimmune disease characterized by positive fluorescent antinuclear antibody test results.

CHAPTER 12

Immunoglobulin E–Mediated Hypersensitivity

In the preceding chapter, the description of how the immune system can turn on its host and cause autoimmune disease became partially understandable, knowing the limits of antibody specificity, the ability of T cells to attack host cells that display novel antigens on their surface, and the manner in which chemical and physical alteration of self-proteins can turn them into self-antigens. In this chapter and the next, a slightly different immunologic confrontation occurs. In the hypersensitivity reactions, the immune system encounters and responds to exogenous antigens and haptens. This is our natural expectation for a system so keenly honed to recognize and protect us against nonself; yet in the hypersensitivities, the events that accompany and follow this confrontation create disease. This is especially discomforting when we realize that most of the antigens involved are not themselves toxic or infectious—in fact, they are usually innocuous except for their hypersensitizing property.

Thus, it is always disturbing to learn that four separate categories of hypersensitivity responses to foreign antigens are well recognized. In the first

category, the potentially lethal anaphylactic reaction, the less serious but
still bothersome allergies, and a few
other conditions are included. These
receive detailed attention in this chapter. The dominant role of IgE, how it
binds to and then later affects mast
cells as it reacts with antigen, and the
numerous products released by mast
cells occupy a large portion of this
chapter.

Classification of the Hypersensitivities

Allergies and hypersensitivities are immunologic reactions of an undesired
sort. The terms **"allergy"** and **"hypersensitivity"** are customarily synonymous, although allergy was originally
defined simply as an unexpected response to antigen. Hypersensitivity
refers to an enhanced reaction to antigen. Hyposensitivity is the opposite of
hypersensitivity. Anergy is also a valid
term and refers to the absence of an
immunologic response when it is
otherwise expected. Allergies begin
with an exposure to antigens (or haptens) and progress to the development
of antibodies or sensitized T cells. The
term "allergen" is often substituted for
"antigen" or "hapten" in discussions of
the hypersensitivities. Upon reexposure to the antigens, the shocking exposure, an allergic reaction, rather
than some immunoprotective function
is expressed.

Dermatologists often classify the allergies as of the **immediate or the delayed type** because it is easy for them
to measure the time course of hypersensitive reactions in the skin (Table
12–1). This is done by injecting a tiny
quantity of the antigen into the skin of
an allergic person. The immediate-type
skin response is evidenced by the development of edema, a spread of this

Table 12–1
**CLASSIFICATION OF THE
HYPERSENSITIVITIES ACCORDING
TO TIME**

	Characteristic
Immediate	
Immune basis	IgE, possibly other immunoglobulins
Cellular basis	Mast cells and basophils
Chemical basis	Histamine, eosinophil chemotactic factors of anaphylaxis, leukotrienes, platelet-activating factor, kinins
Chemotherapy	Antihistamines, adrenergic drugs, cromolyn
Delayed	
Immune basis	T lymphocyte
Cellular basis	Monocyte chemotaxin, macrophage migration inhibitory factor
Chemical basis	Lymphokines
Chemotherapy	Anti-inflammatory drugs, corticosteroids

edema (wheal), and the development of
an erythematous zone around the inoculation site. This is known as the **triple
response**, a response that may take
only 5 to 10 minutes to develop. Delayed-type skin responses progress
over a time frame of many hours or
days and are often maximal 48 hours
after provocation.

The division of allergic reactions into
immediate or delayed types does not
explain the immunologic basis of these
conditions. Classification of allergies
on a sounder immunopathologic basis
divides these reactions into four types
(Table 12–2). **Type I hypersensitivity**
is known both as **anaphylactic and
IgE-mediated allergy**. It is the main
subject of this chapter. The **type II and
type III hypersensitivities**, known as
the **cytotoxic and immune complex
hypersensitivities**, respectively, are

Table 12–2

CLASSIFICATION OF THE HYPERSENSITIVITIES ACCORDING TO THEIR IMMUNOPATHOLOGY

	Anaphylactic	Cytotoxic	Immune Complex	T Cell
Type classification	Type I	Type II	Type III	Type IV
Synonym	Immediate-type hypersensitivity	None	None	Delayed-type hypersensitivity
Immunoglobulin	IgE	IgG, possibly other	IgG, IgM, and others	None
Antigens involved	Heterologous	Autologous or hapten	Autologous or modified	Autologous or heterologous
Complement involved	No	Yes	Yes	No
Major targets	Smooth muscle	Individual cells	Kidney and blood vessels	Varies
Tissue histology	Edema, eosinophilia	Neutrophils	Macrophages	CD4, T lymphocytes, macrophages
Target cells	Mast cells, basophils	RBCs, WBCs, platelets, and others	Varies with site of complex deposit	Varies
Chemical mechanism	Histamine, leukotrienes, ECF-A, and others	Complement cytolysis	Immune complex blockage of tissue or vessels	Interleukins
Examples	Anaphylaxis, hay fever, food allergy	Transfusion reactions, Rh disease, thrombocytopenia	Arthus, serum sickness, pneumonitis	Allergy of infection, contact dermatitis
Desensitization	Yes, build IgG	No	No	Very difficult

dominated by IgG and complement. The **type IV or delayed-type hypersensitivity** has no dependence on immunoglobulins but is instead mediated by T cells.

ANAPHYLACTIC (TYPE I) HYPERSENSITIVITY

The **anaphylactic-type hypersensitivities** *are equivalent to the immediate-type hypersensitivities.* As with all hypersensitivities, there must be an initial exposure to antigen or hapten,

in this instance to stimulate immunoglobulin E formation. After this the individual is described as sensitized and will demonstrate his or her allergy upon reexposure to the antigen. If this is done through an injection of the antigen into the skin, the triple response just described will develop. Histologically, fluid and neutrophils infiltrate the affected area. This relies heavily upon the formation of antigen complexes with immunoglobulin E that has become attached to IgE receptors on the surface of tissue mast cells or basophils. Immune complex formation on the outer membrane of these cells causes them to release several pharmacologic agents from their cytoplasmic granules. Because of the pronounced vasoactive and muscle-contracting actions of these compounds, the blood vessels leak, the surrounding tissue becomes filled with plasma, and erythema develops around this zone. These events are noticed within a few moments, reach their maximum between 10 minutes and 2 hours, and then quickly fade.

If this reaction is provoked by an injection of the antigen into the blood stream, the response may be so massive as to threaten the person's life. The mast cell vasoamines are released from a huge population of these cells, and the high concentration achieved by these compounds causes cerebral edema and collapse. *Constriction of the smooth muscles of the lung can cause death by asphyxiation if not relieved.* This IgE-dependent hypersensitivity reaction is appropriately termed **anaphylaxis** ("ana," without; "phylaxis," protection).

CYTOTOXIC (TYPE II) HYPERSENSITIVITY

Antibodies of the IgG and IgM classes directed against cellular antigens are the aggressors in the type II or cytotoxic form of allergy. When armed with complement these antibodies are cytodestructive to the cells for which they are specific. Thus, antibodies to erythrocytes, white blood cells, or platelets can activate the complement system and cause lysis of these membrane-sensitive cells. Examples of the cytotoxic-type hypersensitivities are blood transfusion reactions, hemolytic disease of the newborn, thrombocytopenia, and certain types of drug allergy. Since these reactions cannot be observed in the skin, it is not conve-

nient to classify them as either immediate or delayed. The time course of these reactions depends upon the amount of antibody involved, the time required for the antibody to reach and then combine with and destroy the target cells, in addition to the sensitivity of the target cell.

IMMUNE COMPLEX (TYPE III) HYPERSENSITIVITY

The third antibody-dependent type of hypersensitivity is referred to as **immune complex allergy**. In the first stage of immune complex allergies, *antibodies of the IgG and IgM class combine with antigens to form soluble immune complexes.* In later stages of the reaction, insoluble serologic precipitates may develop on cell surfaces. These complexes will contain C3b, which will promote deposition on blood vessel walls as part of the immune adherence reaction. Otherwise the soluble aggregates will be removed by the filtration apparatus of the kidney. Glomerulonephritis thus becomes a regular expression of immune complex hypersensitivity. The immune complexes also generate the C4a, C3a, and C5a anaphylatoxins, and the C5a chemotaxin. This causes local edema and an infiltration of neutrophils, which contribute to the local tissue damage. Tissue necrosis seen in the Arthus reaction and allergic pneumonitis depend upon a deposition of immune complexes of sufficient magnitude to occlude minor blood vessels.

DELAYED-TYPE (TYPE IV) HYPERSENSITIVITY

Delayed-type hypersensitivity (DTH) reactions are best observed in the skin. The reaction site develops a thickened, leathery texture (induration) over a period of several days, perhaps not reaching its maximum until 48 or 72 hours after challenge. This contrasts sharply with the time frame of the immediate-type, IgE response. Edema may develop but is not considered a major attribute of pure DTH reactions. In *DTH reactions serum antibodies are not involved; instead, sensitized CD4-positive T lymphocytes react with the antigen* and release lymphokines into the tissues. Some of these lymphokines serve as chemoattractants for monocytes, and others arrest migration of the monocytes as they near the T cell. This accounts for the histologic dominance of monocytes and macrophages in delayed-type skin reactions examined after 48 hours. Earlier neutrophils are also prominent. The prototype of

DTH reactions is the tuberculin reaction, an example of an allergy of infection. The second category of DTH allergy is known as contact dermatitis.

Only type I anaphylactic allergy is considered in this chapter. The other forms of allergy are described in the next chapter.

IgE-Mediated Allergies

In some individuals the injection of antigens or haptens initiates one of the most serious forms of allergy — anaphylaxis, a potentially fatal allergic reaction. The immunologic events that occur in anaphylaxis are similar to those that occur in most food and respiratory allergies but are far more serious. Asthma is related to, yet different from, the purely IgE-dependent respiratory allergies.

ANAPHYLAXIS

Systemic anaphylaxis is the most rapidly life-threatening possibility among the allergic reactions, although the cytotoxic and immune complex reactions can be very serious. Systemic anaphylaxis is an expression of an IgE-based sensitivity to an antigen or hapten that is injected for a second or subsequent time. *The first exposure to the antigen is referred to as the* **sensitizing dose** *and the second exposure as the* **shocking dose**. The shocking dose of antigen normally consists of a *soluble preparation injected by a route that will permit its distribution throughout the body in a very short time;* that is, it is injected into the vascular system either directly or enters from small blood vessels that are ruptured when intramuscular, subcutaneous, or other injections are made. Consequently, anaphylaxis can be avoided by using cellular or insolu-

---

MEMORY CHECK 12-1

Hypersensitivity

1. Is essentially synonymous with allergy
2. Develops because of two exposures to an allergen — first the sensitizing exposure and then the shocking exposure
3. Can be classified as an immediate- or delayed-type reaction
4. May be classified as anaphylactic (type I), cytotoxic (type II), immune complex (type III), or delayed-type (type IV) reactions
5. Of the anaphylactic type relies on an IgE response to the allergen
6. Of the cytotoxic and immune complex type rely on IgG or IgM responses, or both, as well as complement
7. Of the delayed type relies on CD4+ T cells

ble antigens; by careful injections of the antigen into subcutaneous, dermal, or muscular tissues; and by using materials pretested and known to be low-order hypersensitizers. It is also possible to test an individual to determine if he or she has been sensitized to anaphylaxis by previous exposure to an allergen.

The Symptoms of Anaphylaxis

Fatal anaphylaxis in humans is similar to that in guinea pigs that have been used as laboratory models. Within a very few seconds following injection of the shocking dose of antigen, a tingling sensation develops in the throat, a hot "flash" pervades the skin, a shortness of breath soon develops, and laryngo-edema may be noted. This is followed by collapse and *may terminate fatally within minutes* if not treated. Autopsies of persons who have died of anaphylaxis reveal a *marked edema in the respiratory tract* that nearly closes the airway. The lungs are fully inflated. Owing to a powerful contraction of the smooth muscles of the bronchi, the individuals have been able to inspire but not to expire. The lungs, though inflated, contain air from which the oxygen has been consumed and which is no longer life-supporting. The individuals have, in fact, died of asphyxiation.

Temporary Desensitization

If an individual escapes the fatal outcome of anaphylaxis, the return to a normal physiologic state requires less than an hour. Thereafter, the person is *temporarily desensitized* and could without danger receive further injections of the antigen immediately or within the next few days. This is because the body has exhausted its supply of all the chemical mediators of anaphylaxis. Also, all the IgE on the

surface of the mast cells may be saturated with antigen. However, the shocking dose of antigen which provoked the anaphylactic experience may serve as a booster injection and stimulate even higher levels of IgE. These could be responsible for another bout of anaphylaxis at a later time.

Sensitizing Antigens and Haptens

To create the symptoms of systemic anaphylaxis, the antigen must reach the blood stream so that it can be distributed quickly to a large number of basophils and tissue mast cells. A large volume or concentration of antigen is not required for this. Experience and experimental studies have shown that sensitized individuals can be thrown into *anaphylactic shock with microgram quantities of antigen*.

Entry of the antigen into the blood stream need not be by direct intravenous injection. Damage to minor blood vessels during intramuscular, subcutaneous, or other injection routes may initiate anaphylaxis. Ordinary diffusion may be adequate means for low molecular weight antigens to enter the circulatory system in a shock-eliciting dosage. Ocular hypersensitivity testing by placing a drop of antigen in the eye has caused anaphylaxis.

The shocking dose of antigen is invariably given in a soluble form. Cellular, precipitated, or other insolubilized forms of antigen cannot enter the tissues and contact mast cells until they are degraded to a soluble state.

The major anaphylactically active antigens of the past are largely removed from the list of injectable products. A rare case of anaphylaxis may follow an injection of antiserum from a domestic animal, or a protein hormone from a similar source, but the most common source of anaphylaxis is injection with haptens. Insect stings are another important cause.

The insects responsible for anaphylaxis are those in the genus *Hymenoptera*. The common honeybee, the large bumblebee, and several types of wasps and hornets deliver a complicated mixture of antigens when they sting. Phospholipase, phosphatase, hyaluronidase, and mellitin are commonly found in venoms from these insects. Mellitin acts directly on mast cells, but the enzymes function in insect allergy by stimulating IgE. *Anaphylactic death has followed bee stings* in highly sensitized individuals. Veteran beekeepers often develop insensitivity through high levels of protective or blocking IgG.

The *haptenic compounds incriminated in anaphylaxis* represent a special category of these low molecular weight chemicals. These haptens, or their degradation products created in vivo, *all contain a labile chemical grouping that permits them to form covalent bonds with host proteins or polysaccharides*. These haptens have been described as autocoupling or self-reactive haptens. The sensitizing antigen in these hapten-related allergies is the conjugated hapten-antigen product in which the key epitope focuses around the hapten.

One of the most studied of these haptens is allergy to penicillin, but other antibiotics, tranquilizers, sulfonamides, analgesics, and other drug groupings all have their offenders. In the case of **penicillin**, several degradation products have a sensitizing potential. Penicillamine and penicillenic acid have free sulfhydryl groups that are free to bind to proteins with free SH groups. These are active sensitizers but are not as potent as *penicilloic acid–protein complexes*. These are formed by opening of the oxazole ring in penicillenic acid and its reaction with free amino groups of proteins.

Sensitivity Testing — Local Anaphylaxis

An individual can be tested to determine his or her proclivity to respond anaphylactically to an injection of antigen. A person previously sensitized to an antigen will display an immediate-type skin reaction to a highly diluted solution of the antigen. It is advisable not to use a full-strength antigen preparation because exquisitely sensitive individuals have developed severe anaphylactic reactions to antigen preparations of normal strength. *The positive skin test result is a form of local anaphylaxis.*

The Prausnitz-Küstner Test and Schultz-Dale Reaction. Use of the **Prausnitz-Küstner (PK) test** is a second avenue for predetermining an IgE-based allergy. *The PK test is also a form of local anaphylaxis but of the passive type*, arranged by injecting serum from the presumed allergic individual into the skin of a nonallergic volunteer. This is followed several hours later by an injection of the presumed allergen into the same site that received the serum. A positive immediate-type skin reaction is evidence of the allergy in the serum donor. PK testing is infrequently done except with close family members because of the risk of transmitting hepatitis or HIV.

The PK test has also been used to provide support for the concept that **a cell-fixed antibody** is responsible for IgE hypersensitivity. If in the PK test the serum and antigen are injected more or less simultaneously, little or no skin reaction will develop. If several hours intervene between the two injections, then a reaction does develop. The elapsed time period is necessary to allow the transferred IgE to attach to mast cells in the recipient's skin.

Another experiment that demonstrates cell-bound rather than free antibody as the agency of IgE mediated allergy is the **Schultz-Dale reaction**. Strips of intestinal or uterine muscle taken from an allergic animal and ambitiously perfused to remove all traces of blood and free antibody will still contract when exposed to the sensitizing antigen.

RESPIRATORY ALLERGY

Allergy of the respiratory system is often due to an IgE-based sensitivity to inhaled antigens. Familiar symptoms include sneezing; itching or burning of the nose; a nasal discharge; weeping eyes, with red, itching conjunctivae; and inflamed, swollen mucosae. These are the symptoms of anaphylaxis but on a smaller, regional scale. The nasal discharge and weeping eyes are the result of edema. The swollen mucosae and red conjunctivae are examples of both edema and erythema. Because these symptoms are generated in local tissues rather than throughout the body, they are not life-threatening.

Seasonal Allergens

Allergic responses of the upper respiratory tree have been called **atopic** (from "atopy," meaning foreign) because the nature of the antigen, as well as the time and mechanism of the sensitization, may be unknown. Even now, it is not possible to list or describe all of the allergens in precise chemical terms; because of their enormous number, most have escaped study. Antigen E of ragweed is of interest because it is responsible for the naming of the type I allergic antibody as IgE. This stemmed from studies that eventually proved that *an antibody to antigen E was responsible for hay fever, the seasonal allergy to ragweed.* This was the first demonstration of an immunoglobulin as the vehicle for the immediate-type allergies. Prior to the chemical description of IgE, the serum substance responsible for type I allergies was called **reagin**. Reagin was known to be antigen specific, to be transferrable to the skin in PK reactions, and to have the other properties ascribed to IgE.

Most common of the respiratory allergens are to the **pollens** of trees (eg, elm, oak, maple, birch), grasses (blue grass, timothy), weeds (ragweed, thistle, plantain), and spores of fungi. Because plants liberate pollen at specific times during the year, their associated allergies are usually seasonal. In the late summer and early autumn many weeds and grasses pollinate. Atopy at this time of year therefore is known as hay fever. Seasonal or nonseasonal expression of a respiratory allergy is a useful first criterion to determine the source of the allergy.

Nonseasonal Allergens

Molds, dander and feathers, housedust, and certain occupational allergens are constantly present in specific environments and are responsible for the **nonseasonal allergies**. An antigen of contemporary interest is house dust. It was observed from epidemiologic studies that persons allergic to dust from their own environment would also be allergic to dust from other locales where the climate and soil were quite different. This curiosity was resolved when it was determined that microscopic mites in the genus *Dermatophagoides* were common in all the dust samples. This mite dwells in carpets, furniture, bedding, and the like, and allergy develops to its body proteins and waste products wafted into the air during household cleaning.

Asthma

Although related to atopic respiratory allergies, asthma is a different condition. It is characterized by marked wheezing as air enters and leaves the deeper recesses of the lung where the airway is partially obstructed. This is often provoked by breathing cold air, exercise, unusual humidity, and so forth. Asthmatics often display immediate-type skin reactions to respiratory allergens but respond to inhalation of these allergens differently than atopic individuals. *Asthma may represent a response to the late-acting stimuli of respiratory allergy*, with hay fever representing an early response.

FOOD ALLERGY

Allergies to foods are less often atopic than are respiratory allergies because the symptoms immediately follow eating. Allergic individuals can often identify a specific food as the source of their allergy. The symptoms may include inflammation and swelling of the lips and mouth parts, intestinal cramping, gaseous distention or nausea, and diarrhea. Urticarial skin eruptions known as hives also may appear. The foods most frequently responsible for these allergic reactions are chocolate, milk, nuts, shellfish, strawberries, tomato, and egg. Avoidance of the specific food is the simplest escape from these allergies, a solution that may not be possible if the food item is included in a variety of food products. In such

instances skin testing may be required to identify the allergic etiology.

Mechanisms of IgE Allergy

CHEMICAL PROPERTIES OF IgE

Chemistry

IgE shares the typical four-peptide structure of other immunoglobulins in which κ or λ light chains are joined by disulfide bonds to the heavy chain. The heavy chain in this instance is the ϵ chain, which has a molecular weight of approximately 75,000 Mr. The greater molecular weight of the ϵ chain compared with the γ chain is dependent upon a **fourth CH domain**. This gives IgE a molecular weight of approximately 190,000 Mr (Table 12–3). IgE *does not produce visible serologic reactions* in vitro with antigen as do IgG and IgM and is heat-labile. IgE in combination with antigen is *unable to acti-*

MEMORY CHECK 12–2

Examples of IgE-dependent hypersensitivity include

1. Systemic anaphylaxis
2. Many forms of local anaphylaxis
   a. Direct skin tests
   b. PK tests
   c. Food allergies
   d. Respiratory allergies
   e. Schultz-Dale reaction

Table 12–3
PROPERTIES OF IMMUNOGLOBULIN E

Chemical Properties

Molecular weight	190,000
Sw,20 value	8.2
Electrophoretic mobility	1
Carbohydrate content (%)	11.7
Concentration (mg/dL) of serum	0.1–1.0
Amount of serum immunoglobulins (%)	<1
Half-life (days)	2.3
Rate of synthesis (μg/kg of body weight/day)	2.3
Heavy chain constant domains	4

Biological Properties

Does not pass the placental barrier

Responsible for anaphylactic-type allergies

Binds to receptors on mast cells and basophils

vate *the complement system.* Heat inactivation of IgE requires 56°C to 60°C for 30 or more minutes. IgE is present in serum at very low concentrations during normal health—only 0.1 to 1 mg/dL. IgE represents less than 1% of the total immunoglobulins. The half-life and rate of synthesis of IgE are approximately the same: about 2.5 days and 2.5 μg per kg per day, respectively.

Quantitation

Because of the low serum level of IgE in healthy persons, and even in some allergic persons, it is necessary to use sensitive serologic procedures for its quantitation. It is possible to measure the total amount of IgE present in a serum sample by radial immunodiffusion or nephelometric methods, and these methods are often preferred because they are inexpensive. Radioimmunoassay (RIA) and enzyme-linked immunosorbent assay (ELISA) procedures are slightly more sensitive. Two of the RIA methods are RIST and RAST.

RIST

Historically, the **radioimmunosorbent** test (**RIST**) is important because it was the only sensitive assay procedure available until the mid-1980s. ELISA modifications of the RIST method are also available to quantitate IgE. The details of RIA and ELISA are discussed in Chapter 14. Briefly, an anti-IgE is attached to the surface of a well in a microtiter tray and a serum sample containing IgE is added. After the IgE and anti-IgE have reacted, the well is rinsed. Thereafter, a radiolabeled anti-IgE is added. After the reaction between the isotopically labeled anti-IgE and IgE is complete, the excess antibody is removed by rinsing. The amount of radiolabel left in the well is an index of the quantity of IgE in the serum sample. *RIST thus measures total serum IgE.*

RAST

The **radioallergosorbent test** (RAST) *defines how much of the total IgE is specific for a certain allergen.* In RAST selected allergens are adsorbed to separate wells of a microtiter plate. The patient's serum is added and its IgE is allowed to react with the allergens. Allergen-bound IgE is then removed by gentle washing. Thereafter, radiolabeled antibody specific for human IgE is added, and any excess is washed away after a brief incubation. Quantitation of the isotopically labeled antibody in any given well is a measure of the IgE present for the chosen allergen. By using a panel of allergens, the breadth of a person's allergy can be determined.

CELL-BOUND IgE

Immunoglobulin E, like the other immunoglobulins, is secreted from plasma cells and distributed through the blood. These circulating immunoglobulins enter into an equilibrium state between the blood and the tissues. When IgE enters the tissues it has a unique capacity to attach to the outer membrane of tissue mast cells. In the circulation some of the IgE binds to basophils.

Mast Cells and Basophils

Mast cells are widely distributed throughout the body and are especially numerous in connective tissue, near blood vessels, and in the lung. Mast cells have a diameter of 10 to 15 μ and are literally filled with basophilic granules, 0.5 to 2.0 μ in diameter. *All* mast cells are not alike—**T-type mast cells** are so designated because they contain the enzyme tryptase. T_C **mast cells** contain both tryptase and chymase. Tryptase and chymase are similar in substrate specificity to trypsin and chymotrypsin. As yet, there is no evidence that tryptase and chymase contribute to allergy. The T_C mast cell may contribute more to IgE-dependent allergies than the T-type cell because it contains more histamine. On the other hand, the T-type mast cell is more numerous in the lung, the human organ most affected by anaphylaxis.

Superficially, basophils resemble mast cells in their content of granules, the presence of histamine in these granules, and in having an outer surface attractive to IgE.

Fc Receptors for IgE

Receptor molecules on basophils and mast cells are designed to combine with the Fc region of IgE. The **major receptor, Fc$_e$RI**, has a higher affinity for IgE than the Fc$_e$RII receptor. The RI molecule consists of three peptides, α (the outermost), β (a transmembrane peptide), and two molecules of γ that are disulfide bonded to each other and situated most internally. The α, β and γ peptides are noncovalently associated with each other. The evidence indicates that *amino acids in the CH2 – CH3 juncture in the Fc region of IgE bind to* the α peptide of the RI receptor.

Less is known about **the RII receptor,** *also known as the CD23 protein.* It is apparently a single peptide of 50,000 Mr but this has been contested. Its role in anaphylactic-type allergy is uncertain because it does not bind IgE very well. Its presence on B cells, T cells, eosinophils, and platelets further clouds its physiologic role, and suggests that RII may have multiple functions.

MEMORY CHECK 12-3

◆

IgE differs from other immunoglobulins

1. Except IgM by having four CH domains
2. Except IgD and IgA by failing to activate complement
3. Except IgD by being at a very low concentration in blood
4. By being more heat labile
5. By failing to produce visible serologic reactions with antigen
6. By having Fc receptors on mast cells and basophils

IgE Bridging

When two molecules of IgE on the mast cell or basophil surface combine with the same molecule of antigen, a process leading to degranulation begins (Fig. 12 – 1). **Antigen bridging of two IgEs is** compatible with the high number of RI receptors per mast cell, probably exceeding 500,000. Antigen fractions containing a single epitope and simple haptens are incapable of initiating degranulation because they can react only with a single arm of a single IgE molecule.

SECOND-MESSENGER PATHWAYS

The bridging of IgE by antigen is the first message that initiates the process of mast cell degranulation. The mechanism of degranulation is complex, the order of the reactions is uncertain, and it appears there are *two major pathways. The first of the pathways* to be described involves cyclic 3′, 5′ adenosine monophosphate, better known as

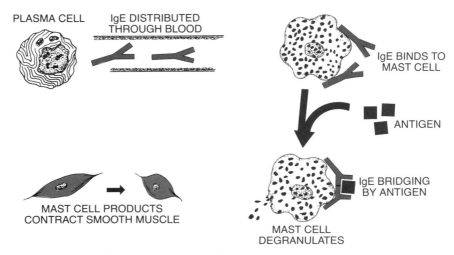

Figure 12–1. After IgE is released from plasma cells, it enters the blood and then the tissues, where it attaches to mast cells. When two Fc$_\epsilon$R-bound IgE molecules are bridged by antigen, mast cell degranulation follows. These granule products have many properties, including the contraction of smooth muscle, which is contributory to anaphylaxis.

cyclic AMP (cAMP). *The second scheme involves* **phosphatidyl inositol.** Both systems are associated with an early influx of Ca²⁺ into the cell.

Phosphatidyl Inositol Pathway

One hypothesis of mast cell degranulation relies on **G proteins** and **Ca²⁺ ions** (Fig. 12–2). In this instance, the G proteins stimulate the conversion of **phosphatidyl inositol (PI)** through several stages in which it acquires additional phosphate groupings. The first important new product is PI diphosphate. Removal of inositol triphosphate from PI diphosphate by **phosphorylase C** produces **diacylglycerol (DAG)** and eases the entry of calcium into the cell. Under the influence of Ca²⁺, protein kinase A is activated and this contributes to degranulation. Meanwhile, **lysophatidyl choline (LPC)** is being produced, first by methylation of PI and then by the action of **phospholipase A2** to remove a fatty acid. DAG and LPC are both known to behave like lipid solvents, and as such could fuse

the lipids of the granule membrane to lipids in the cell membrane, thereby prompting exocytosis.

Cyclic AMP Pathway

The initiator of the cAMP pathway is believed to be a G protein located at the foot of the IgE receptor (Fig. 12–3). This **G or guanosine-dependent protein** is activated by a serologic reaction on the cell surface and *activates the enzyme adenylate cyclase. A marked increase of intracellular cAMP occurs,*

MEMORY CHECK 12–4

♦

Mast cell degranulation involves

1. Cyclic AMP formation
2. G protein activation
3. Calcium ion influx
4. Protein kinase activation
5. Phosphatidyl inositol metabolism
6. Fusogen formation

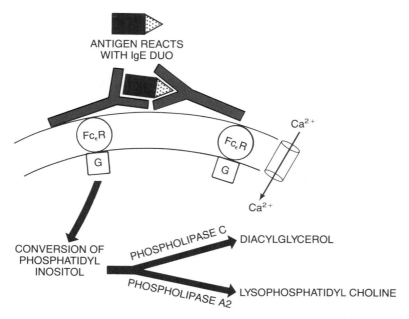

Figure 12–2. An alternative mechanism for mast cell degranulation is similar to that depicted in Figure 12–3, but involves the liberation of the fusogens diacylglycerol and lysophosphatidyl choline after G protein activation of phosphatidyl inositol degradation.

and phosphate derived from the conversion of adenosine triphosphate (ATP) to cAMP is used by *protein kinase A to* phosphorylate the mast cell granules. This is believed to labilize the granule surface. *An influx of Ca^{2+}* is also instrumental in the activation of protein kinase A. Calcium may also be needed to alter the integrity of the granule and outer mast cell membranes, thereby encouraging degranulation. Degranulation continues if a phosphodiesterase degrades just enough cAMP to keep its concentration at the degranulating threshold. Inhibitors of the phosphodiesterase that allow the level of cAMP to exceed this threshold impair degranulation.

Figure 12–3. One biochemical mechanism of mast cell degranulation involves the activation of G proteins by the serologic reaction on the mast cell surface. The G protein activates adenylate cyclase, which then allows an influx of Ca^{2+} into the cell and protein kinase C activation. This destabilizes mast cell granules, allowing the release of histamine and other mediators.

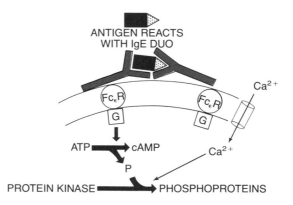

Table 12-4
MEDIATORS AND MODERATORS OF TYPE I HYPERSENSITIVITY AND
THEIR CONTROL

Mediator	Description	Primary Activity	Antagonist
Histamine	From histidine, mol wt 111	Contraction of smooth muscle	Antihistamine
Eosinophil chemotactic factors of anaphylaxis	From mast cells, mol wt about 350, Val Gly Ser Glu and Ala Gly Ser Glu	Attraction of eosinophils	None known
Leukotrienes C, D, and E	Fatty acids, mol wt about 400	Prolonged contraction of smooth muscle	Aryl sulfatase; indomethacin
Bradykinin and related kinins	From plasma kininogens, mol wt about 1000	Slow contraction of smooth muscle	None known
Platelet-activating factor	Substituted phosphorylcholine	Aggregates platelets	Phospholipases A, C, and D
Serotonin	From tryptophan, mol wt 171, and aromatic amine	Contraction of smooth muscle	Methysergide

MEDIATOR RELEASE

A number of vasoactive compounds called spasmogens because of their effect on smooth muscle are released during anaphylactic-type allergic reactions (Table 12-4).

Histamine

The primary toxic agent released from the human mast cell is **histamine** (Fig. 12-4). Chemically, histamine is a simple molecule with a molecular weight of 111. It is formed when the mast cell enzyme histidine decarboxylase removes a carboxyl group from histidine. The mast cell stores histamine in an ionic complex with heparin at a level of about 10 to 15 $\mu g/10^6$ cells. **Heparin** is an acidic, sulfated polysaccharide that binds ionically with the basic histamine molecule. During type I allergic reactions, *both histamine and heparin are released from mast cell granules.* This is noted as the histamine-induced rapid contraction of smooth muscle

and a prolonged blood clotting time due to heparin.

When histamine contracts smooth muscles of the vascular system, particularly the venules, alteration of the permeability of the blood vessels allows fluid to flow from the vessels into the tissues, causing edema — cerebral edema causes the person to collapse. Constriction of the smooth respiratory musculature prevents normal breathing. In its severest form, this reaction is responsible for anaphylactic death.

Leukotrienes

When **arachidonic acid (icosatetraenoic acid)** is released from lipids present in the mast cell membranes, enzymes begin a series of transformations through the lipoxygenase pathway that produce several vasoactive compounds. These compounds, the leukotrienes, are more potent in muscle contraction than histamine, but the muscles contract more slowly than

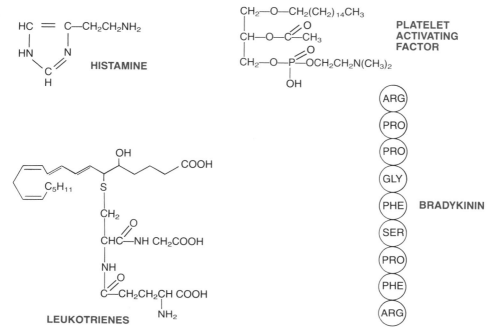

Figure 12–4. Major contributors to anaphylaxis are histamine, the leukotrienes, platelet activating factor, and bradykinin, among other agents.

when exposed to histamine. This accounts for the earlier designation of the leukotrienes as the slow-reacting substances of anaphylaxis (SRS-A).

The first metabolite of arachidonic acid is the unstable leukotriene A, an unsaturated 20-carbon fatty acid like its predecessor. Leukotriene A is stabilized and converted to **leukotriene C (LTC)** by the addition of glutathione. Successive losses of glutamic acid and glycine yield **leukotrienes D and E (LTD and LTE)**. These three stable leukotrienes have a common activity on smooth muscle. Because of their protracted effect on muscle these compounds are considered very important in asthma (Fig. 12–5).

Platelet-Activating Factor

Another molecule released from mast cells and basophils engaged in anaphy-

lactic degranulation is 1-0-alkyl-2-acetyl-glyceryl-3-phosphorylcholine, also known as the **platelet-activating factor (PAF)**. PAF causes platelets to undergo the platelet release reaction, which is characterized by aggregation or clumping of the platelets (thrombocytes) and a secretion of several molecules including serotonin, arachidonic acid, and derivatives of the prostaglandins. PAF's contribution to anaphylaxis is uncertain, but it is known that anaphylaxis is accompanied by a transient thrombocytopenia.

Eosinophil Chemotactic Factors of Anaphylaxis

A fourth activity that contributes to type I hypersensitive reactions is produced by a duo of molecules with an identical pharmacologic activity. These are the **eosinophil chemotactic**

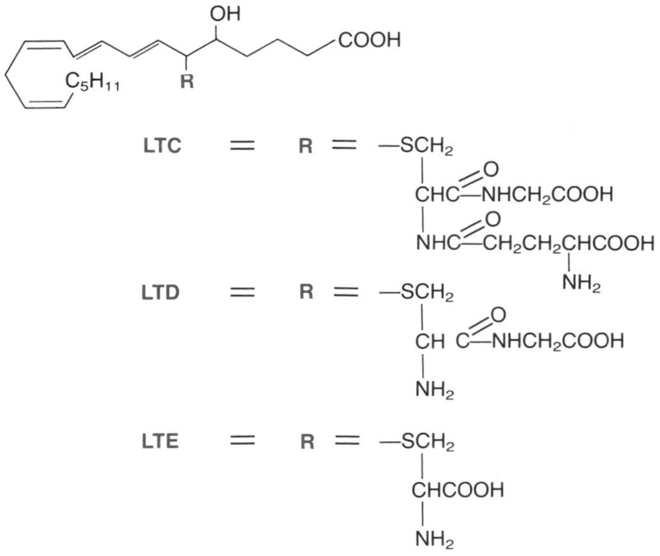

Figure 12-5. Differences in the R group account for the slight differences among LTC, LTD, and LTE.

factors of anaphylaxis (ECF-A). ECF-A activity is present in two low molecular weight peptides that have the amino acid sequences Val Gly Ser Glu and Ala Gly Ser Glu. The exact origin of these tetrapeptides in mast cells is uncertain. These factors stimulate the chemotactic entrance of eosinophils into the arena where the mast cells are degranulating. It is known that allergy resulting from intestinal parasitism, hay fever, or other IgE-based allergies is accompanied by an intense eosinophilia of blood and of nasal and ocular secretions.

Serotonin

Serotonin is a molecule present in human platelets but not in basophils or mast cells. This molecule has the same pharmacologic action as histamine— namely, a rapid contraction of smooth muscles and an increase in vascular permeability. Because the human mast cell and basophil are devoid or contain only traces of serotonin, it is believed that serotonin does not play a significant role in human anaphylactic reac-

tions, although it may do so in other species.

Kinins

Bradykinin, a peptide consisting of only nine amino acids, is a potent vasodilating agent with many of the properties of histamine. As its name indicates, bradykinin provokes a prolonged or protracted contraction of muscle. Bradykinin does not originate from mast cells but rather from a series of proenzyme-enzyme conversions that degrade two high molecular weight serum proteins known as kininogens. Within the core of each of these is the nonapeptide bradykinin.

The kinin pathway begins with an activation of the **Hageman factor** or other enzymes when immune complexes are formed. These proteolytic enzymes convert serum **plasminogen proactivator to plasminogen activator**. Plasminogen activator converts **plasminogen to plasmin**. Subsequently, plasmin converts **prokininogenase (prekallikrein)** into the enzyme kininogenase. Then **kinin-**

ogenase, **also called kallikrein**, acts upon the high molecular weight **kininogens** to release the low molecular weight bradykinin. In these transformations, 10 and 11 amino acid kinins may also be formed.

Prostaglandins

Several **prostaglandins** are formed when arachidonic acid is metabolized by the **cyclooxygenase** pathway. Prostaglandin D_2 is derived from mast cells and can produce wheal and flare reactions in the skin. Prostaglandins E, F_2, and I_2 are all powerful vasodilators. Because of uncertainties regarding the concentration, location, and kinetics of prostaglandin formation, their role in IgE hypersensitivities remains uncertain.

Although the immediate hypersensitivity response is easily separated from delayed-type reactions, it is divisible into an early and a late phase. The early phase, which occurs within minutes of allergen exposure, is highly dependent upon mast cells and their mediators—histamine, the leukotrienes, kinins, and possibly prostaglandin D_2. The late phase, which begins 3 to 4 hours later, is related to mast cells only in the ability of mast cell products to attract basophils, eo-

sinophils, and neutrophils into the reaction site. Then a second wave of histamine release from basophils and additional kinin and leukotriene activity is noted. Prostaglandin D_2, which is present in mast cells but not in basophils, does not reappear.

Control of IgE Allergy

CHEMICAL METHODS

The identification of several mediators of anaphylaxis encouraged the development of a battery of antagonists. Owing to the specificity of these antagonists, no single molecule can prevent all the symptoms of anaphylaxis (Table 12–4).

Antihistamines

Regulation of the IgE-mediated allergic reactions is based primarily upon a chemical moderation of the pharmacologic effects of the mast cell mediators described earlier. As a consequence of this, **antihistamines** are the most commonly used drugs. A large number of antihistamines is available but all of them are limited to a single mode of action. These compounds do not affect histamine release from mast cells nor basophils but they do block histamine-induced effects on capillary permeability and smooth muscle. Antihistamines function much better when they can attach to receptors on smooth muscle prior to histamine, which they cannot easily displace. This is rarely the case in human allergies, in which treatment usually follows evidence of the allergic reaction. Consequently, the effect of antihistamines is often less successful than anticipated. One must weigh the benefit of antihistamines against the known side effects of large doses of these drugs—particularly the sedative or soporific effect—and the knowledge

---

MEMORY CHECK 12–5

The major vasoactive mediators of type I allergies are

1. Histamine
2. Leukotrienes C, D, and E
3. Platelet-activating factor
4. Eosinophil chemotactic factors
5. Bradykinin
6. Serotonin
7. Prostaglandins

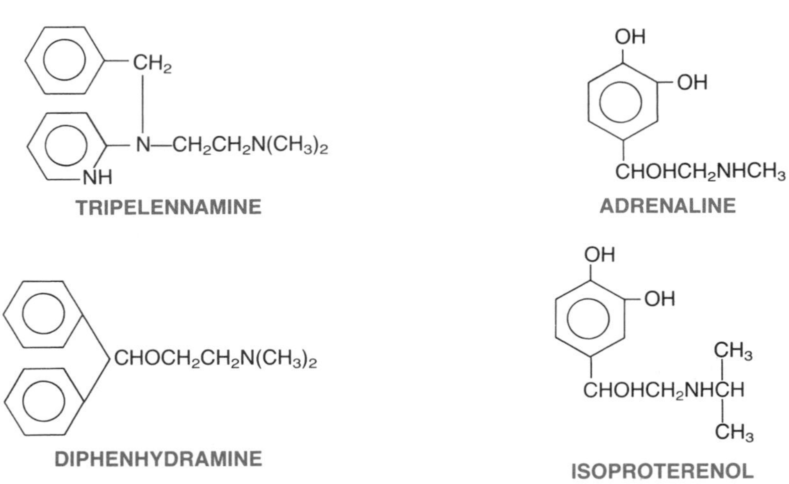

Figure 12–6. The structure of two antihistamines (*left*) shows how little they mimic the structure of histamine. Two adrenergic drugs are shown at right.

that other agents in addition to histamine contribute to the allergy (Fig. 12–6).

Adrenergic Drugs

The **adrenergic drugs** represented by adrenalin and other **catecholamines** are potent bronchodilating and smooth muscle–relaxing molecules. The pharmacologic activity of these drugs is to reverse the action of histamine and certain of the other mediators of the anaphylactic reaction. The adrenergic drugs also attach to specific receptors on mast cells and stabilize these cells against further degranulation, thus slowing histamine release. As a consequence of the dual activity of relaxing smooth muscle and stabilizing granules in mast cells, adrenergic drugs are considered the most effective compounds available to moderate the anaphylactic reaction.

Cromolyn

A compound known by various names, but available under the name **cromo-** **lyn** sodium, also has the rather unusual property of *stabilizing mast cells* against degranulation. This drug thus prevents the escape of histamine, the leukotrienes, and the other pharmacologic mediators from mast cells. Cromolyn sodium is highly insoluble in body fluids and must be aspirated as a fine dust into the lungs, from which it is absorbed.

Relaxation of smooth muscle by **methylxanthines** such as caffeine, theophylline, and theobromine has encouraged their use as **bronchodilators**. These compounds also function at the mast cell level by increasing the concentration of cAMP and stabilizing mast cell granules.

IMMUNOLOGIC METHODS

When skin tests indicate a person is allergic to an injectable, ingestable, or inhalant allergen, it is possible to produce an **immunologic desensitization**.

This can be accomplished by injecting tiny quantities of the allergen over an extended period of time, during which *the dose is gradually increased*. The injections must be monitored carefully to ensure that toxic quantities of vasoactive mediators are not released by the antigen as it reacts with IgE present on mast cells. When such symptoms are not observed, it indicates that the person can tolerate a larger antigen dose. These larger doses serve as booster doses of the antigen and cause an increased formation of all immunoglobulins. Most important of these is the increase in the quantity of circulating IgG. The next time the allergic individual encounters antigen, the circulating *IgG serves as a blocking antibody*, combines with antigen, and removes it from the circulation. These immune complexes are then ingested and degraded by phagocytic cells. Elimination of the antigen in this way prevents its entrance into tissues where the IgE-coated mast cells reside. As a consequence of the high blood levels of IgG, the person is desensitized to the allergy. It is now clearly proven that the *desensitization can be correlated exactly with the level of the serum IgG-blocking antibody that is formed*. Such treatment is used to prevent allergic reactions to ragweed pollen, bee stings, grass pollens, and other inhalant allergens.

Anaphylactoid Reactions

Nonimmunologic events that cause mast cells to discharge the same pharmacologic agents they release during anaphylactic reactions are termed **anaphylactoid reactions**. Nonantigens such as radiocontrast dyes used in the diagnosis of kidney or heart disease may bind directly to the surface of mast cells and force their degranulation. Alternatively these agents may activate the complement cascade and cause C3a, C4a, and C5a to be formed. These anaphylatoxins then activate mast cells. Aggregated proteins including gamma globulins used in passive immunotherapy are known to cause anaphylactoid reactions by the second mechanism.

References

Holgate, ST (ed): Mast Cells, Mediators and Disease. Kluwer Academic Publishers, Dordrecht, Netherlands, 1988.

Ishizaka, K: Regulation of IgE biosynthesis. Hosp Pract 24(9):51, 1989

Levine, L (ed): Arachidonate metabolism in immunologic systems. Prog Allergy 44:1, 1988.

Metzger, H: Molecular aspects of receptors and binding factors for IgE. Adv Immunol 43:277, 1988.

Proud, D, and Kaplan, AP: Kinin formation: Mechanisms and role in inflammatory disorders. Annu Rev Immunol 6:49, 1988.

QUESTIONS AND ANSWERS

1. All of the following are derived from mast cells *except*
   A. Histamine
   B. Bradykinin
   C. Platelet-activating factor
   D. Eosinophil chemotactic factors of anaphylaxis
   E. Leukotriene C

Answer B

Bradykinin is a peptide released by an enzymatic attack upon plasma kininogens. This is a complicated process that involves several proenzyme-enzyme transformations. The other agents listed are released by mast cells during degranulation.

2. Which of the following will degranulate mast cells with IgE on their surface?
   A. Fab from an IgG specific for IgE (anti-IgE)
   B. F(ab')2 from an IgG specific for IgE (anti-IgE)
   C. Fc from an IgG specific for IgE (anti-IgE)
   D. IgE specific for IgG (anti-IgG)
   E. None of the above

Answer B

Two molecules of IgE on the surface of mast cells must be bridged by antigen in order to trigger mast cell degranulation. This bridging can also be accomplished by other divalent reagents that will combine with IgE. The F(ab')2 molecule is the only agent listed that fulfills this requirement.

3. Adrenergic drugs are often superior to antihistamines in controlling anaphylactic-type allergies because adrenergic drugs
   A. Stabilize mast cells
   B. Relax smooth muscle
   C. Tend to stimulate formation of cAMP
   D. Activate G proteins
   E. All of the above

Answer E

Adrenalin and other beta-adrenergic drugs unite with their specific receptor on mast cells. This activates the G proteins and adenylate cyclase to form cAMP. The accumulation of cAMP impedes mast cell degranulation. Beta-adrenergic drug receptors on smooth muscle cause smooth muscle to relax. All answers are correct.

4. The best method of avoiding a second allergic reaction to a food is
   A. To be desensitized
   B. To take antihistamines immediately after eating the food
   C. Simply to avoid eating that food
   D. To have RIST assays to monitor the level of the sensitivity; if low, eat the food
   E. To eat the food only after it is well cooked

Answer C

It is expensive and troublesome to be desensitized to a food, when a food allergy can usually be controlled by avoiding eating that food. Drug treatments may modify the reaction but antihistamines will not neutralize the leukotrienes or kinins, for example. Allergies develop to natural and to heat-denatured proteins, so cooking would be useful only when the allergy is to a raw food. RIST assays are expensive and would not determine the degree of one's sensitivity to a particular allergen.

5. Skin testing of a known penicillin-sensitive individual will not always produce an immediate-type skin reaction. These failures can be explained most logically by which of the following mechanisms:
   A. Monovalent penicillin derivatives react with IgE before multivalent derivatives can
   B. Penicillin allergy is due to metabolic derivatives of penicillin, not penicillin per se
   C. The formation of increased levels of beta-lactamase by the allergic person
   D. Individuals readily develop antibodies to histamine, to the leukotrienes, and so forth
   E. Individuals develop increased levels of histaminase after having an anaphylactic-type reaction

Answer A

Beta-lactamase is not an enzyme of the blood, and histaminase does not behave as an adaptive enzyme. Mediators of anaphylaxis, such as histamine, the leukotrienes, and so on, are not antigenic and are not autocoupling haptens. Answers C, D, and E are untenable. Penicillin allergy is indeed directed against its derivatives but this is not related to the problem. These derivatives would also appear after skin testing with penicillin. Unchanged penicillin or monovalent derivatives can combine with IgE but cannot bridge two antibody molecules. Their binding would prevent bridging by multivalent reactants. The only correct answer is A.

Case Study: The Red Man Syndrome

Don M., a 37-year-old industrial engineer, developed peritonitis and septicemia following emergency surgery for a ruptured appendix. Because of a known allergy to penicillin and the antibiotic sensitivity of the organisms isolated from his blood, vancomycin was chosen instead of penicillin as the preferred antibiotic for therapy. Accordingly, 1 g of vancomycin was infused with 500 mL of 5% glucose regulated by an infusion pump at 10 mL/min. Within 5 minutes after the infusion was begun, Don M. developed an intense erythematous rash that spread from his neck to his face and scalp and very shortly to his upper chest and upper arms. Intense pruritus was associated with the evolution of this rash. The infusion was stopped immediately. The patient's blood pressure was 98/57, a drop from the previous reading of 122/78. Respiration was normal but the pulse was elevated to 74 per minute from the normal 60. Within 5 minutes after halting the infusion, and before any treatment could be given, the rash began to clear, and within 30 minutes no outward sign of the incident persisted.

Questions

1. Is the known allergy to penicillin related to this reaction to vancomycin?

2. Assuming that the red man syndrome is an allergy to vancomycin, what treatment would you suggest?

3. Assuming that the red man syndrome is not an IgE-dependent allergic reaction, what treatment would you suggest?

4. Why did the red man syndrome clear spontaneously upon cessation of the infusion?

Discussion

Don's previous allergy to penicillin is unrelated to this incident with vancomycin. Penicillin and vancomycin both inhibit the synthesis of bacterial cell walls but are vastly different in structure; thus, no cross-related allergic reactions are possible.

If the red man syndrome is an allergic reaction it must be a type I, IgE-dependent reaction based on the symptoms, which are clearly anaphylactic in nature. An allergic basis of the reactions requires an earlier sensitization of which there was none in Don's medical history. However, in many instances patients are unaware of precisely which antibiotics have been used to treat earlier infections. If this is an IgE-based reaction, adrenalin and antihistamines should be part of the therapy.

Though there is no evidence that the red man syndrome is an allergic reaction, the treatment nevertheless should be antihistamine and adrenalin. Treatment is a response to symptoms, and the symptoms are those of mast cell mediators. Histamine is a proven part of the red man syndrome, probably released by the direct binding of vancomycin to mast cells.

Spontaneous relief from mild anaphylactic reactions is expected. The body has many moderators of this reaction, most of which are enzymes. Decomposition of histamine, leukotrienes, and so on, by these enzymes will reduce their concentration below pharmacologically significant concentrations.

GLOSSARY

adrenergic drugs Drugs that constrict blood vessels and relax smooth muscles; synonym of catecholamine.

anaphylactoid reaction A reaction similar to anaphylaxis except that it is not created by antigen-antibody reactions.

anaphylaxis ("ana," without; "phylaxis," protection) A detrimental reaction to a second exposure to antigen in which vasoactive substances are released from mast cells.

antihistamine A drug that is a competitive inhibitor of histamine.

atopy An IgE-dependent allergy often arising from an unknown exposure to an antigen.

blocking antibody An IgG that prevents the action of IgE, formed during desensitization against atopic allergies.

bradykinin A specific peptide of nine amino acids formed during anaphylaxis, and derived from the plasma protein kininogen.

catecholamine An adrenergic drug.

cromolyn A mast cell-stabilizing drug.

desensitization Elimination or reduction of allergic sensitivity, usually through a programmed course of antigen treatment.

ECF-A Eosinophilic chemotactic factor of anaphylaxis.

histamine A specific spasmogenic compound released from mast cells during anaphylaxis.

kinins Peptides that possess vasodilating and muscle-contracting activity.

leukotriene A derivative of arachidonic acid released during anaphylaxis.

LT A leukotriene.

PAF Platelet-activating factor.

platelet-activating factor A substituted glyceride that causes degranulation of platelets.

Prausnitz-Küstner (PK) test A test for immediate hypersensitivity performed in a healthy person who has been passively sensitized by IgE from the allergic individual.

prostaglandin A derivative of arachidonic acid released during anaphylaxis.

reagin Older name for IgE.

Schultz-Dale reaction In vitro anaphylaxis, a response of IgE-sensitized uterus or gut when exposed to antigen.

serotonin 5-hydroxytryptamine.

CHAPTER 13

◆

Cytotoxic, Immune Complex, and Delayed-Type Hypersensitivity

The potentially dangerous IgE-based hypersensitivities are described in the previous chapter. The focus of this chapter is on two immunoglobulin-dependent, plus the immunoglobulin-independent, delayed-type hyersensitivities. The **cytotoxic and immune complex allergies**, the two antibody-mediated allergies, also known as the **type II and type III hypersensitivities**, are caused predominantly by an IgG response to an antigen, although other immunoglobulins may play a minor role in these reactions. **Delayed-type hyersensitivity (DTH)**, the **type IV hypersensitivity**, relies on the response of previously sensitized CD4-positive T cells.

Unlike the IgE-dependent type I allergies, the conditions described in this chapter are rarely life-threatening, though they may cause considerable discomfort. Many of the most common examples of cytotoxic hypersensitivity can be avoided by careful work in the hematology laboratory. The immune complex hypersensitivities can often be avoided once their origin has been identified. The DTH conditions are either easily avoided (contact dermatitis) or of no consequence to health (allergy

279

of infection). Because of these differences from type I hypersensitivity, desensitization is seldom attempted for the hypersensitivities described in this chapter.

The two examples of cytotoxic hypersensitivity included in this chapter both involve blood groups—the ABO and the Rh systems. In the section on immune complex hypersensitivity, serum sickness, the Arthus reaction, and immune complex pneumonitis—a natural expression of the Arthus reaction—are described. The chapter ends with a section on delayed-type hypersensitivity exemplified by allergy of infection and contact dermatitis.

Cytotoxic Hypersensitivity

On a daily basis the alloantigens of human erythrocytes are more a part of medical practice than most other antigens. Hardly a patient entering a hospital escapes routine blood-grouping tests. Most forms of hemolytic disease of the newborn, most blood transfusion problems, and certain medicolegal situations demand the attention of immunohematologists. Erythrocyte antigens and their antibodies are important in tissue transplantation immunity, although they are not considered histocompatibility antigens per se. Antibodies that react with and destroy cellular antigens, usually with the aid of complement, are responsible for the cytotoxic hypersensitivities. The antibodies are usually IgG, with some contribution by IgM and possibly by other immunoglobulins.

THE ABO BLOOD GROUP SYSTEM

Discovery

Karl Landsteiner received a Nobel prize in medicine and physiology in 1930 for his discovery some 30 years earlier of the ABO blood group system. Landsteiner collected the erythrocytes and serum from the blood of several of his laboratory associates, incubated each red blood cell suspension with each serum, and observed the mixtures for hemagglutination. He never observed a person's serum to agglutinate his own erythrocytes, but he did observe hemagglutination in a number of the reciprocal mixtures. From these results he established the four ABO blood groups.

The ABO Groups

The **four blood groups** are A, B, AB, and O. Individuals with blood group A have an antigen on their erythrocytes, arbitrarily assigned the letter A; those with group B blood have a different antigen, given the letter B, on their erythrocytes. The serum of an individual from one of these groups will clump the red blood cells of a person in the other group, and the serum from an individual in either of these groups will clump the cells of a person in a third, the AB group. These reactions are compatible with the presence of an antibody, anti-B in group A sera and anti-A in group B sera. Persons having blood group AB possess both of the corresponding antigens on their red blood cells, which are agglutinated by both sera. Group AB persons lack both anti-A and anti-B. A person in the fourth group, group O, has neither the A nor the B antigen but has both anti-A and anti-B in the serum. Sera from a group O individual will agglutinate the red blood cells of a person in any of the other three groups (Table 13–1).

Subgroups of group A are known. The two most frequent of the A subgroups are A_1 and A_2, and these are present in a ratio of about 4:1. It has recently been recognized that slightly different but cross-reacting antigens account for the A_1 and A_2 specificities.

Table 13–1
HUMAN ABO BLOOD GROUPS

| Blood Group | % | Antigen on RBC | GENETIC POSSIBILITIES | | Antibody in Blood |
			Homozygous	Heterozygous	
A	42	A	AA	AO	Anti-B
B	10	B	BB	BO	Anti-A
AB	3	A and B	—	AB	Neither anti-A nor anti-B
O	45	Neither A nor B	OO	—	Both anti-A and anti-B

The Polysaccharide Precursor

The major human blood group, the ABO blood group system, is founded on the chemistry of two antigens, the A and B antigens. The **immunodominant portion** of the A and the B antigens is a **terminal oligosaccharide** located on a protein anchored in the red blood cell membrane. The A and B antigens arise from a precursor substance that serves as a core for other erythrocyte antigens as well. In fact, there are two variations in the structure of the core, one of which is a D-galactosyl β-1,3-N-acetyl-D-glucosaminyl β-1,3-D-galactosyl β-1,3-N-acetyl-D-galactosamine. The other tetrasaccharide core is composed of exactly the same four sugars, but the galactose-acetylglucosamine bond is a β-1,4 linkage rather than a 1,3 linkage. In either case this polysaccharide is the immunodominant portion of a large glycoprotein molecule. It is typical of many terminal units of large molecules to have a high antigenic potency.

The H Substance

An additional monosaccharide, fucose, is added to the terminal galactose of the precursor to create the pentasaccharide known as the **H substance**. The fucose is linked to the final D-galactose unit of the precursor molecule by an α1,2 bond. The H substance is present on all human erythrocytes and is the immediate precursor to the A and B antigens. To form *the A antigen,* an *N-acetyl-D-galactosamine is attached* by an α1,3 bond to the end galactose, *and the B antigen is formed by adding a D-galactose by an α1,3 bond* to this same galactose of the H substance (Fig. 13–1). The A and B antigens are either present independent of each other (groups A and B), together (group AB), or not formed from the H substance (group O). Biochemically, a group O person can be described as lacking the requisite galactosyl transferase to form the B antigen and lacking the galactosylamino transferase needed to form the A antigen. Obviously individuals with blood group AB have both of these enzymes, and those with A or B have one or the other of the transferases.

Inheritance of ABO System

The distribution of the ABO antigens varies from one ethnic or racial group to another, but in the United States average figures are 45% group O, 42% group A, 10% group B, and 3% group AB. American blacks are about 28% group A and 20% group B, with a similar incidence of O and AB as in the population as a whole.

Synthesis of the A or B antigens is a genetic characteristic. Group O persons are homozygotic and are genotypically OO, whereas AB persons are genetically AB heterozygotes. Group A and B persons may be either homozygotes (AA and BB) or heterozygotes

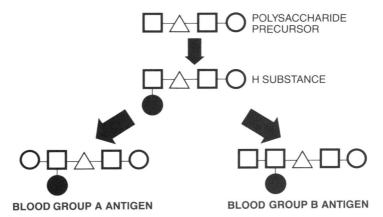

POLYSACCHARIDE PRECURSOR

H SUBSTANCE

BLOOD GROUP A ANTIGEN

BLOOD GROUP B ANTIGEN

Figure 13-1. The derivation of the H substance from the polysaccharide precursor is affected by the addition of a fucose. The A antigen is formed by adding N-acetyl-D-galactosamine, and the B antigen by adding D-galactose to the H substance. The open circles represent N-acetyl-D-galactosamine, the open square D-galactose. The dark circle and triangle represent fucose and N-acetyl-D-glucosamine, respectively.

(AO or BO). Inheritance of these genes is apparently by simple mendelian genetics, a fact that is of considerable importance in forensic medicine. The antigens appear early in fetal life as soon as the red blood cells are formed, and may be found in a soluble form in the body fluids of approximately 78% of the population. Secretion of soluble A, B, or H substances into saliva, serum, urine, gastric juice, and so forth, is regulated by the dominant secretor (Se) gene.

Origin of the Antibodies

One of the uncertainties concerning the ABO blood group system regards the origin of these **alloantibodies**. These antibodies (usually of the IgM class) are barely detectable in the sera of newborn infants but increase rapidly in titer during the first few months of life. This fact has been used to evaluate the maturation rate of the "bursal equivalent" in infants. Because there is a stepwise development of these antibodies, it has been suggested that inapparent immunizations in infancy may

be responsible for the production of anti-A and anti-B. Many intestinal bacteria that are a part of the normal flora, *Escherichia coli*, *Klebsiella*, and certain intestinal pathogens in the genera *Salmonella* and *Shigella* have **polysaccharide antigens that cross-react** with the human A and B antigens. According to this hypothesis, all infants are exposed to these bacteria and thus to both the A and B antigens. Group A persons form only anti-B and not anti-A, because their own A antigen has conferred a specific immunologic tolerance on them that prevents a response to the A antigen. Similar logic explains the formation of the B antibodies. Because group AB persons have both antigens, they form neither anti-A nor anti-B.

Blood Grouping

The goal of a blood transfusion is to provide the exact antigenic type of blood that the recipient has. It is difficult to achieve this goal, but it can be closely approached in terms of the major antigens if certain hemagglutination tests, called the major and minor cross match, are performed. The **major cross match**, now renamed the **compatibility test**, is performed by mixing the serum of the recipient with the red blood cells of the donor. If hemagglutination occurs, this blood cannot be given to the recipient for the obvious reason that he or she has antibodies capable, with complement and phagocytosis, of destroying the administered cells. In the **minor cross match** the recipient's red blood cells are incubated with serum of the donor and observed for agglutination. Again, if hemagglutination occurs the donor's blood should not be given because it contains antibodies capable of attacking the recipient's erythrocytes. A positive minor cross match destroys the earlier concept that group O persons are universal donors and group AB persons are universal recipients. Group O blood contains both anti-A and anti-B and can only match with group O blood. Such blood is sometimes transfused in emergency situations on the assumption that the antibodies will be diluted beyond their reactive titer in the recipient (Fig. 13–2).

It is also desirable to determine ex-actly which of the major blood group antigens are on the donor's erythrocytes even if they are not agglutinated by the recipient's serum. For example, if the donor were Rh-positive, group A, and the recipient were Rh-negative, group A, the compatibility test would predict a safe transfusion. That would be true in the first instance, but the transfusion would immunize the person to the Rh antigen, with potentially serious results in the next transfusion or in an eventual Rh-positive pregnancy. (The Rh antigen system is described later.)

Transfusion Reactions

When the recipient of a blood transfusion receives blood that contains antigens serologically reactive with his or her antibodies, the person will quickly develop severe chills, nausea, low back pain, hemoglobinuria, and jaundice. The concept that these transfusion reactions rely almost exclusively on lysis of the donated red blood cells by complement and antibody has been challenged. Recent studies have demonstrated a significant removal of the mismatched erythrocytes by macro-

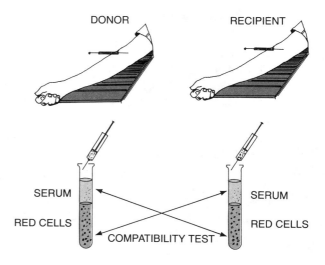

Figure 13–2. The acceptability of blood for transfusion is based on cross-matching cells and serum from the donor and the recipient. The most important of these crosses is the compatibility test, the mixture of donor cells with the recipient's serum. If no hemagglutination occurs, the transfusion is usually successful.

phages in the spleen. It is within the macrophages that cytolysis occurs. Phagocytosis and red cell destruction in the spleen account for the low back pain observed in **transfusion reactions**.

Forensic Medicine

Medicolegal decisions associated with the *identification of parents, of other kinships*, and of potentially *misidentified babies* in the newborn nursery may be resolved by knowledge of the inheritance of blood group antigens. These problems can only be solved by exclusion and not by inclusion. For example, if a rape victim gave birth to a group O child, an AB man cannot be implicated as the father because he would transmit either the A or B characteristic to the child. Because of the possibility of heterozygous group A and B men as well as group O men transmitting the O gene, they are potential fathers if the mother is group O. These men (group AO, BO, and OO) would include 97% of all males, and the proof of any one of them being the

father cannot be determined by blood group analysis. The AB male can be excluded, however.

At present, the reliance of forensic medicine on the ABO and other blood group systems to solve medicolegal problems is diminishing. Identification by means of the HLA antigens is much more exact because so many more antigens are involved (see Chapter 9).

THE Rh SYSTEM

Discovery

The **Rh factor** was originally described as an *antigen common to 85%* of all human erythrocytes (in those who are therefore defined as Rh-positive persons), and to the erythrocytes of the rhesus monkey. It is now known that the human and rhesus antigens are not identical but are strongly cross-reactive. Naturally occurring *Rh alloantibodies are not present in that 15% of the population that is Rh negative*. Antibodies to the Rh antigens develop from overt immunizations. The Rh-negative person does not automatically have Rh antibodies in his or her serum. Consequently, the Rh system could not be discovered by cross-testing human red blood cells and sera. The Rh system was discovered by hemagglutination testing of rabbit antimonkey red blood cell sera with human erythrocytes.

Nomenclature Systems

It is now clear that there is a *battery of Rh antigens*, not just a single antigen. At first it was believed there were six of these Rh antigens; now the number is in excess of 45. The evolution of new antigen discoveries prompted changes in the nomenclature for these antigens.

The alphabetic designation of the original six Rh antigens, which used both lowercase and uppercase letters

---

MEMORY CHECK 13 – 1

The ABO blood group

1. A antigen is built by adding acetylgalactosamine to the H substance
2. B antigen is built by adding galactose to the H substance
3. Antibodies are developed through immunization with cross-reactive antigens
4. Is being replaced by HLA for forensic purposes
5. Compatibility test could result in recipient immunization to donor red cell antigens

(C, D, E, c, d, e), has gradually fallen into disfavor. It is being replaced by the Wiener nomenclature system, in which Rh in uppercase or lowercase letters, supplemented by subscripts and superscripts, is employed. The move to adopt a new naming system stems in part from the fact that Wiener's hypothesis for the inheritance of the Rh antigens, which used his nomenclature, has proved more acceptable to geneticists than other hypotheses. Examples of Wiener's system include Rh_O, rh′, hr′, Rh^A, and so on. In this system, Rh_O is equivalent to D of the original six antigens, which is equivalent to Rh-positive (Table 13–2).

Immunoglobulins directed against the Rh antigens do not differ significantly from antibodies against other red blood cell antigens, except that, as mentioned, the alloantibodies arise from known immunizations and do not occur "naturally." One source of human anti-Rh antibodies is the Rh-negative person who has been immunized by a blood transfusion with Rh-positive blood. For simplicity, Rh-positive in this discussion refers to the Rh_O (D) antigen. All humans possess one or another of the Rh antigens; thus, everyone could be described as "Rh-positive." However, the D antigen,

which is one of the most potent Rh antigens, is accorded the honor of being referred to as "the Rh factor." Another route of immunization is through the exposure of an Rh-negative mother to the blood of her Rh-positive child during birth. In some studies, as many as 50% of the mothers were shown to have fetal erythrocytes in their circulation shortly after delivery. Abortion under similar circumstances (Rh-positive child and Rh-negative mother) could also be an immunizing experience.

Hemolytic Disease of the Newborn

When a pregnant, Rh-negative woman has circulating anti-Rh_O simultaneously with an Rh_O-positive fetus, the stage is set for the development of **erythroblastosis fetalis**, now more frequently referred to as **hemolytic disease of the newborn (HDN)**. The Rh-positive child must inherit the Rh_O antigen from the father, since the mother is Rh-negative. Such marriages were once described as Rh-incompatible because only this type of mating can lead to Rh-positive children. If the father is homozygous, all children would be Rh-positive; if he is heterozygous, statistically 50% of the children would be Rh-positive and at risk for HDN. HDN is an alloimmune disease caused by the placental transmigration of maternal IgG that is specific for the Rh-positive fetal erythrocytes (Fig. 13–3). Usually this means anti-Rh_O, but HDN caused by maternal IgG specific for other erythrocyte antigens can occur. Simple ABO incompatibilities seldom lead to neonatal hemolytic disease unless the mother has been hyperimmunized and has a high level of IgG. In the absence of overt immunization, the usual ABO allohemagglutinin

Table 13–2
SIMPLIFIED CLASSIFICATION OF
HUMAN Rh BLOOD GROUP*

Fisher-Race Designation	Wiener Designation
C	rh′
D	Rh_O
E	rh″
c	hr′
d	—
e	hr″

*Approximately 50 additional antigens are classified as Rh antigens.

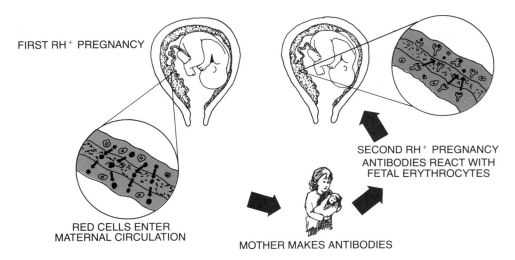

FIRST RH$^+$ PREGNANCY

SECOND RH$^+$ PREGNANCY
ANTIBODIES REACT WITH
FETAL ERYTHROCYTES

RED CELLS ENTER
MATERNAL CIRCULATION

MOTHER MAKES ANTIBODIES

Figure 13–3. Hemolytic disease of the newborn (HDN) is caused by immunization by fetal erythrocytes of an Rh$^-$ mother at birth. In a subsequent pregnancy anti-Rh$^+$ antibodies enter the fetal circulation and cause HDN.

is an IgM that cannot transgress the placental barrier.

When maternal anti-Rh$_O$ IgG enters the fetal circulation and combines with Rh positive erythrocytes, the presence of complement and phagocytic cells ensures destruction of the fetal erythrocytes. Immature erythrocytes (erythroblasts) enter the circulation from the bone marrow to compensate for the loss of the mature red blood cells, creating the condition of erythroblastosis fetalis. This may terminate the pregnancy in a stillbirth or a live abortion, or in milder cases the child may not give much evidence of the disease until the first hours after birth during its physiologic adjustment period.

Coombs' Testing

Indirect Coombs' Test. To determine if the mother has antibodies against Rh antigens that might lead to HDN, it is only necessary to incubate a portion of her serum with Rh-positive cells and observe for hemagglutination. A negative test result does not necessarily

mean that Rh antibodies are absent. Because nonagglutinating antibodies are potentially destructive in vivo, a determination for their presence is mandatory. This is accomplished by the **indirect Coombs' test**, which requires two incubation steps. The first of these is the incubation of *maternal serum* with known Rh-positive cells, and in the absence of hemagglutination at this stage, a second incubation with antihuman gamma globulin is conducted. A positive result after this second incubation is proof that the mother has anti-Rh globulins that could cause HDN (Fig. 13–4).

Direct Coombs' Test. In the case of the newborn infant who is developing jaundice or has other signs of hemolytic disease, the **direct Coombs' test** is used. *Erythrocytes of the neonate* are exposed to *antihuman gamma globulin* and observed for hemagglutination. If hemagglutination occurs, the infant's red blood cells are coated with antibody and are at risk for immunolysis. In the direct Coombs' test, only one incubation period is necessary because

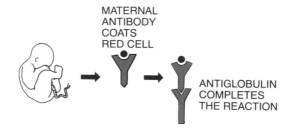

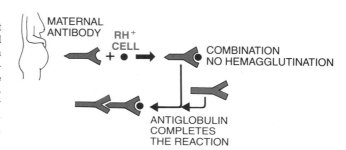

Figure 13–4. In the direct Coombs' test (*upper panel*) fetal erythrocytes coated in vivo with maternal antibody are agglutinated by the antiglobulin. In the indirect test (*lower panel*), maternal antibody is reacted with Rh+ erythrocytes, which are then agglutinated by antiglobulin in a subsequent incubation.

the first incubation was performed in vivo.

Rh Immunoprophylaxis

The problem, of course, is what medical steps should be taken if the indirect Coombs' test result were positive. In the case of a positive direct Coombs' test result, an exchange transfusion may be indicated, but positive indirect tests, especially when noted early in a pregnancy, constitute a difficult medical problem. As with most situations, the prevention is simpler than the cure, and the prevention of Rh immunization of women is a superb example of how basic immunologic studies led to a practical solution of a serious medical situation. The passive administration of an antiserum to an antigen, simultaneous with the antigen itself, blocks the formation of antibodies to that antigen—a form of **immunoglobulin-induced immunosuppression**. To

this knowledge was added the information that blood group O, Rh-negative mothers had fewer infants with hemolytic disease than statistics would predict. It was surmised in these situations that the natural maternal anti-A and anti-B combined with any A-positive, Rh-positive or B-positive, Rh-positive fetal erythrocytes and hastened their removal from the maternal circulation without antibody formation. Evidence was already accumulating that most maternal immunizations with Rh antigens occurred at childbirth; therefore, if anti-Rh_O were administered just after birth, it should prevent maternal sensitization to the antigen. This was tested, and proved a tremendous success. In one study 173 mothers were given the antibody and only one became immunized at delivery. In the control group of 176 mothers not given anti-Rh_O, 38 developed anti-Rh_O. *Administration of anti-Rh_O is now considered a regular part of perinatal care. It* must be given at the first and every succeeding pregnancy; once the woman has formed the antibodies (which is also possible from mismatched blood transfusions or abortions), anti-Rh$_0$ gamma globulins are ineffective in preventing later episodes of HDN.

MEMORY CHECK 13–2

In the Rh system

1. "Natural" immunization is not responsible for anti-Rh antibodies; immunization requires exposure to Rh-positive blood
2. Rh$_0$ or D is equivalent to the original Rh antigen
3. The direct Coombs' test detects maternal antibody on the child's red blood cells
4. The indirect Coombs' test detects maternal Rh antibodies
5. Sensitization to HDN can be prevented by treatment with anti-Rh$_0$ at each delivery of an Rh-positive child

Immune Complex Hypersensitivity

The immune complex hypersensitivities share with several other immunologic phenomena an inappropriate name. The type I and type II hypersensitivities are based on the formation of a complex between an antigen and an antibody, as much as the type III immune complex allergies. The difference is only that the **type III hypersensitivities** begin with a *soluble, cell-free immune complex*. These complexes in themselves are not particularly distressing from the viewpoint of good health.

The seriousness of immune complex diseases can be related to the ratio of antigen to antibody in the circulating complex. Mononuclear phagocytic cells, especially of the liver and spleen, efficiently clear the blood of complexes in which the proportion of antibody exceeds that of antigen, but when complexes in the zone of *antigen excess* are formed, *clearance is incomplete*. Whether the complex contains an excess of antigen and would thus favor the development of an immune complex disease is related to the phase of antibody production and to the number of antibody-binding sites on the antigen. Thus, the early phase of antibody production to a soluble antigen with numerous binding sites would favor the deposition of immune complexes on cell membranes rather than phagocytic elimination.

Most of the tissue injury from immune complexes follows their deposition on the *walls of the blood vessels* or their removal by the *filtration apparatus of the kidney*. The generation of C5a by complexes that contain IgG or IgM is responsible for the chemotactic appearance of granulocytes which then displace endothelial cells to reach the immune deposits. Proteinuria develops as a result of kidney damage. Inflammation is not entirely restricted to the scene of immune complex deposition but may be seen elsewhere when sufficient amounts of the C3a, C4a, and C5a anaphylatoxins are released.

SERUM SICKNESS

Serum sickness is a condition that formerly developed in 50% of the humans who received injections of bovine or horse antitoxin against tetanus, gas gangrene, or other toxins for prophylactic or therapeutic purposes. Antitoxin therapy is less frequently practiced today because of the superiority of active immunizations with toxoids to prevent these diseases. **Serum sickness** still occurs in transplant recipients who receive *foreign animal sera* (antilymphocyte globulin) as part of their immunosuppressive regimen. A serum sickness–like syndrome may also follow injections of other materials including penicillin and other drugs.

Primary Serum Sickness

Ordinary serum sickness is an allergic reaction that is accompanied by the development of marked edema, especially about the face, neck, and joints; joint pain; and hives; in addition to malaise and fever. These symptoms of serum sickness do not present themselves until about 5 to 10 days after the injection of a substantial quantity of antigen or autocoupling hapten. It should be recalled that this is the time normally required before circulating antibodies are detectable in the blood. Because of the magnitude of the dose of antigen previously injected, antigen and antibody coexist in the circulation and can form immune complexes. These immune complexes deposit on the walls of blood vessels and are often trapped in the kidney, where they cause **immune complex nephritis**. These complexes, via the chemoattraction of neutrophils, may cause damage wherever they deposit.

The C3a, C4a, and C5a anaphylatoxins that arise from the complement system during its activation cause the release of histamine from mast cells. Likewise, kinins are generated from the blood proteins. These vasoactive compounds are responsible for the edema seen in serum sickness. The immune complexes and neutrophils are responsible for the tissue destruction seen in this form of allergy.

It should be noted that in serum sickness the sensitizing and shocking doses of antigen are one and the same.

It is the magnitude of antigen used that allows it to persist until antibody appears in the bloodstream.

Accelerated Serum Sickness

An accelerated form of serum sickness can develop in a person previously sensitized to an antigen, when the antigen is given for a second time. **Accelerated serum sickness** appears within 2 or 3 days after the antigen injection. This early appearance of the symptoms is due to the function of the second antigen exposure as an anamnestic booster that causes a sharp outpouring of immunoglobulin G into the blood over the subsequent few hours or days. Within a briefer time than in primary serum sickness, a sufficient quantity of immune complexes is available to express the symptoms of serum sickness.

THE ARTHUS REACTION

When a soluble antigen is injected repeatedly into the skin of an individual, ultimately high levels of circulating IgG are produced. If the quantity of antigen injected into the skin is sufficiently large, it will diffuse through the local tissues and enter the vascular bed, where it can combine with this antibody. This results in the formation of an antigen-antibody complex of such magnitude that physical precipitation occurs (Fig. 13–5). This precipitate may be so extensive that blockage of the small venules draining the surrounding area deprives the local region of proper gas exchange, prevents a proper supply of nutrients and disposal of waste products, and results in death of the neighboring tissues. The **necrotic lesion** that appears is known as the **Arthus reaction**.

The influence of the Arthus reaction on modern medical practice has been simply to eliminate repeated intrader-

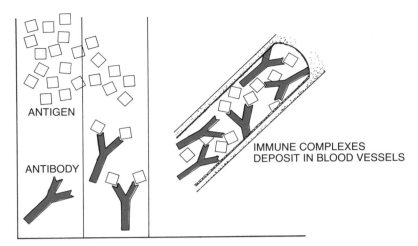

ANTIGEN

ANTIBODY

IMMUNE COMPLEXES
DEPOSIT IN BLOOD VESSELS

Figure 13-5. In immune complex disease, a large dose of antigen is followed by an outpouring of antibody. As the immune complex of antigen and antibody accumulates, it will bind C3b. The complex may deposit on blood vessel walls or physically occlude the smaller vessels.

mal injections of antigen into the skin wherever possible. For example, booster injections of the vaccine against pneumococcal pneumonia are not recommended for fear of provoking an Arthus reaction. However, injections of drugs that can function as autocoupling haptens or which can be converted to autocoupling haptens in vivo can provoke the Arthus reaction. Particulate or cellular antigens are not involved in Arthus reactions.

IMMUNE COMPLEX PNEUMONITIS

A human ailment referred to variously as **immune complex pneumonitis, allergic pneumonitis**, or **hypersensitivity pneumonitis** is a natural expression of the Arthus reaction. This condition is one in which persons exposed to *atmospheres heavily laden with antigens* develop a pneumonitis. Since this is often associated with specific occupations or avocations, a number of synonyms have been applied to the disease to reflect this. Thus, we have such

terms as **farmer's lung, bird fancier's lung, pigeon breeder's lung, cheese washer's disease**, and so forth, as descriptive terms for conditions that share a common immunologic base (Table 13-3).

Individuals who regularly inhale antigen-loaded air are being immunized by one of the most efficient routes known. After a period of time, high levels of IgG are achieved in the circulation, and when antigen is again inhaled deeply in to the lung, Arthus reactions develop deep within the alveoli. These small areas of necrosis develop slowly over several hours after the inhalation of the antigen and, as a consequence of this, the symptoms of the illness are not at first associated with the person's occupation or hobby. However, a medical history and physical examination will usually uncover the nature and source of the antigen. For farmer's lung, the most common antigen is spores of *Thermoactinomyces* fungi that grow in silage and moldy hay. These or other molds are associated with **mushroom worker's lung, bagassosis, malt worker's lung,**

Table 13-3
VARIETIES OF IMMUNE COMPLEX PNEUMONITIS

Disease	Source of Antigen	Antigen
Farmer's lung	Moldy hay	*Thermoactinomyces vulgaris*
Mushroom worker's lung	Compost	Thermophilic actinomycetes
Bird fancier's lung	Dry bird droppings	Avian proteins
Pigeon breeder's lung	Pigeon dander or droppings	Pigeon proteins
Bagassosis	Moldy bagasse	Thermophilic actinomycetes
Maple bark pneumonitis	Maple bark dust	*Cryptostroma corticale*
Malt worker's lung	Moldy barley	*Aspergillus clavatus*
Wheat weevil disease (miller's lung)	Infected flour	*Sitophilus granarius*
Sequoiosis	Moldy sawdust	*Graphium* species
Humidifier allergy	Humidifier, hot tub water	*Thermoactinomyces*
Suberosis	Cork dust	*Penicillium* species

maple bark pneumonitis, and cheese washer's disease. Bird fancier's lung and pigeon breeder's lung arise from sensitization to antigens in bird droppings and dander, which are wafted into the air by the beating wings of the birds.

MEMORY CHECK 13-3
◆
Immune complex hypersensitivity is

1. Highly dependent on the activity of neutrophils
2. Often expressed as a glomerulonephritis
3. Responsible for allergic pneumonitis
4. Related to high IgG titers

Delayed-Type Hypersensitivity

Cell-mediated hypersensitivity as a synonym for CD4[+] T cell–dependent hypersensitivity is a misnomer and fortunately is falling into disuse. The term

arose before it was not known that T cells secrete peptides, the interleukins, that are responsible for their specific kind of hypersensitive response and other immune functions. Unlike the immunoglobulin products of B cells, interleukins rarely achieve high titers in the blood. Consequently, the transfer of a T-cell hypersensitivity from an allergic person to a nonallergic individual required the transfer of living T cells. It is currently possible to effect successful transfers of DTH with concentrates of T-cell culture fluids or with extracts of the T cells.

ALLERGY OF INFECTION

The Prototype Tuberculin Reaction

The prototype of allergies of infection is the **tuberculin skin reaction**. The tuberculin skin reaction was discovered by Robert Koch in his early studies of tuberculosis at the end of the last century. Koch found that the intradermal injection of concentrated culture filtrates of *Mycobacterium tuberculosis* into tuberculous guinea pigs caused a gradual reddening and thickening of the skin around the injection site. These features developed over 24 to 72 hours and were usually maximal at 48 hours, after which they gradually disappeared. Similar injections into normal guinea pigs were innocuous. Later it was found that injections of these culture filtrates into human beings would produce a similar kind of skin reaction if the person had tuberculosis or had recovered from an earlier infection with the tubercle bacillus. Thus, positive tuberculin skin test reactions are not diagnostic of a concurrent infection but will detect the allergy that results from the infection. Remember that allergy is defined as any unexpected response to an antigen or hapten.

Old Tuberculin and Purified Protein Derivative

The original preparation of Koch is known as **old tuberculin (OT)**. OT is prepared from a culture medium in which *M. tuberculosis* has grown for several weeks. The bacteria are heat killed and removed by filtration. The culture fluid is then evaporated to one-tenth its original volume, reclarified, tested for potency, and used as OT. The active factor in OT is a peptide — **purified protein derivative (PPD)** — with a molecular weight of only 2000 that can be precipitated with trichloroacetic acid. After being returned to solution and passing potency tests, it too is used in skin testing. Other peptides contained in OT may also have some activity in eliciting the delayed-type hypersensitivity reaction. Because these peptides are all below the threshold of antigenicity, repeated skin testing will not convert a person to a positive reactor status.

DTH Tests and Infectious Disease

Many infections may induce a **delayed type of dermal hypersensitivity**, ranging from the submicroscopic viruses to the large animal parasites. Skin testing reagents are available for a large number of bacterial infections, including tuberculosis, leprosy, diphtheria, brucellosis, and streptococcal infections. These are infrequently used for diagnostic purposes but are used for epidemiologic studies to evaluate the range of disease or to detect the presence of disease in certain areas. The reagents used in testing for viral diseases are often the materials that comprise the vaccines, as is the case in mumps. Skin tests for viral diseases use intact viral particles rather than purified proteins. Tests for DTH reactions to viral infections are uncommonly used in medicine (Table 13–4).

The reagents used to skin test for the fungal diseases are highly cross-reactive and can only be diagnostic of a previous or concurrent infection when coupled with other information. For example, if a person's test result was negative last month but is positive now, the conclusion of an active, current disease is logical. In addition, many of the fungal testing reagents stimulate the formation of circulating antibodies, and, because the presence of these antibodies is often critical in diagnosing fungal infections, the fungal skin testing reagents should be used only under special circumstances. Such products as blastomycin, coccidioidin, and histoplasmin fall into this category.

A more recent use of these skin testing reagents has been to evaluate the function of the T-cell system. This is possible because certain dermatophyte and yeast (*Candida albicans*) infections are almost universal, and a fail-

Table 13-4

SKIN TESTS FOR DELAYED-TYPE HYPERSENSITIVITY TO INFECTIOUS DISEASE

Disease	Name of Test	Reagent
Tuberculosis	Mantoux, Vollmer, Tine, and so on	Old tuberculin (OT) or its purified protein derivative (PPD)
Leprosy	Lepromin (Mitsuda)	Extract of lepromatous tissue
Glanders	Straus reaction	Mallein
Diphtheria	Moloney	Diphtheria toxoid
Brucellosis	Brucellergen	Heat-killed organism
Tularemia	Foshay	Bacterial protein antigen
Streptococcal infection	—	Streptokinase-streptodornase
Viral Diseases		
Lymphogranuloma	Frei	Inactive virus
Smallpox	—	Vaccinia virus
Mumps	—	Mumps virus vaccine
Fungal Diseases		
Histoplasmosis	Histoplasmin	Concentrate of mycelial culture medium
Coccidioidomycosis	Coccidioidin	Concentrate of mycelial culture medium
	Spherulin	Concentrate of yeast culture medium
Blastomycosis	Blastomycin	Concentrate of mycelial culture medium
Candidiasis	Candidin, oidomycin	Concentrate of yeast culture
Epidermophytosis	Trichophytin	Concentrate of mycelial culture medium

ure to express a delayed-type hypersensitive reaction to their products means a failure of T cells rather than a lack of infection.

Tissue Histology

The cellular morphology of delayed-type hypersensitivity skin reactions in humans has been thoroughly analyzed. There is a greater participation of basophils and mast cells in these reactions than is generally recognized. Early in the development of the reaction there is an infiltration of basophils from the vascular system and a piecemeal degranulation of these cells. Fixed tissue mast cells also degranulate, and this is followed by an increase in vascular permeability as the products of these granules influence the vascular bed. This is further exemplified by vascular compaction, extravasation of erythrocytes, and fibrin deposition as the clotting mechanism is activated. The peak intensity of the reaction is between the second and fourth days. By this time a significant infiltration of macrophages dominates the histology of the erythematous, indurated reaction site.

Interleukins in DTH Reactions

Specific products of the CD4$^+$ lymphocyte are known to contribute to the DTH reaction. Primary among these are the **T-cell chemotaxin** and the **macrophage migration inhibition factor (MIF)**. The T-cell chemotaxin secreted by sensitized T cells upon recontact with antigen is a peptide of only 12,500 molecular weight. Distribution of this protein through the blood allows it to attract monocytes. These monocytes enter the reaction site and encounter MIF (32,500 molecular weight), and their mobility is arrested. In this locale the monocytes transform into macrophages and encounter other T cell products such as IFN-γ. This further activates the macrophages that become hyperphagocytic and engulf and destroy antigen, thereby gradually returning the tissue site to its normal histology.

Transfer Factor

An additional product of the DTH T cell should be mentioned here because it is able to effect a cell-free transfer of DTH from a positive reactor to an unsensitized recipient. The product responsible for this is antigen-specific, unlike the interleukins. That is, if the donor's reaction is DTH-positive to PPD but not to histoplasmin, that person's T cells or T-cell extracts will transfer only sensitivity to PPD. **Transfer factor (TF)**, as the product is called, has been elusive and difficult to characterize. It is a nonantigenic, polypeptide-polynucleotide complex in the molecular weight range of 700 to 4000. It is not a DNA and does not permanently transform the response specificity of recipient T cells, although the acquired sensitivity has a duration of several weeks or months. This reagent, TF, has been useful in treating chronic

mucocutaneous candidiasis (see Chapter 8).

CONTACT DERMATITIS

Intermittent or constant dermal contact with a wide selection of chemicals may induce the form of T-cell–dependent hypersensitivity known as **contact dermatitis**. Such chemicals are present as dyes in leather, elastic, or cloth products; as cosmetics and hair dyes; as staining reagents, and as a multitude of other products. A number of chemicals found in various industries such as the rubber industry, the detergent or cosmetic industry, and the photographic and plastic industries, also contain chemicals that are hypersensitizing. Contact dermatitis is often associated with the specific area of the body in contact with the sensitizing reagent, such as the allergy that develops beneath a watchband, necklace, or bracelet, or on other areas of the body where cosmetics or certain clothing items come in regular contact. These products cause a delayed-type skin reaction of the chronic type in which there is usually a dry, scaly, thickened erythematous zone at and around the site of contact with the offending chemical. The anatomic distribution of these rashes is often helpful in eliminating other possible diagnoses such as skin infections or parasite infestations. The specific chemicals responsible for many of these reactions include formaldehyde; various metals such as mercury, nickel, and copper; special dyes such as potassium dichromate or paraphenylenediamine; and others. A complete listing of chemicals is not possible simply because of its magnitude.

Contact dermatitis also arises from exposure to natural plants such as **poi-**

son ivy, sumac, poison oak, primrose, mango, or others. In virtually every instance, these allergies are attributable to low molecular weight chemicals present on the leaves or other parts of these plants. Poison ivy allergy, for example, is a delayed-type hypersensitivity to substituted **urushiols** produced by the plant. The urushiols contain quinone groups, which can be reduced to hydroxyl groups. By a removal of a hydrogen atom, covalent coupling of these compounds to skin or tissue proteins forms neoantigens. The hypersensitivity that develops against these neoantigens is the actual cause of the allergic reaction. The urushiols produced by these plants are not directly toxic and cause no reaction upon first exposure to normal skin.

MEMORY CHECK 13–4
◆

Delayed-type hypersensitivity

1. Exists as an allergy of infection or contact dermatitis

2. Is a T-cell nonantibody–dependent allergy

3. Skin histology is related to the chemotaxin and migration inhibition factor released by T cells

4. DTH cell is a CD4-positive MHC class II–restricted T cell

5. Is transferable with transfer factor

References

Dahl, MV: Clinical immunodermatology, ed 2. Year Book Medical Publishers, Chicago, 1988.

Daniele, RP (ed): Immunology and Immunologic Diseases of the Lung. Blackwell Scientific Publications, Oxford, 1988.

Harmening, D, Calhoun, L, and Polesky, HF (eds): Modern Blood Banking and Transfusion Practices, ed 2. FA Davis, Philadelphia, 1989.

Middleton, E, Jr, et al (eds): Allergy, Principles and Practice, ed 3. CV Mosby, St Louis, 1988.

Norris, DA (ed): Immune Mechanisms in Cutaneous Disease. Marcel Dekker, New York, 1989.

Turgeon, ML: Fundamentals of Immunohematology: Theory and Technique. Lea & Febiger, Philadelphia, 1989.

QUESTIONS AND ANSWERS

---

1. The direct Coombs' test, as used to evaluate erythroblastosis fetalis, is a measure of
   A. Maternal Rh_O (D) antibody
   B. Maternal Rh_O (D) antigen
   C. Infant Rh_O (D) antigen
   D. Infant Rh_O (D) antibody
   E. Paternal Rh_O (D) antigen

Answer A

In the direct Coombs' test, red blood cells of newborn infant are incubated with antihuman gamma globulin. Hemagglutination is a positive test result and usually indicates the presence of maternal anti-Rh_O (D) on the child's erythrocytes. In rare instances, the maternal antibody could be directed against some other antigen.

2. Prevention of Rh hemolytic disease is based on
   A. The administration of maternal erythrocytes to the infant
   B. Passive immunization of the child with anti-Rh sera
   C. Neutralization of existing maternal anti-Rh globulins with excess antigen
   D. Steroidal immunosuppression, which normally accompanies childbirth
   E. None of the above

Answer E

Hemolytic disease of the newborn is preventable by anti-Rh_O passive immunization of the mother after the delivery of every Rh_O-positive child. This applies equally to abortion and natural delivery. As indicated in the answer to question 1, rare instances of HDN may be caused by other antigen-antibody systems.

3. Farmer's lung is an example of
   A. An IgG-related allergy
   B. An Arthus-type reaction
   C. An immune complex disease
   D. An allergic disease in which mold spores are often the offending antigen
   E. All of the above

Answer E

IgG is the primary antibody involved in Arthus reactions, which are examples of immune complex allergy. Farmer's lung customarily develops from the IgG response to mold spores in silage or hay.

4. Transfer factor is frequently considered different from an interleukin because
   A. It is not a protein
   B. It is antigen specific
   C. It contains nucleic acid–like properties
   D. It has a lower molecular weight than interleukins
   E. All of the above

Answer E

Interleukins are not antigen specific, and all of them appear to be low molecular weight proteins. Transfer factor is unlike the interleukins in all the respects listed in the question.

5. The major aspects of a dermal DTH reaction are caused by
   A. Mast-cell degranulation
   B. The activities of interleukins (lymphokines)
   C. Direct toxicity of agents applied to the skin
   D. The formation of immune complexes in the skin
   E. Lysis of T cells by cytotoxic antibody

Answer B

Mast cells are not extensively involved in DTH reactions, even though they do participate in these reactions. Interleukins, particularly the chemotaxins and migration inhibitors, have a central role. Contact dermatitis is an allergic, not a toxic, reaction. Antibody and CTLs are not essential for DTH reactions.

Case Study: The Skin Rash

Fred B. was a 75-year-old victim of a heart attack. Because of severe bursitis in a hip joint and low blood pressure, he had been taking aspirin and some "blood pressure pills" for several years. Antiarrhythmic drugs were added to the treatment regimen after his heart attack. His unusual toxic response to the experimental antiarrhythmic drugs under evaluation to regulate his ectopic heart contractions required the implantation of a pacemaker. At this time, he was also started on quinidine. Within 4 days, his ECG patterns had again stabilized and he was discharged. Six days later, Fred was readmitted with a light erythematous, intensely itching rash on his trunk, arms, and legs.

Questions

1. What is the probable etiology of Fred's dermatitis?

2. Are patients with heart disease more apt than others to develop a "skin rash"?

3. Why was Fred re-admitted to the hospital for a simple skin rash?

4. What is the recommended therapy in instances of this sort?

Discussion

Fred's dermatitis is almost certainly the result of a drug allergy. It is a hypersensitivity of the delayed type and is a T-cell–dependent allergy. Because Fred had been taking aspirin for his bursitis and other medications for low blood pressure for a long time, it is unlikely that they contributed to his present condition. The time required for the development and expression of a delayed hypersensitivity is 5 to 14 days; therefore, the search should be for some potential allergenic event occurring within that time frame.

Local anesthetics used during pacemaker implantation may be allergenic. Because such drugs were used only once in Fred's treatment, it is not likely that they are responsible for the current expression of his allergy. Chemical compounds used in the preparation of plasticware and in the plastics themselves may be released after implantation of catheters, pacemakers, dialysis tubing, and the like, but these are low-potency allergens. The most likely cause of allergy in Fred's case is quinidine, one of a family of compounds known to be potent allergens and known to be associated with the development of autoimmune hemolytic disease and thrombocytopenia.

Fred was readmitted to the hospital not because of the dermal allergy but because of an important aspect of the treatment. The treatment required removal of the inciting drug from the list of medications and its replacement with another antiarrhythmic drug, which meant that his ECG had to be monitored during this transition. An oral antihistamine and topical corticosteroids were used to alleviate the skin irritation. (Although the irritation would normally clear a few days after withdrawal of the quinidine, this treatment accelerates the process.)

GLOSSARY

allergy of infection   An allergy of the delayed type, caused by an infection.

Arthus reaction   A necrotic, dermal reaction caused by antigen-antibody precipitation.

cell-mediated hypersensitivity   Delayed-type hypersensitivity.

contact dermatitis   A delayed-type hypersensitivity to cutaneously applied allergens.

Coombs' test   An antiglobulin test to detect the presence of a nonhemagglutinating antibody on the surface of erythrocytes.

delayed-type hypersensitivity (DTH)   A form of allergy expressed by T lymphocytes and not involving immunoglobulins.

DTH cell   The $CD4^+$ T cell responsible for delayed-type hypersensitivities.

erythroblastosis fetalis   Hemolytic disease of the newborn due to the acquisition of maternal antibodies specific for fetal erythrocyte antigens.

HDN   Hemolytic disease of the newborn; see Erythroblastosis fetalis.

immune complex pneumonitis   An alveolar Arthus reaction with many synonyms.

OT   Old tuberculin.

PPD   Purified protein derivative of tuberculin.

serum sickness   An allergic reaction caused by the presence of antigen at the time that antibody is being formed.

transfer factor (TF)   A polynucleotide-polypeptide complex that can transfer DTH hypersensitivities.

tuberculin   A concentrate of the growth medium of *Mycobacterium tuberculosis* used to test skin for delayed hypersensitivity to this organism.

urushiols   Catechols found on poisonous plants, responsible for contact dermatitis.

Diagnostic Serology

In this chapter, a large array of serologic tests are described. Several of these are merely qualitative and reveal only the presence, not the quantity, of an antigen or antibody. Many of these tests are equally suitable with haptens or antigens. Others require antigens and are unsuitable with haptens. Certain of these tests are used to aid the diagnosis of infectious or autoimmune disease. Still others are useful in evaluating other conditions such as drug abuse, as well as endocrinologic function and antibiotic therapy. These are some of the features to keep in mind as the nine major variations of diagnostic serology are described in this chapter. These nine major serologic tests are the ligand-binding assays, including radioimmunoassays, enzyme-linked assays, and fluorescent antibody methods; nephelometric tests; precipitation tests; immunodiffusion tests (of which there are several variations); agglutination tests; flocculation; complement fixation; flow cytometry; and neutralization. These are described in this order after a general description of the serologic reaction.

The Serologic Reaction

THE DILUTION SERIES

The combination of an antigen in vitro with its specific antibody usually results in a physical change that is easily detected and serves as evidence of the serologic reaction. This physical change is not observed when the two reagents are in improper concentrations or proportions. To guard against the possibility of missing a serologic reaction, a **dilution series** of the antiserum is normally prepared, and each dilution is tested for its ability to react with a fixed concentration of antigen. In some instances this is reversed and the concentration of the antigen is varied and tested against a constant amount of antiserum. The dilution series is a crude means of estimating the amount of antibody in an antiserum. The greatest dilution at which an antiserum (or antibody) will produce a positive test is known as its **titer**, and comparisons of antiserum titer are useful in evaluating the relative potency of antisera when the two sera are tested under identical conditions.

There is a considerable difference in the ability of an antibody to detect tiny traces of antigen or hapten. Radioimmunoassays, enzyme-linked immunosorbent assays, neutralization, and complement fixation tests are usually considered the most sensitive (Table 14–1).

ZONES OF THE REACTION

In the first tubes of the dilution series, the excess of immunoglobulin compared with antigen favors the formation of **soluble aggregates**. This zone is known as the **prozone**. The prozone is followed by a series of several tubes in which steadily increasing amounts of the serologic product are formed, and then an additional few tubes in which the product dwindles in amount. At the far right of the dilution series no serologic product will be visible be-

Table 14–1
RELATIVE SENSITIVITY OF SEROLOGIC TESTS

Highly Sensitive
Radioimmunoassay
Enzyme-linked immunosorbent assay
Hemolysis
Complement fixation
Passive agglutination

Intermediate Sensitivity
Neutralization
Hemagglutination
Bacterial agglutination
Nephelometry

Low Sensitivity
Qualitative fluid precipitation
Immunodiffusion
Immunoelectrophoresis

cause of the excessive dilution of antibody; this area is known as the **postzone**.

PHASES OF THE REACTION

The serologic reaction occurs in **two phases**. The *first is* **combination**, in which antigen and antibody associate with each other but do not form a visible product. Combination of antigen with antibody depends upon a complementarity of the hypervariable regions of the L and H chains of the antibody with epitopes of the antigen. This is largely an **ionic association**, though **hydrogen bonding** and even hydrophobic groups influence this event. These bonds are infirm and are dissociable even though the equilibrium constant favors combination. Ultimately dissociation and recombination of the serologic complexes continues until the equilibrium state is reached. Eventually a **latticework** of alternating antigen and antibody molecules will develop in what is termed the **aggregation phase** of the serologic reaction. Because a hapten is essentially a single epitope, it can react with only one molecule of antibody and no latticework can be formed. Serologic reactions with soluble complete antigens result in precipitation, cellular or particulate antigens in agglutination, or, in the case of erythrocytes, hemagglutination.

MEMORY CHECK 14-1

1. Serologic reactions occur in two stages
   a. Stage one: Combination; it occurs immediately but is invisible
   b. Stage two: Aggregation; it requires time for dissociation and recombination to form a visible latticework
2. Dilution series will identify prozone, postzone, and titer

---

Ligand-Binding Assays

A **ligand** is any *molecule that forms a complex with another*. In the field of serology, haptens and antigens are considered as ligands that react with antibodies, and vice versa. Because the binding of antigen and antibody with each other frequently results in a visible reaction and reactions involving haptens do not, "ligand-binding" is often reserved to describe serologic reactions involving haptens.

RADIOIMMUNOASSAY

By careful radioiodination of antigens or immunoglobulins, the serologic be-havior of these proteins is not altered, and their release of beta or gamma particles is a sensitive detector of their location. This is the basis of radioimmunoassays (RIAs).

Solid-phase RIA

Solid-phase procedures can be varied for specific purposes, but to determine the quantity of an antigen in a preparation of unknown concentration the following protocol could be used. First the wells in the multiconcavity plate are rinsed with antiserum specific for the antigen to be quantitated. Many protein antigens bind nonspecifically to plastic or glass surfaces. This is sometimes described as coating with the **capture antibody**. Then the wells are rinsed with a **blocking protein** such as gelatin or bovine serum. The blocking protein will adsorb to the surface of the well not previously coated with antibody, and this will prevent the nonspecific attachment of antigen used in the third rinse. The fourth rinse is of a radiolabeled antibody specific for the antigen. After a brief incubation the excess antibody is removed by washing, and the amount of isotope bound to the concavity is a measure of the amount of antigen in the preparation.

Because an antibody is useful for antigen capture and another antibody is used for antigen quantitation, this is an example of a **double antibody** procedure. In this form of **solid-phase RIA**, haptens cannot be measured because they have no epitope remaining for combination with the second antibody. It is necessary to prepare a standard curve using different known concentrations of antigen. Only by comparing the experimental system against the standard can the quantity of antigen in the unknown be determined.

Competitive Inhibition RIA

Competitive inhibition assays also require preliminary experiments to produce a standard curve. For example, to measure the quantity of human growth hormone (HGH) in a serum sample, it is necessary to have anti-HGH adsorbed to the surface of concavities, block the surface with gelatin, and then add various amounts of radiolabeled HGH to the different concavities. After incubation and rinsing, the amount of label bound to the different wells is recorded and plotted.

After this standard determination to measure HGH bound to antibody (Fig. 14–1), a known quantity of isotopically labeled HGH is mixed with the unknown sample of HGH and added to the antibody-containing concavities. Because the two forms of HGH have an equal opportunity to attach to the fixed antibody, some of the radiolabeled HGH will be left free and can be rinsed from the concavity. Quantitation of the free HGH is used to calculate the amount of competing HGH. Conversely, the reduced amount of labeled HGH bound to the well is measured and used to calculate the amount of HGH in the sample.

In the simplest calculation, it can be seen that 100 molecules of IgG, because of its serologic valence of 2, will bind 200 parts of labeled HGH in the preliminary titration. If 200 parts of HGH in an unknown sample are mixed with 200 parts of isotopically labeled HGH, then 100 parts of labeled and 100 parts of unlabeled HGH will attach to the fixed antibody. Thus, a failure of 50% of the isotope to bind to the anti-HGH indicates that the unknown contained the same quantity of HGH as the known. Note that with necessary pre-

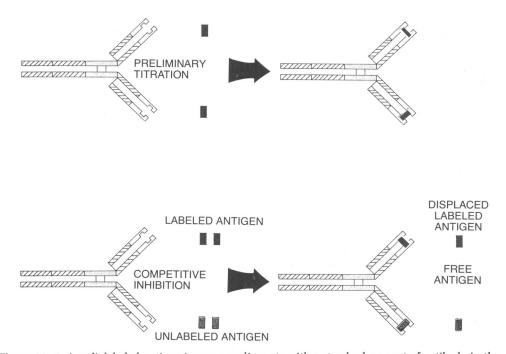

Figure 14–1. A radiolabeled antigen (*upper panel*) reacts with a standard amount of antibody in the preliminary titration. In the competitive inhibition assay (*lower panel*), the amount of isotopically labeled antigen unable to react with antibody is a measure of the unlabeled antigen added.

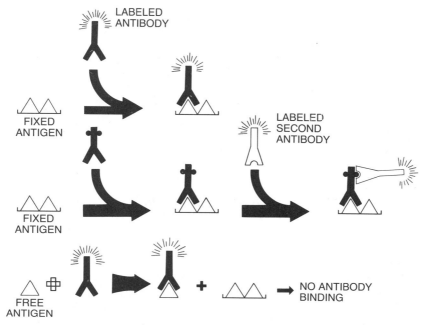

Figure 14-2. There are several variations to radioimmunoassay (RIA) tests. In the direct RIA test (*upper panel*), a radiolabeled antibody, used in excess, attaches to fixed antigen. The amount of antibody fixed quantitates the antigen. To measure the amount of an antibody (*middle panel*) it is first reacted with antigen and subsequently with an isotopically labeled antibody. Here the amount of labeled antibody bound quantitates the first antibody. Soluble antigen reacts with antibody to block fixation of the antibody to a fixed preparation antigen (*lower panel*). This is the basis for inhibition or blocking tests used to measure the amount of antigen in a solution.

titrations, **competitive inhibition RIA** is equally useful for antigens and haptens.

Applications of RIA

Regardless of the experimental technique used (Fig. 14-2), the great advantage of all RIA procedures is their high sensitivity. Only enzyme-linked immunosorbent assays (ELISA) approach RIAs in the ability to detect trace amounts of antigen (hapten). Commercially available RIA kits may detect as little as 1 nanogram (a billionth of a gram) or 1 picogram (10^{-12} gram, or a trillionth of a gram) of antigen. This is obviously of great significance in following or determining the blood level of certain hormones or

therapeutic agents that seldom exceed a few micrograms per milliliter.

RIA procedures have the disadvantage of relatively great expense in terms of the radioisotope-counting equipment and the small but unavoidable hazard associated with radioisotopes. These features obviously have not been a serious handicap to the clinical application of RIA, although many are being replaced by enzyme-linked immunoassays. RIA procedures currently in use for monitoring cardiovascular function include assays for digoxin, digitoxin, renin (angiotensin), and aldosterone. Reproductive functions can be estimated by RIA methods for follicle-stimulating hormone (FSH), leuteinizing hormone (LH), human placental lactogen (HPL), testosterone, estrogen, and progesterone; hematopoietic function by vitamin B_{12}, folic acid, and immunoglobulin methods; and various metabolic functions by RIA for insulin, thyroxine (T_4), triiodothyronine (T_3), adrenocorticotropic hormone (ACTH), cortisol, parathormone, HGH, and thyroid-stimulating hormone (TSH). RIA kits are available to quantitate opiates, barbiturates, amphetamines, and other abused drugs. Hepatitis virus, AIDS virus, and other infectious agents have also been detected by RIA (Table 14–2).

ENZYME-LINKED IMMUNOSORBENT ASSAY

The possibility to develop **enzyme immunoassays** was created when it was

discovered that enzymes could be covalently linked to immunoglobulins through a conjugation process that did not damage the catalytic site of the enzyme nor the idiotypic region of the immunoglobulin. The enzyme marker on the immunoglobulin must be stable under storage and the conditions of its use. It should be of low molecular weight so that it will not create steric effects that would interfere with the reaction of the immunoglobulin with the antigen or hapten.

In general, ELISA and RIA techniques are quite similar and are of essentially equal sensitivity. In certain circumstances, ELISA methods may be even more sensitive than RIA methods. In the latter, when the radionucleide emits the γ or β particle, it is then less radioactive or inactive and cannot be

Table 14–2
PARTIAL LIST OF BIOLOGICALLY IMPORTANT ANTIGENS AND HAPTENS DETERMINED BY RIA OR ELISA

Hormones
Insulin
Human chorionic gonadotropin (HCG)
Human placental lactogen (HPL)
Thyrotropin
Follicle stimulating hormone (FSH)
Adrenocorticotropic hormone (ACTH)
Luteinizing hormone (LH)
Parathyroid hormone (PTH)
Calcitonin
Glucagon

Enzymes
C1 esterase
Plasmin
Carboxypeptidase
Trypsin
Chymotrypsin
Elastase

Tumor Antigens
Alpha fetoprotein
Alpha hepatoprotein
Carcinoembryonic antigen

Viruses
Hepatitis B
AIDS virus
Rubella virus
Hog cholera virus
Rabies virus
Cytomegalovirus
Mouse leukemia agent

Bacterial Antigens
Group A streptococci
Cholera toxin
Streptolysin O

Interleukins
Interleukin 1
Interleukin 2
Interferons
Interleukin 4

Immunoglobulins
IgG   IgD
IgE   IgM
IgA κ chains
        λ chains

measured again as a radioisotope. In ELISA, the enzyme catalyzes a change in a substrate molecule, but the enzyme is not itself consumed in this process. The enzyme molecule continues to act on more substrate and gives off more signals in the form of enzyme end-product. In this way ELISA is more sensitive than RIA.

Basic Procedures

In solid-phase ELISA tests, an antibody with specificity for an antigen is coated on the surface of wells in a microtiter plate and the surface is blocked with an extraneous protein (Fig. 14–3). Thereafter, the antigen, perhaps insulin in a patient's serum, is allowed to react with the antibody to insulin. This is followed by addition of an **enzyme-labeled conjugate of anti-insulin**, which reacts with the antigen. Following these serologic reactions, an enzymatic reaction is generated by adding the enzyme's substrate. Conversion of the substrate to product is then quantitated spectrophotometrically or colorimetrically. For example, if the anti-insulin is labeled with **alkaline phosphatase**, the conversion of the colorless enzyme substrate, p-nitrophenyl phosphate, to the yellow product, p-nitrophenol, can be determined easily. The amount of product formed under prescribed assay conditions is an index of the amount of enzyme-linked antibody present, which is a reflection of the amount of antigen present. When this is compared with the amount of chromogen formed in tubes that contain known amounts of antigen (ie, the standard curve), the concentration of antigen in the unknown sample can be determined.

Notice that in this procedure, as well as by the RIA technique, the antigen could be an immunoglobulin. To measure the amount of IgG in a human serum, one would first coat the wells with antihuman IgG, block the wells, add the serum sample containing IgG, and follow this with either a radiolabeled anti-IgG or an enzyme-labeled anti-IgG and enzyme substrate. In this *immunologic sandwich* all three layers are globulins.

As might be expected, there are several variations of ELISA tests, one of which permits quantitation of haptens, equally as well as antigens (competitive inhibition ELISA). One variation uses an antigen labeled with an enzyme that becomes inactive when it

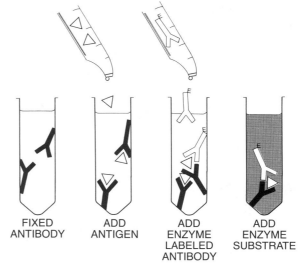

Figure 14–3. In one variation of the ELISA test, antibody is bound to a surface and then reacts with antigen. The bound antigen is reacted with an enzyme-labeled antibody whose function is demonstrated by adding enzyme substrate.

FIXED ANTIBODY　　ADD ANTIGEN　　ADD ENZYME LABELED ANTIBODY　　ADD ENZYME SUBSTRATE combines with antibody. Blockade of the antibody with unlabeled antigen and the concomitant decrease in the ability of the antibody to quench enzyme-labeled antigen is used to quantitate the unlabeled antigen.

Choice of Enzymes

Because the enzyme label is the critical portion of ELISA methods, selection of the label is very important. The primary criteria are that the enzyme must be stable under the conditions used for storage, cross-linking, and assay; have a high specific activity or substrate turnover number; and be inexpensive. Equally important is that the enzyme must be absent from the antigen or antiserum preparation to be used in the serologic tests; otherwise, false-positive test results would ensue. False-negative results could stem from the presence of enzyme inhibitors or inactivators in the serologic reagents. Appropriate controls must be incorporated into the tests to identify these potential problems.

Numerous enzymes have been used in ELISA tests. The most commonly used are **horseradish peroxidase** and alkaline phosphatase. Enzyme activity is usually determined spectrophotometrically. Alkaline phosphatase is easily detected by the color change associated with cleavage of p-nitrophenyl phosphate as the substrate. The oxidizing activity of the H_2O_2 formed by glucose oxidase is its measure of concentration. Peroxidase is measured by its ability to change the color of o-dianisidine. Other enzymes have equally simple colorimetric or spectrophotometric quantitation methods.

Cross-Linking Reagents

Glutaraldehyde is a common cross-linker used to join the enzyme to the antibody. The reaction proceeds through the dialdehyde portion of the molecule and amino groups on the reactants. Dimaleimide, another **cross-linking agent**, bridges proteins through their —SH groups.

FLUORESCENT ANTIBODY METHODS

To prepare a fluorescent antibody (FAB), a fluorescent dye is covalently linked to the antibody in such a way as to preserve the properties of the dye and antibody in the conjugate. The fluorescent antibody technique uses the physiochemical properties of certain dyes, referred to as **fluors** or **fluorochromes**. Fluors respond to short-wavelength light and emit a longer-wavelength light. Typically fluors absorb ultraviolet or short blue wavelengths (200 to 400 nm), and emit light in the visible range.

The first fluorochromes chosen were **fluorescein** and a rhodamine such as lissamine rhodamine B. Fluorescein emits a green or yellow-green light, and rhodamine an orange-red light. More recently, pigmented proteins used by algae in photosynthesis have been introduced because they are much more sensitive than organic fluors. Phycoerythrin, one of the algal phycobiliproteins, fluoresces with 10 to 30 times the intensity of fluorescein and has both an absorption and an emission spectrum different from those of the fluors used previously. Double staining with fluors of different emission spectra is possible when two or more antigens are to be identified.

Direct Method

Fluorescent antibodies are **histochemical reagents** that react with and identify antigens that are then viewed by **fluorescent microscopy**. An antigen such as the rabies virus in brain tissue from a rabid animal is fixed on a regular microscopic slide. Thereafter, the slide is flooded with a fluorescent antibody specific for rabies virus. This is allowed to combine with the antigen during a brief incubation period and the excess of the antibody is then removed by washing. The slide is then examined under a fluorescent microscope assembly. The rabies virus is present wherever fluorescence characteristic of the fluor is seen.

Fluorescence Microscopy. Fluorescence microscopy is more demanding than ordinary light microscopy because objects are always much dimmer in the former technique. A conventional microscope of good quality can be used. There is no need for quartz optics. The usual physical arrangement is depicted in Figure 14–4. A high-pressure lamp emitting ultraviolet and short wavelength blue light is needed. The light is filtered by the primary filter to remove wavelengths longer than 450 to 500 nm. A front-surfaced mirror diverts the light into a darkfield condenser. A **darkfield condenser** is preferred because it is easier to see a point of colored light on a black field than against a bright white background. When the light coming through the condenser strikes the fluorescent antibody on the specimen slide, the fluor emits visible light. This visible light, possibly mixed with stray ultraviolet rays, progresses up the tube of the microscope to the observer. A secondary filter will remove stray ultraviolet light that might damage the observer's eyes. Because the objects are often only faintly visible, this

technique should be performed in a darkened room. For the same reason, a monocular microscope may be preferred.

The Blocking Test. FAB procedures are subject to errors due to spontaneous **background fluorescence** or **nonspecific binding** of the labeled antibody to materials on the slide. These false-positive reactions are best controlled by the blocking test. The **blocking test** is important because it provides (1) the most useful control for the direct test and (2) a method of demonstrating antibody in a patient's serum without the time and expense of attaching a fluor to every serum specimen to be tested.

In the first application, the antigen preparation is first reacted with an unlabeled portion of antiserum. Combination of the antigen with these antibodies will block its combination with the subsequently applied fluorescent antibody. A serologic test for syphilis is an example of the second application. If a patient's serum blocks fluorescent antibody staining of *Treponema pallidum*, the etiologic agent of syphilis, then the patient has antibodies against this pathogen and possibly syphilis.

Indirect Method

Unfortunately, it is expensive and troublesome to keep a large battery of labeled antisera in reserve for direct fluorescent antibody staining, and this led to the development of the indirect

Figure 14–4. This is the microscopic arrangement for fluorescent antibody assays. Visible light is blocked from entering the microscope. Filters allow only light of the chosen wavelength to enter. A darkfield condenser prevents this light from progressing through the microscope. Only visible light emitted by objects on the microscope stage can be seen.

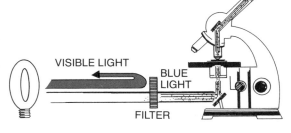

fluorescent antibody procedure. This is especially advantageous in human medicine where one needs to identify antibodies only in human sera rather than in several species of animals, as in veterinary medicine.

The first step in the **indirect** procedure is the same as in the direct procedure: fixation of an antigen to a slide. For example, in the indirect fluorescent antibody test for syphilis, spirochetes that cause syphilis are fixed on the slide. The patient's serum is then flooded onto the slide. If antibodies are present they will attach to the spirochetes. Excess serum proteins are removed by washing. Next, a second antibody—an antiglobulin prepared by immunizing goats with human

gamma globulin and then labeled with a fluor—is used. This reagent will react with the patient's antibody bound to the spirochetes. As in the blocking variation to the direct test, this reaction indicates a possible diagnosis of syphilis.

The indirect fluorescent antibody procedure is an example of the second antibody, **antiglobulin**, or immunologic sandwich technique. In the example described, the globulin in the patient's serum functions both as an antibody and as an antigen. By varying the first antigen used, a broad range of antibodies in patient sera can be evaluated with only one fluorescent reagent, a fluorescent antihuman globulin (Fig. 14–5).

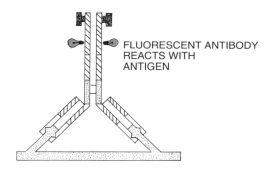

FLUORESCENT ANTIBODY REACTS WITH ANTIGEN

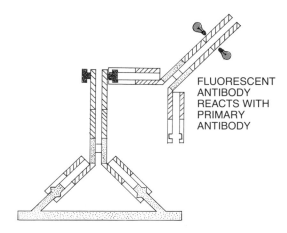

FLUORESCENT ANTIBODY REACTS WITH PRIMARY ANTIBODY

Figure 14–5. In the direct FAB procedure (*upper panel*), a fluorescent antibody reacts with the antigen. In the indirect method (*lower panel*), the second antibody is labeled with a fluor and reacts with the first antibody.

Modifications for Electron Microscopy

A variation of the labeled antibody as a histochemical reagent is the use of **ferritin-labeled antibody** in electron microscopy. Ferritin is a protein of 465,000 Mr that bears about 23% of its weight as iron. This iron is localized in distinct micelles that are opaque to electrons, thus permitting the localization of a ferritin-labeled antibody under an electron microscope. Recently immunoglobulins labeled with microscopic particles of gold have been used in electron and in visible microscopy as histochemical reagents. Enzyme-linked immunoassays that produce electron opaque products can also be applied to electron microscopy.

OTHER ANTIBODY DETECTORS

The second antibody or antiglobulin reactions to improve the sensitivity of serologic reactions have proved so popular and practical that several variations on that theme have been developed. The first of these made use of **protein A**; the second was built upon the high affinity of the **avidin-biotin** complex.

Protein A

Protein A binds to human IgG and IgM although it does not bind well to subclass IgG3. Consequently, any label applied to protein A, whether an isotope, enzyme, fluor, colloidal gold, or other, creates a tracer for IgG and IgM. This eliminates the immunization, purification, and testing of labeled antiglobulins because protein A is easily purified from the bacterium *Staphylococcus aureus*, where it exists as a surface protein of 42,000 Mr. A labeled protein A could be used to amplify a test in which solid-phase antigen is used to capture an IgG or IgM and a labeled protein A detects capture of the antibody. Proteins from other microorganisms are being investigated as substitutes for second antibodies.

Avidin-Biotin

A generation ago it was recognized that a protein in egg white would bind very tightly to the vitamin biotin. This egg protein bound so tightly that it was named avidin. Immunologists have designed serologic procedures based on this ability of avidin to bind four molecules of biotin (see Fig. 14–6 and Fig. 14–7). Several modifications of the

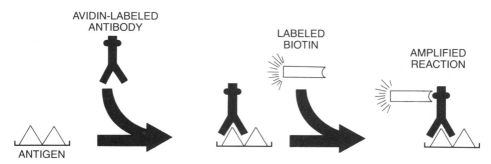

Figure 14–6. Avidin-biotin enhancement of a serologic reaction is illustrated by an avidin-labeled antibody bound to antigen. Avidin then reacts with biotin. The biotin may be isotopically or enzymatically labeled to amplify the serologic reaction.

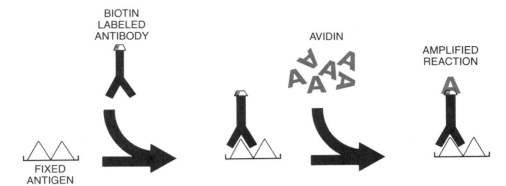

Figure 14–7. This illustrates a radiolabeled avidin binding to a biotin-labeled antibody as an enhancement procedure. Here again the avidin molecule, indicated by the letter *A*, could be isotopically or enzymatically labeled.

avidin–biotin system exist. For example, an avidin-labeled antibody could be combined with an antigen in solid phase. Thereafter, an enzyme-linked biotin could be used to amplify the primary reaction. Conversely, a biotin-labeled antibody could be reacted with antigen and an enzyme-labeled avidin could then be used to amplify the primary reaction. Radioisotopic, fluor, gold, or other labels can be applied to the avidin-biotin system.

Streptavidin, a protein recoverable from *Streptomyces avidinii*, has all the properties of avidin while being less subject to spontaneous precipitation with proteins; it has replaced avidin in many procedures.

Nephelometry

When antigen and antibody molecules combine, the first immune complexes that form are soluble. If the concentration of the reactants is low, large aggregates (precipitates) cannot develop. Nevertheless, the extent of small complex formation can be determined by **nephelometry**. Nephelometry differs from colorimetry by measuring the amount of light reflected at an angle from a light beam rather than the amount of light absorbed by a solution. This has provided a very sensitive and rapid (the combination phase of the serologic reaction occurs instantaneously) means of quantitating antigens. For use in nephelometry, the reagents must be crystal clear; otherwise,

---

MEMORY CHECK 14–2

◆

Ligand assays

1. Are able to measure either haptens or antigens

2. Are among the most sensitive serologic tests available

3. Exist in three major forms — RIA, ELISA, and FAB methods

4. By RIA and ELISA are most commonly performed as solid-phase and competitive inhibition tests

5. By FAB are either direct or indirect methods; blocking test is important

6. By double antibody, protein A, and avidin-biotin techniques increase the sensitivity of these tests

excessive background reflection prevents interpretation of low readings against the background.

Antisera are available to quantitate the level of human IgG, IgM, IgA, complement components C3 and C4, transferrin, α1 antitrypsin, and ceruloplasmin in serum by nephelometry. Nephelometry is replacing many immunodiffusion tests.

Precipitation

When a completely soluble antigen reacts with its antibody in an antiserum, precipitation takes place. This precipitation may occur directly from the fluid state or may take place in a gel matrix where the two reactants have combined. The latter are referred to as immunodiffusion tests because the antigen and antiserum are often required to diffuse toward each other from separate origins in order to reach precipitating proportions.

MEMORY CHECK 14–3
◆

Nephelometry
1. Measures the combination phase of the serologic reaction
2. Is a rapid test with increasing clinical application

Precipitation
1. Cannot measure haptens and uses soluble antigens
2. Is primarily used as a qualitative test

Immunodiffusion Tests

Immunodiffusion tests are designed so that one or both of the serologic reactants diffuses through a gel. The advantage of **immunodiffusion tests** is

that they can identify the number of antigen-antibody systems functioning in a mixture of several systems, can determine the serologic identity of an antigen or antibody with another antigen or antibody, and in some variations of the test can quantitate one of the reactants. The diffusion of antigen and antibody molecules can occur by simple diffusion or can be accelerated by electrophoresis, in which case it is referred to as immunoelectrophoresis.

OUCHTERLONY-TYPE IMMUNODIFFUSION

The **Ouchterlony immunodiffusion test** is prepared so that an antigen and an antibody in an immune serum diffuse toward each other and precipitate in the space between their two reservoirs. If multiple antigens are present in a solution, then multiple lines of precipitate will appear (Figs. 14–8 and 14–9). To identify an antigen as *serologically identical* to another, the unknown and known antigens are diffused from separate reservoirs in a triangular arrangement with a third well containing antibody specific for the known antigen. When the precipitation lines form, there will be a *fusion of the lines* from the reservoirs at an intercept that will form a perfect arc in a *reaction of identity*. The third type of Ouchterlony *reaction is one of nonidentity*. This occurs when two unrelated antigens are diffused against an antiserum containing antibodies to each and the two lines of precipitation completely intersect each other.

RADIAL IMMUNODIFFUSION

Technique

When an antigen diffuses through a gel that contains its specific antibody, a ring of precipitate develops around the

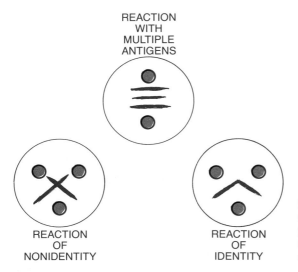

REACTION
WITH
MULTIPLE
ANTIGENS

REACTION
OF
NONIDENTITY

REACTION
OF
IDENTITY

Figure 14–8. The advantage of the Ouchterlony test to detect multiple antigens (*upper*), nonidentical antigens (*left*), and identical antigens (*right*) is depicted by the different precipitation patterns.

well. This is known as **radial quantitative immunodiffusion**. At the end of the diffusion process, when the size of the immunoprecipitation ring has stabilized, the area within the ring (or any parameter of the area) is proportional to the concentration of antigen. Because the radius and diameter of a circle are proportional to its area, one of these measurements is usually taken. When the diameters of immunoprecipitation rings produced by several concentrations of antigen are plotted against antigen concentration, a straight line is produced. From this, the concentration of antigen in unknown

solutions can be determined with accuracy.

Applications

Radial immunodiffusion is in current use for the quantitation of IgG, IgM, IgA, IgD, transferrin, complement components C3 and C4, $\alpha 1$ trypsin inhibitor, lysozyme, ceruloplasmin, alpha fetoprotein, albumin, and haptoglobin, among others. Such tests rely on the availability of monospecific antisera for these antigens. Because of variations in the potency of these antisera,

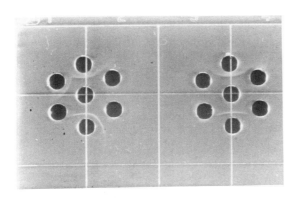

Figure 14–9. These immunodiffusion plates contain antibody to hepatitis B virus in the center well and patient sera in the outer wells. The presence of a precipitate is evidence of a hepatitis virus in the patient's specimen. (See color figure after Table of Contents.)

standards should be included with each determination.

IMMUNOELECTROPHORESIS

An electrophoretic separation of molecules that differ in ionic charge, though having similar diffusion coefficients, increases the probability that different antigens will produce separate precipitation arcs in a subsequent immunodiffusion assay. This is the basis of **immunoelectrophoresis (IEP)**, an electromotive variant of immunodiffusion. A further advantage of some IEP methods is that the results are often available more quickly because the diffusion has been accelerated by the electromotive force.

Ordinary Immunoelectrophoresis

In the simplest IEP method, an antigen mixture is separated by electrophoretic displacement from its origin in a well cut in an agarose gel. Resulting from inequalities in this displacement caused by differences in electrical charge, the antigens in the mixture are moved to different positions in the gel. Now an antiserum containing antibodies to one or more of the antigens is placed in a trough cut along the edge of the gel. Simple diffusion of the reactants allows each antigen-antibody system to form its own precipitation arc much as in the Ouchterlony test (Fig. 14–10). Ordinary immunoelectrophoresis is a qualitative method, but it

may have semiquantitative applications when dilutions of an antigen are examined in parallel with standards.

Immunoelectrophoresis is most often applied clinically for the analysis of serum proteins. The use of specific antisera against IgG, IgA, or IgM or against κ- or λ-type light chains identifies the molecules bearing these specific antigenic determinants. The intensity of the precipitation arc can be used as a crude quantitative estimate of the concentration of these proteins and can assist in the diagnosis of hypoglobulinemias or hyperglobulinemias, although the more precise radial immunodiffusion procedure is a more secure basis for such diagnoses.

Counterimmunoelectrophoresis

Counterimmunoelectrophoresis is a double immunodiffusion test in which an electric force is applied to accelerate the convergence and combination of antigen and antibody. A major restriction is that the antigen and immunoglobulin must carry opposite ionic charges at the pH of the buffering system employed. Movement of gamma globulins at pH 8.6 is largely by **endosmosis** rather than electrophoresis; therefore, the test is limited to antigens with an acidic isoelectric point. Fortunately, viruses, polysaccharide capsules of bacteria, nucleoproteins, and several other antigens fulfill this restriction. These antigens, when present in patient specimens such as urine or spinal fluid, are electrophoresed from one well in an agarose gel toward a

Figure 14–10. After electrophoretic separation of albumin, α, β, and γ globulin, their location and relative concentration can be determined by immunodiffusion.

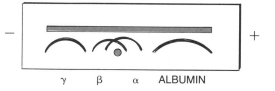

well containing antibody. Combination of the reagents in the gel is followed by precipitation. Because the identity of the antigen in patient materials is usually unknown, the specimen is electrophoresed against several antisera of differing but known specificity. For example, antisera are available that are specific for the capsular antigens of *Neisseria meningitidis*, *Streptococcus pneumoniae*, and *Haemophilus influenzae*. Counterimmunoelectrophoresis with these antisera will identify capsular antigens of these organisms in spinal fluid within an hour after the sample is received. Rapid serodiagnosis of this sort is useful in establishing the etiology of meningitis.

WESTERN BLOTTING

Western blotting has proved very useful for quantitating antigens and for following antigens through stages of purification. Many variations of Western blotting are available, the simplest being dot blotting. To determine the concentration of an antigen by dot blotting, several dilutions are prepared and a drop of each is dotted in a known place on a strip of nitrocellulose paper. This treated paper binds protein antigens very tightly. Thereafter, the dotted paper is immersed in antibody specific for the antigen. If this is a radio- or enzyme-labeled antibody, quantitation is affected by the usual RIA or ELISA methods. It is also possible to employ the second antibody technique, again with isotope or enzyme-labeled antibody to enhance the sensitivity of the procedure.

If Western blotting is preceded by electrophoresis, the proteins must be transferred to the nitrocellulose paper. This can be accomplished by simple diffusion or electrophoresis to the paper placed on top of the gel. Western blotting of electrophoretic gels is a sensitive means of locating and quantitating a single antigen in a mixture of antigens. This technique is used to identify the AIDS virus in human specimens.

MEMORY CHECK 14–4

Immunodiffusion
1. The Ouchterlony test is qualitative and radial immunodiffusion is quantitative.
2. Ouchterlony reactions of nonidentity, identity, and partial identity produce complete intersection, complete fusion, and spurred lines.
3. Radial immunodiffusion is a commonly used quantitative procedure.

Immunoelectrophoresis
1. Ordinary IEP is qualitative and good for serum immunoglobulins and Bence Jones proteins.
2. Counterimmunoelectrophoresis is an electrophoretic variant of the Ouchterlony test.
3. Western blotting can be either a qualitative or a quantitative procedure. It is used to identify the AIDS virus.

Agglutination Tests

The aggregation of cellular antigens by antibody is called **agglutination**. Bacteria were among the first antigens used in agglutination tests.

BACTERIAL AGGLUTINATION

Agglutination of pathogenic bacteria by antisera is one of the oldest serologic tests available to the clinical laboratory; it was advanced as an aid to the diagnosis of bacterial infections by Widal in 1896. The reference to bacterial agglutination as the **Widal test** is gradually falling into disuse. The diagnostic advantage of the agglutination test can be achieved from either of two directions: (1) unknown bacteria can be identified by known antisera maintained in the laboratory or (2) antibodies in a patient's serum can be identified by using known bacteria. The latter, the analysis of patient sera for **febrile agglutinins** as an index of the bacterial etiology of a disease, is not as frequently used now as it was earlier. The former application, however, is still practiced.

One might anticipate that most fevers of infectious origin should be diagnosed by recovery and cultivation of the infectious agent, but this is not always the case. A complete bacteriologic identification of these organisms relies on their ability to ferment various carbohydrates and to form specific end-products from their metabolism of amino acids, as well as on other biochemical tests. This is time consuming, expensive, and often frustrated by an inability to make an exact identification because of a deviation of one or more tests from that produced by typical strains. Accordingly, once biochemical tests have indicated the probable identity of an organism, agglutination tests are used to complete the identification.

PASSIVE AGGLUTINATION

The physical adsorption or covalent bonding of soluble antigens to inert carriers such as latex or polystyrene spheres converts soluble (precipitating) antigens to a form suitable for agglutination tests. Clumping of these particles with specific antisera is referred to as **passive** or **indirect agglutination** (or

passive hemagglutination, if the carrier is an erythrocyte). "Passive" is used because the particle is not the antigen per se. Conversion of precipitation tests to passive agglutination tests is of great benefit because test results are available more quickly and less antigen (or antibody) is needed to achieve a positive result (ie, passive agglutination tests are more sensitive than precipitation tests).

Applications of passive agglutination tests in clinical serology include those used to identify antibodies that develop during histoplasmosis, cryptococcosis, and haemophilus or neisserial infections. In these instances, antigens of the specific pathogen are adsorbed onto latex spheres. If the patient has had an immunologic experience with the pathogen, his or her antibodies will passively agglutinate the particle. By reversing the process and placing antibody on the spheres, one can seek antigens in patient materials such as the capsular antigens of *Cryptococcus neoformans, H. influenzae, N. meningitidis,* or *S. pneumoniae* in spinal fluid.

PASSIVE AGGLUTINATION INHIBITION

One of the most frequently applied passive agglutination tests is actually an inhibition test used for the serologic diagnosis of pregnancy. Kits are available commercially for personal use, often containing a latex particle coated with human chorionogonadotropic (HCG) hormone and antiserum for the hormone. Mixture of these two reagents results in passive agglutination. Preincubation of urine containing HCG with the antiserum will saturate the antibody so it cannot agglutinate the particle. This test result is positive for pregnancy; it is a positive **passive agglutination inhibition test** result. If

HCG is not present in the urine, then the particles are agglutinated, and the test result is negative.

Flocculation

Flocculation tests used in medical microbiology are special tests in which the antigen, originally in true solution, is converted to a colloidal state. These colloidal particles, microscopic or submicroscopic in size, are approximately the dimensions of bacteria. When these antigen particles are mixed with their specific antiserum, a serologic reaction in all respects like agglutination is observed.

Serologic tests for syphilis (STSs) take many forms, but the preparation of one type of "antigen" embodies the admixture of cholesterol and lecithin with an alcoholic extract of beef heart (cardiolipin). One form of this test depends on the coating of this cardiolipin onto particles of charcoal. Antibodies to the spirochete of syphilis will flocculate (agglutinate) these tiny particles. This test shows a good agreement with true cases of syphilis, but because the antigen is a nonspecific antigen in the sense that it has no antigenic relationship with *Treponema pallidum*, serologic tests for syphilis rely on a second test using specific treponema-derived antigens, such as fluorescent antibody tests.

Complement Fixation

Complement fixation tests are complicated, tedious to perform, require labile reagents, and may even be difficult to interpret. For this reason, complement fixation tests are declining in popularity. The complement fixation test is founded on two critical properties of the complement system: its participation with certain immunoglobulins to produce immunolysis and its ability to participate in a serologic reaction even though not required for that reaction. In the performance of the test an awareness of the heat lability of complement and its presence in all sera is important.

The discussion of complement fixation tests is simplified if the test is fragmented into its two overlapping halves —the **test system** and the **indicator system**. The test system is composed of an antigen and a patient's serum or dilutions of the serum believed to contain an antibody reactive with that antigen. When the test is designed to detect syphilis, the complement fixation test is known as the Wassermann test. The serum sample is held at 56°C for 30 minutes to destroy its complement. To the antigen and the serum a predetermined amount of complement in the form of normal guinea pig serum is added and an incubation period is allowed. If the serum does contain antibodies, they will bind both the antigen and the complement (Fig. 14–11).

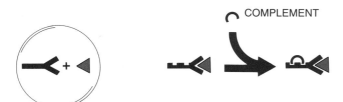
COMPLEMENT

Figure 14–11. In the complement fixation test, the combination of an antibody with antigen causes a change in the structure of the antibody so that it can activate the complement system represented by the letter *C*.

Then, when the indicator system of sheep red blood cells and an antibody directed against these cells (hemolysin) is added, there is no complement remaining to lyse the red cells during a second incubation period. Conversely, if the patient's serum were devoid of antibody, there could be no serologic reaction in the test system and complement would be free to catalyze the hemolytic reaction of the indicator system. The interpretation of the complement fixation test is that lysis is a negative test result and no lysis is a positive result.

NEUTRALIZATION

The principle of **neutralization tests** rests on the ability of an appropriate antiserum to diminish or abolish some biologic property of the antigen other than its antigenicity—its toxicity, its infectivity for cells or laboratory animals, or its enzymatic activity.

The antistreptolysin (ASO or ASTO) test is a neutralization test. Streptolysin is a hemolytic agent produced by group A streptococci and is also antigenic. Antibodies that appear in a person's serum as the result of an infection with group A streptococci will neutralize this hemolytic property. Hyaluronidase and deoxyribonuclease (DNAase) are two additional enzymes used in neutralization tests to aid the diagnosis of streptococcal infections.

Flow Cytometry

The enumeration and identification of cells, previously a laborious microscopic exercise, has been revolutionized by developments in flow cytometry. In this highly automated technique, a large population of partially purified cells is entered into a stream of fluid that is passing out a small orifice. Cells exit through this port in single file. As the cells pass before a beam of light, detectors record the interruptions in this beam as the number of cells in a unit volume. Light scattered from the path of the beam and witnessed by other detectors determines the cell size. Previous selective staining of the cells allows the cell content of DNA, RNA, polysaccharide, or other chemicals to be determined.

Fluorescent antibodies have been applied extensively to flow cytometry because they can detect a specific marker on the cell surface. It is possible to use two different fluorescent antibodies simultaneously, if their fluors emit light of different wavelengths. For example, with antibodies specific for CD3 and CD4, the total number of T cells and the number of T_H and T_{DTH} cells in a population can be determined. This procedure has been useful

---

MEMORY CHECK 14–5

1. Bacterial agglutination tests are used to identify bacteria isolated from patients.

2. Passive agglutination inhibition is a sensitive test, used in pregnancy kits, and other conversions from precipitation tests.

3. Flocculation is akin to agglutination and is used as a primary diagnostic aid for syphilis.

4. Complement fixation is rarely used, and the test and indicator systems, are the key to its understanding, complement is always fixed.

5. Neutralization of viruses and bacterial enzymes is used to diagnose infections. The ASTO and anti-DNAase tests are examples.

in analyzing lymphocytes in patients with autoimmune disease, immunodeficiency conditions, leukemia, infectious diseases such as AIDS, and other immune system abnormalities.

A research modification of flow cytometry enables cells with a specific marker to be sorted from the remaining cells. These exceptionally purified cells can then be analyzed for their ability to cooperate with other cells in the immune response, to respond to specific antigens, to repopulate immunodeficient individuals, and to participate in any number of immunologic experiments.

References

Bjerrum, OJ and Heegaard, NHH (eds): CRC Handbook of Immunoblotting of Proteins. CRC Press, Boca Raton, FL, 1988.

Catty, D (ed): Antibodies: A Practical Approach. Vols 1 and 2. IRL Press, Oxford, 1988, 1989.

Day, ED: Advanced Immunochemistry. Wiley-Liss, New York, 1990.

Dunbar, BS: Two-Dimensional Electrophoresis and Immunological Techniques. CRC Press, Boca Raton, FL, 1988.

Langone, JL and Van Vunakis, H (eds): Immuno-chemical techniques. Parts B and C. Methods Enzymol 72; 73:1, 1981.

Larsson, L-I: Immunocytochemistry: Theory and practice. CRC Press, Boca Raton, FL, 1988.

Maggio, ET (ed): Enzyme-immunoassay. CRC Press, Boca Raton, FL, 1980.

Sternberger, LA: Immunocytochemistry, ed 3. John Wiley & Sons, New York, 1986.

Van Vunakis, H and Langone, JL (eds): Immuno-chemical techniques. Methods Enzymol 70:1, 1980.

Vogel, C-W (ed): Immunoconjugates. Oxford University Press, Oxford, 1987.

Weir, DM (ed): Handbook of Experimental Immunology, ed 4. Vols I–IV. Blackwell Scientific, Oxford, 1986.

Widmann, FK: An Introduction to Clinical Immunology. FA Davis, Philadelphia, 1989.

QUESTIONS AND ANSWERS

1. The following diagram of an Ouchterlony immunodiffusion test indicates
   A. The antigen preparation contains at least three antigens
   B. Antiserum A contains at least two antibodies
   C. Antiserum B contains at least one antibody
   D. Both antiserum A and B contain IgG
   E. All of the above

1 = anti IgG
2 = antiserum A
3 = antigen
4 = antiserum B

Answer E

All statements are true. Antiserum A indicates the antigen is a mixture of at least two antigens. Antiserum B contains an antibody that reacts with a third antigen, inasmuch as the precipitation line it forms with antigen completely intersects those formed by antiserum A. Anti-IgG produces a reaction of identity with both antisera.

2. Which of the following will fail to precipitate an antibody to a digitoxin–bovine serum albumin conjugate?
   A. Digitoxin–bovine serum albumin
   B. Digitoxin
   C. Bovine serum albumin
   D. Digitoxin–human serum albumin
   E. All of the above, except A

Answer B

Antisera to a hapten-antigen conjugate will normally precipitate with the original antigen (answer A), any multideterminant component of the conjugate (answer C), and the hapten conjugated to a different antigen (answer D), assuming more than one digitoxin per mole of human albumin. Digitoxin will react with the antibody but not precipitate, owing to its haptenic nature. Thus, answer E is incorrect.

3. If IgG has an antigenic valence of 15, then
   A. A maximum of 30 antibody molecules would attach to a single molecule of IgG because it has a *serologic* valence of 2
   B. Indirect fluorescent antibody tests will be essentially 15 times more sensitive than direct fluorescent antibody tests
   C. Monomeric IgA, essentially the same size as IgG, must also have an antigenic valence of 15
   D. All subclasses of IgG must have the same antigenic valence
   E. κ and λ chains must have no epitopes

Answer B

Answer A is incorrect because the number of Fab units (the serologic valence) of IgG has no relationship to its valence as an antigen. Assuming that no steric hindrance occurs, answer B is correct. Answer C is incorrect because antigenic valence does not rely on size alone; for this reason answer D is also incorrect. Both κ and λ chains (Bence Jones proteins) are antigenic, have epitopes, and may contribute to the antigenic valence of IgG.

4. In complement fixation tests, complement is
   A. Always fixed in the indicator system
   B. Always fixed
   C. Fixed only by IgG
   D. Fixed only by IgM
   E. Inactivated at 56° C for 30 minutes prior to use in the test

Answer B

Answer B is correct because in positive complement fixation tests, complement is fixed in the indicator system. In negative test results it is fixed in the test system. Both IgG and IgM activate the complement system (see Chapter 6). Complement in the sera used in complement fixation tests is heat inactivated, which is not the case for the complement source itself.

Case Study: Pneumococcal Vaccine

The children in the sixth grade of Washington Grade School had served as volunteers in one of the earliest pneumococcal vaccine trials. The vaccine tested at that time contained capsular polysaccharide from each of three serotypes of *Streptococcus pneumoniae*. Each child received a 0.25-mL subcutaneous injection, followed 2 months later by an identical repeat injection of the vaccine. Each injection contained 100 μg of capsular polysaccharide per milliliter of each pneumococcus type. Blood samples were collected three times: first, for a preimmunization sample, then 2 weeks after the first immunization, and finally 2 weeks after the second immunization.

Questions

1. What techniques are suitable for measuring antibodies to capsular polysaccharide antigens?

2. What are the relative merits of these procedures?

3. What results would you anticipate from this vaccine trial?

Discussion

Several techniques can be used to measure anticapsular antibodies and among these passive hemagglutination is one of the simplest to perform and least expensive. Counterimmunoelectrophoresis has also been used, as have other immunodiffusion techniques. RIA, ELISA, and blotting procedures have also been devised for this purpose.

By nature's own design, polysaccharide antigens attach spontaneously to erythrocytes, thus facilitating preparation of an antigen for use in passive hemagglutination assays. Passive hemagglutination tests are simple to perform and are very sensitive, requiring as little as 0.006 μg of antibody protein per milliliter of serum to produce a positive test result. Among the disadvantages of passive hemagglutination are that the antigen is not covalently bound to the carrier and that it can dissociate from the carrier, resulting in an antigenless erythrocyte. This can be prevented by the use of coupling reagents.

RIA and ELISA tests are so much alike that they can be described together. Both are exceptionally sensitive and may require less than 0.006 μg of antibody protein per milliliter to produce a positive test result, depending upon the variation of the test chosen. Both can be adapted to measure either IgG or IgM. For example, in RIA, the pneumococcal polysaccharide solid phase could be reacted with the volunteer's serum and either with radiolabeled anti-IgG or anti-IgM, depending upon which immunoglobulin was of interest. The RIA and ELISA tests are more time consuming and more expensive and require more sophisticated equipment than passive hemagglutination.

In this trial, the pretest sera evidenced low titers in the range of 1:100 to 1:150 against each of the three sera tested individually. The postprimary immunization titers ranged from 1:750 downward to 1:450, and did not increase after booster immunization. These results indicate that children have low quantities of antibody to pneumococci from subclinical infections but that immunization is successful, within limits. The failure to improve antibody titers to polysaccharide antigens is typical of the IgM response to T-cell–independent antigens.

GLOSSARY

agglutination Aggregation of a cellular or particulate antigen by an antiserum containing antibodies to one or more surface antigens.

antiglobulin test A test to determine the presence of one globulin (antibody) by using a second globulin (antibody) with a serologic specificity for the first.

avidin/streptavidin Proteins from egg white and streptomyces, respectively, that bind firmly to biotin.

counterimmunoelectrophoresis Electrophoresis of antigen and antibody toward each other through a gel.

double antibody technique Often an antiglobulin procedure, but sometimes varied so that two antibodies react with the same antigen.

ELISA Enzyme-linked immunosorbent assay.

enzyme-linked immunosorbent assay A serologic test that uses an enzyme-labeled reagent.

FAB Fluorescent antibody.

flocculation 1. A specific type of precipitation that occurs over a narrow range of antigen concentration. 2. Aggregation of colloidal particles in a serologic reaction, as in syphilis serology.

fluorescent antibody An immunoglobulin conjugated to a fluorescent dye for use in ultraviolet microscopy.

hemagglutination The agglutination of erythrocytes, especially by antiserum.

immunodiffusion The diffusion of soluble antigens and antibodies toward each other and their precipitation in gel.

immunoelectrophoresis An electrophoretic displacement of antigen(s) or antibodies followed by immunodiffusion.

Ouchterlony test An immunodiffusion test based on diffusion of both antigen and antibody through gels.

passive hemagglutination Hemagglutination resulting from antibodies directed toward antigens adsorbed to the erythrocyte surface.

postzone Failure of a serologic reaction to occur in extreme dilutions of antibody.

protein A A protein on the surface of *Staphylococcus aureus* that binds IgG.

prozone Failure of a serologic reaction to occur in a high concentration of antibody.

radial immunodiffusion A quantitative immunodiffusion test of antigen moving through a gel containing antibody.

radioimmunoassay A serologic test in which one of the reagents is labeled with a radioisotope.

RIA Radioimmunoassay.

solid-phase radioimmunoassay   A radioimmunoassay in which one of the reactants is bound to a surface.

titer   The greatest dilution of antigen or antibody that will produce the desired result in a serologic test.

Western blotting   The serologic reaction of an antigen in a gel with an overlaid antibody.

Widal test   A bacterial agglutination test used to diagnose infectious diseases.

Final Examination

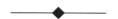

1. Immunoglobulin class switching is influenced by:
   A. IL-2
   B. IL-4
   C. IL-6
   D. TNFα
   E. IFNγ

2. An antigenic determinant site (epitope) of a protein is
   A. Always a linear sequence of amino acids
   B. Always a nonlinear, conformational arrangement of amino acids
   C. Variable, depending upon the genetic basis of different hosts to recognize different determinants
   D. Normally considered to be the same as the valence of an antigen
   E. Always hidden within the structure of a protein and exposed during antigen processing

3. Which of the following is *not* true of antigens?
   A. All antigens require T-cell assistance to initiate an antibody response.
   B. Antigens are resistant to hydrolytic attack by macrophages.
   C. Antigens may be the same as tolerogens.
   D. Host control of antigenicity is expressed through immune response genes.
   E. Superantigens link MHC proteins and the T-cell receptor for antigen.

4. Which of the following is the most active phagocyte?
   A. Basophil
   B. Eosinophil
   C. Lymphocyte
   D. Neutrophil
   E. Langerhans' cell

5. Which aids the maturation of T lymphocytes?
   A. M-CSF
   B. G-CSF
   C. GM-CSF
   D. IL-3
   E. IL-2

6. Which of the following is considered an integrin?
   A. Mac1 (CR3)
   B. IL-3
   C. FcγRI
   D. CR1
   E. MHC class II protein

7. Which of the following is genetically and structurally related to TNFα?
   A. IL-1
   B. IL-3
   C. ELAM-1
   D. C5a
   E. LT

8. Which is the initial event in phagocytosis?
   A. Oxidative burst
   B. Chemotaxis
   C. Phagolysosome formation
   D. Opsonization
   E. IL-1 release

9. The human equivalent to the bursa of Fabricius is
   A. Bone marrow
   B. Spleen
   C. Lymph nodes
   D. Thymus
   E. None of the above

10. Which of the following is *not* found on the surface of B lymphocytes at any stage of development?
    A. CR2
    B. IgM
    C. IgD
    D. TCR
    E. FcγR

11. The response of B lymphocytes to antigen includes
    A. Maturation of plasma cells
    B. Class switching
    C. Activation by IL-4
    D. Alterations in phosphatidylinositol metabolism
    E. All of the above

12. A powerful mitogen for B cells is
    A. Lipopolysaccharide
    B. Anti-IgM
    C. Protein A
    D. Pokeweed mitogen
    E. All of the above

13. A strong correlate of T_H cells is
    A. CD2
    B. CD3
    C. CD4
    D. CD8
    E. None of the above

14. The T-cell receptor for antigen is physically associated with
    A. LFA-3
    B. CD3
    C. IL-2R
    D. The concanavalin A receptor
    E. MHC class I protein

15. A thymic hormone is
    A. A peptide that stimulates T cells
    B. Any mitogen for T cells
    C. Able to bind directly to TCR1 and TCR2
    D. The same as an interleukin
    E. Exemplified by IFNγ

16. T_{H1} cells are known to secrete
    A. IL-2
    B. IL-3
    C. IFNγ
    D. GM-CSF
    E. All of the above

17. The immunoglobulin with the largest molecular weight is
    A. IgG
    B. Secretory IgA
    C. IgE
    D. IgM
    E. Serum IgA

18. Isotype refers to
    A. Characteristics of the immunoglobulin H chain
    B. Antigenic differences due to variations in allelic genes
    C. The difference in κ and λ chains
    D. Unique amino acids in the combining site of an antibody
    E. None of the above

19. Papain digestion of IgG will
    A. Destroy its idiotypic determinants
    B. Cleave each H chain at one site
    C. Produce the $F(ab')_2$ and Fc fragments
    D. Cleave the H chains in the CH3 domains
    E. Will produce two L and two H chains

20. The hypervariable regions of an immunoglobulin are
    A. Major contributors to the antigen binding site(s) of an antibody
    B. Found in both L and H chains
    C. Contributors to idiotypic determinants
    D. The same in IgG and IgM produced by a cell after it switches from IgM synthesis
    E. All of the above

21. A hybridoma
    A. Normally produces an antibody to a single determinant of an antigen
    B. Is derived from a cell that produced an M protein in its original state
    C. Is a composite of a plasma cell and a B cell
    D. Can be grown either in vivo or in vitro
    E. All of the above

22. The 7/9 and 12/23 rules
    A. Apply to C gene selection during immunoglobulin class switching
    B. Apply to both V_κ and V_λ alignment with the JC gene pair
    C. Refer to the number of amino acids in the hypervariable domains of immunoglobulins
    D. Indicate where the splice site between C genes and J genes is located
    E. None of the above

23. A difference between secreted IgD and membrane IgD is
    A. The presence of SC in secreted IgD
    B. The location of splice sites in mRNA for the two forms of IgD
    C. The presence of slightly larger H chains in secreted IgD
    D. Related to the different V genes selected in their H chains
    E. The presence of SC and J chain in secreted IgD

24. Which of the following is both an anaphylatoxin and a chemotaxin?
    A. C3a
    B. C4a
    C. C5a
    D. desArg C3a
    E. desArg C5a

25. Enzyme activity is *not* present in
    A. Activated C1r
    B. Activated C1s
    C. Factor D
    D. Properdin
    E. Ana INH

26. C3b contributes to
    A. Opsonization
    B. Immune adherence
    C. The alternative complement pathway
    D. C5 convertases of both the classic and the alternative pathways
    E. All of the above

27. The primary toxic activity of phagocytes is dependent upon
    A. Lysosomal hydrolases
    B. Granzymes
    C. Oxidative metabolism
    D. Lysozyme
    E. Defensins

28. The oral (Sabin) vaccine against poliomyelitis
    A. Is clearly better than the Salk, killed vaccine
    B. Is potentially able to immunize all members of a household passively after active immunization of a single member
    C. Cannot revert to the wild, virulent type
    D. Is a good model for the development of an AIDS vaccine
    E. Is composed of only one antigenic form of the virus

29. Recombinant vaccines
    A. Are the same as synthetic vaccines
    B. Can be developed in either viral or bacterial hosts that accept DNA of a pathogen
    C. Are probably unsuitable for the virus of AIDS
    D. Utilize the 7/9 and 12/23 rules
    E. Stimulate only B cells and not T cells

30. Which of the following is *not* expressed as a sex-linked disease?
    A. Bruton's disease
    B. Chronic granulomatous disease
    C. Wiskott-Aldrich syndrome
    D. Selective IgA deficiency
    E. All of the above are sex-linked

31. The biochemical basis of chronic granulomatous disease is
    A. Lack of NADPH oxidase
    B. Myeloperoxidase deficiency
    C. Excess production of superoxide dismutase
    D. Loss of cytochrome b
    E. The same as in actin deficiency

32. Adenosine deaminase deficiency can be treated successfully by
    A. Transfusion with normal red blood cells
    B. Thymus grafts
    C. Purine nucleotide phosphorylase injections
    D. Transfer factor injections
    E. None of the above

33. The antigenic determinant most contributory to allograft rejection is the
    A. α peptide of the MHC class II protein
    B. $\beta 2$ microglobulin
    C. $\alpha 1$ and $\alpha 2$ sectors of MHC class I proteins
    D. HLA-C determinant
    E. A class III MHC gene product

34. Bone marrow purging
    A. Can be accomplished with complement and antibody
    B. Is possible with immunotoxins
    C. Is an avenue to prevent GVH disease after bone marrow grafting
    D. With anti-CD8 immunotoxins will help prevent GVH disease
    E. All of the above

35. Cyclosporin A
    A. Acts on T cells before and after their activation
    B. Acts primarily to block IL-2 synthesis
    C. Is the new name for agent FK506
    D. Use does not lead to a higher risk for infectious disease
    E. Cannot be used to impede GVH disease

36. Oncogenic virus(es)
    A. Produce TSTAs that are antigenically the same from one tumor to another
    B. May be either DNA or RNA viruses
    C. Include HTLV I and HTLV II
    D. Can produce penile and plantar warts
    E. All of the above

37. Carcinofetal antigens
    A. Are responsible for cancers in fetal and newborn infants
    B. Have been associated only with cancers of the digestive tract
    C. Are useful in cancer diagnosis and prognosis
    D. Are not produced in normal animals after birth
    E. Are always useful in diagnosing spina bifida

38. The tumor marker protein produced in Waldenström's macroglobulinemia is
    A. The Epstein-Barr virus
    B. Related to activation of genes resulting from chromosome-8 and -14 translocations
    C. CEA
    D. IgM
    E. Usually restricted to the Bence Jones protein

39. Which of the following is associated with an immune response to a receptor?
    A. Myasthenia gravis
    B. Multiple sclerosis
    C. Systemic lupus erythematosus
    D. Rheumatic fever
    E. Nezelof's syndrome

40. The escape from self-tolerance that then allows an autoimmune state to develop
    A. Is actually a quite common event
    B. Always results in severe disease
    C. Cannot be used to explain the etiology of multiple sclerosis
    D. Involves only T_H cells and not other T-cell subsets
    E. None of the above

41. The primary event in the etiology of most autoimmune diseases is
    A. Due to cross-reactive antigens
    B. Excessive T_H cell activity
    C. Related to excess MHC class II protein expression
    D. The development of hapten-self antigen complexes
    E. Not known

42. Antihistamines
    A. Relax smooth muscle
    B. Block mast cell degranulation
    C. Block basophil but not mast cell degranulation
    D. Also inhibit leukotrienes
    E. None of the above

43. The high-affinity receptor for IgE
    A. Binds the Fab regions of IgE
    B. Consists of three peptides: α, β, and γ
    C. Also binds IgM, since IgE and IgM have four CH domains
    D. Reversibly exists as $Fc_\epsilon RI$ and $Fc_\epsilon RII$
    E. Is present on mast cells, basophils, B cells, T cells, and so on

44. Vasoactive amines derived from arachidonic acid include
    A. Histamine
    B. PAF
    C. ECF-A
    D. LTC and LTD
    E. Phosphatidylinositol

45. Which of the following is an example of an immune complex hypersensitivity?
    A. Hemolytic disease of the newborn
    B. Poison ivy dermatitis
    C. Allergic pneumonitis
    D. Penicillin allergy
    E. Anaphylaxis

46. Transfer factor is not a true interleukin because
    A. Transfer factor is antigen specific
    B. Transfer factor acts only on T cells and interleukins act on T and B cells
    C. Transfer factor is larger than the interleukins and is structurally more like antibody
    D. It is not produced by a white blood cell
    E. It causes allergies; it does not prevent them

47. In the Rh system,
    A. The antibodies are formed as the result of bacterial colonization of the intestine
    B. Rh$^+$ mothers are more likely to have infants affected by HDN than are Rh$^-$ mothers
    C. Antigen D is considered one of the most potent
    D. HDN can be prevented even if anti-Rh globulin is not given at the first Rh$^+$ pregnancy
    E. The H substance serves as the Rh-precursor molecule

48. The blocking test in FAB serology
    A. Is useful as a negative control
    B. Is useful in identifying antibody in an unknown serum
    C. Requires addition of the blocking antibody before the standard antibody
    D. Is also useful in other types of serologic tests
    E. All of the above

49. Amplification of serologic tests is possible with
    A. Protein A
    B. Avidin–biotin systems
    C. Secondary antibody procedures
    D. ELISA methods
    E. All of the above

50. In Western blotting
    A. An antigen is usually detected in an electrophoretic gel by an antibody
    B. ELISA procedures are not possible
    C. Large quantities of antigen are needed to yield a positive test result
    D. The antigen must have an ionic charge opposite to that of antibody
    E. None of the above

51. Which of the following is a characteristic of Burkitt's lymphoma?
    A. It is a B-cell proliferative disease.
    B. Its etiologic agent enters cells via the CD4 protein.
    C. It is always fatal.
    D. It is associated with chromosome 6/14 translocations.
    E. It is the precursor condition to infectious mononucleosis.

52. Which of the following is true of T-cell–dependent antigens?
    A. They induce tolerance easier than T-cell–independent antigens.
    B. They generate an immune response dominated by IgM.
    C. They are structurally more complex than T-cell–independent antigens.
    D. Their anamnestic response is feeble.
    E. All of the above

53. The antigen receptor
    A. On B cells is an immunoglobulin
    B. On T cells consists of two peptides
    C. May be an immunoglobulin on macrophages
    D. On T cells reacts with superantigens
    E. All of the above

54. Exposure to a hapten alone may cause antibody formation if
    A. It is processed by macrophages
    B. A complex with self-proteins occurs in vivo
    C. The hapten is applied to the skin
    D. The individual is treated simultaneously with IL-1
    E. The hapten is, in fact, an agretope

55. The granulocytopenia that follows treatment with a cytotoxic drug such as methotrexate
    A. Includes a serious loss of neutrophils, monocytes, lymphocytes, and erythrocytes
    B. Could be treated logically with GM-CSF
    C. Would not affect antigen presentation if macrophages are unaffected
    D. Occurs because only granulocytes are sensitive to methotrexate and other cytotoxic drugs
    E. Occurs because these drugs typically form hapten-protein complexes on granulocyte surfaces

56. Which of the following is *not* produced by macrophages?
    A. TNFα
    B. Singlet oxygen
    C. DR protein
    D. Formyl peptides (fMet peptides)
    E. Cachectin

57. Phagocytosis
    A. On blood vessel surfaces is enhanced by ELAM-1
    B. Is accompanied by a burst in oxidative metabolism
    C. Is stimulated by derivatives of arachidonic acid
    D. And intraphagocytic exposure to defensins is lethal to bacteria
    E. All of the above

58. The peripheral blood
    A. Ratio of T cells to B cells is about 2:1 in healthy individuals
    B. Usually contains 3% to 5% of its cell population as plasma cells
    C. Is a rich source of J chain
    D. Is considered the site of B-cell maturation into plasma cells
    E. Is devoid of C1 INH in healthy individuals

59. The stage of immunoglobulin synthesis first detectable in immature B cells is the
    A. Synthesis of IgM
    B. Synthesis of μ chains
    C. Alignment of L chain genes
    D. Presence of surface IgM
    E. Dual synthesis of IgM and IgD

60. The primary effect of IL-4 on B cells is
    A. To promote expression of 20 α steroid dehydrogenase
    B. To stimulate Tac antigen synthesis
    C. To block plasma-cell formation
    D. Improve class switching to IgE synthesis
    E. The same as the effect of LPS on these cells

61. A major characteristic of a secondary response to a T-cell–dependent
    antigen such as tetanus toxoid is
    A. A sharp decrease in the amount of IgM in the blood
    B. That it cannot be repeated
    C. That it frequently causes anaphylaxis
    D. A marked elevation of IgM in the blood compared with the primary
       response
    E. That new germinal centers appear in lymphoid tissue

62. B lymphocytes
    A. Differ from macrophages by having surface FcγR
    B. Differ from T lymphocytes by being phagocytic
    C. Differ from T lymphocytes by lacking an antigen receptor
    D. Respond to many lymphokines that also stimulate T cells
    E. Respond only to T-cell–independent antigens

63. A B-cell hybridoma
    A. Is the same as a B-cell plasmacytoma
    B. Is the fusion product of two B cells
    C. Is not influenced by interleukin 6
    D. Is unable to grow in vitro without the addition of IL-1 to the culture
       medium
    E. Is typically exposed to antigen in vitro to stimulate antibody formation

64. The T-cell receptor
    A. Consists of the α/β and γ/δ peptides on each T cell
    B. Is known also as leukocyte functional antigen 3 (LFA-3)
    C. Recognizes a small peptide of a protein antigen, not the entire antigenic
       molecule
    D. Is surface IgM and/or IgD
    E. Is the DR protein

65. Antigen-presenting cells include all of the following *except*
    A. Helper T cells
    B. Macrophages
    C. Langerhans' cells
    D. B cells
    E. Dendritic cells

66. Interferon gamma is
    A. Not produced by T cells
    B. Best known for its immunoregulatory function
    C. Able to use the same cell receptor used by IFNα
    D. Not produced in response to exposure to antigens
    E. Produced by all T-cell subtypes

67. Suppressor T cells
    A. Are unlike other T-cell subsets, since they are CD8 positive
    B. Must be in physical contact with the T$_H$ cells they regulate
    C. Secrete one or more soluble factors that control T$_H$ cells
    D. Regulate T$_H$ cells via their other role as cytotoxic T cells
    E. Are more numerous in blood than CD4-positive cells

68. An anti-antibody system that regulates antibody production is known as the
    A. Allotypic network
    B. Epitopic network
    C. Idiotypic network
    D. Agretopic network
    E. Feedback inhibition system

69. Specific regions in an antibody that make up its antigen-combining site are the
    A. Variable domains
    B. Hypervariable regions
    C. Constant domains
    D. Hinge region
    E. Disulfide bonds

70. The synthesis of J chain
    A. Occurs only in IgM-synthesizing plasma cells
    B. Occurs in all plasma cells
    C. Occurs in mucosal cells
    D. Occurs in plasma cells that make polymeric immunoglobulins
    E. Is characteristic of all plasmacytomas

71. κ chains differ from λ chains by
    A. Failing to establish an S–S linkage to H chains
    B. Having a molecular weight of approximately 22,000
    C. Also existing as Bence Jones proteins
    D. Possessing allotypic markers
    E. Failing to combine with α chains

72. Which of the following reacts with another member of the immunoglobulin supergene family?
    A. IgA
    B. FcγRI
    C. MHC class II protein
    D. TCR (α/β)
    E. All of the above

73. An infant boy with recurrent bacterial infections of the skin that lack an infiltration of neutrophils
    A. May lack CR3 on his neutrophils
    B. May be granulocytopenic
    C. Could have a genetic predisposition to these infections
    D. May have hyperimmunoglobulinemia E
    E. May have all of the above (all the above are true)

74. The enzymatic site in the C3 convertase of the alternative complement pathway is
    A. Properdin
    B. Factor I
    C. Bb
    D. C1,4b,2a
    E. C3b or a C3b-like molecule

75. The ability of C4b to attach directly to antigen is due to
    A. Activation of its internal thioester bond
    B. A unique chemical structure also found in C3b
    C. The activation of a chemical grouping when C4a is removed
    D. A unique chemical grouping not found in C5b
    E. All of the above

76. Which of the following is an example of naturally acquired passive immunity?
    A. Previous infection
    B. Maternally derived antibody in a newborn infant
    C. Protection derived from normal bacterial flora
    D. The opsonic role of C3b
    E. Phagocytosis

77. Hyperimmune gamma globulin
    A. Is effective in preventing hemolytic disease of the newborn
    B. Injections provide naturally acquired passive immunity
    C. Injections also activate T-cell–dependent immunity
    D. Is primarily effective as a therapeutic, not a prophylactic agent
    E. None of the above

78. The preferred treatment of Bruton's (sex-linked) agammaglobulinemia is
    A. Bone marrow grafts
    B. Combined bone marrow and thymus grafts
    C. Injections of pooled human gamma globulin
    D. Injections of B-cell growth factor
    E. Injections of lymphocyte colony stimulatory factor (L-CSF)

79. Which of the following is considered a phagocytic cell deficiency disease?
    A. DiGeorge's syndrome
    B. Ataxia telangiectasia
    C. Chronic mucocutaneous candidiasis
    D. Hyperimmunoglobulinemia E
    E. Paroxysmal nocturnal hemoglobinuria

80. The metabolic fault in common variable immunoglobulin deficiency is
    A. In immunoglobulin class switching
    B. A failure to produce B cells
    C. A failure to produce T cells
    D. The same as in Bruton's agammaglobulinemia
    E. In the nucleotide salvage pathway

81. A haplotype consists of or refers to
    A. The genes that control a single HLA specificity, for example, HLA-A or HLA-DP
    B. All the allotypic specificities in half the members in one family
    C. The genes found in one child but not other children in the same family
    D. The specificities transmitted to a person from one parent
    E. Half of the genes on human chromosome 6

82. Histocompatibility testing may be accomplished by
    A. Microcytotoxicity tests
    B. Primed lymphocyte reactions
    C. One-way mixed lymphocyte reactions
    D. T-cell transformation caused by alloantigenic B cells
    E. All of the above

83. Which of the following is/are antigenically identical in all persons?
    A. $\beta 2$ microglobulins
    B. HLA-A peptides
    C. Complement molecule C3
    D. DP proteins
    E. $\alpha 1$ sector of HLA-B peptides

84. First-set transplant and tumor rejection are accomplished in some circumstances by
    A. LGL cells
    B. Antibody to blood group antigens
    C. Preformed antibody to HLA antigens
    D. Only answers B and C
    E. Answers A, B, and C

85. Burkitt's lymphoma may develop from
    A. An HIV infection
    B. An infiltration of tumor-infiltrating lymphocytes
    C. Activation of an myc gene by chromosome translocation
    D. The production of a carcinoembryonic antigen
    E. A loss of immune tolerance

86. Hairy-cell leukemia is best described as a
    A. Tumor of the hair follicles
    B. Malignancy of B cells
    C. Chronic lymphoblastic leukemia
    D. Malignancy of T cells
    E. Synonym for Hodgkin's disease

87. A unique chemical type of enzyme is an important antigen in
    A. Bullous pemphigoid
    B. Rheumatoid arthritis
    C. Poststreptococcal glomerulonephritis
    D. Systemic lupus erythematosus
    E. Hashimoto's hypothyroiditis

88. An important autoantigen in rheumatoid arthritis is
    A. The Gm determinant
    B. IgM
    C. Joint tissue
    D. Group A streptococci
    E. The HLA-DR protein

89. Seasonal allergies are
    A. Limited to exposures to plant pollens
    B. Dependent upon T_{DTH} cell activities
    C. Sometimes referred to as atopic allergies
    D. Often caused by house dust
    E. Illustrated by farmer's lung

90. Mast-cell degranulation is associated with
    A. Antigen bridging of surface IgE molecules
    B. Activation of protein kinase
    C. Activation of G proteins
    D. An influx of calcium
    E. All of the above

91. RAST
    A. Measures total plasma IgE
    B. Is performed in an allergic patient's skin
    C. Requires numerous antigens (allergens) in order to provide useful information
    D. Measures cell-bound IgE
    E. Is the required allergen sensitivity test

92. Pigeon breeder's disease is
    A. A seasonal allergy
    B. Dependent upon an IgE response to pigeon antigens
    C. Immunologically similar to farmer's lung
    D. An example of a delayed-type hyersensitivity
    E. Best treated with antihistamines

93. In the ABO blood groups system, the A and B antigens are
    A. Totally different chemicals
    B. Nonantigenic in a group O person
    C. Similar to cross-reacting antigens in enteric bacteria
    D. Altered slightly in vivo to produce the RhD antigen
    E. Formed from separate precursors

94. The failure of an adult to exhibit a hypersensitivity response to
    dermatophytes or yeasts suggests
    A. A loss of T-cell function
    B. The person has a macrophage deficiency disease
    C. That transfer factor is nonantigenic in that person
    D. The person could never develop serum sickness
    E. The individual has tuberculosis

95. Which of the following complement deficiencies is most associated with
    an increased incidence of serious infectious diseases?
    A. C1 INH
    B. C3
    C. Paroxysmal nocturnal hemoglobinuria
    D. C2
    E. C9

96. Nephelometric tests for antigen detection
    A. Are highly sensitive
    B. Require a pure, clean antibody solution
    C. Are rapid
    D. Can measure only soluble antigens
    E. All of the above

97. Which of the following is best adapted to detect multiple antigens in an
    antigen preparation?
    A. Bacterial agglutination
    B. Radial immunodiffusion
    C. Immunoelectrophoresis
    D. Ouchterlony tests
    E. Fluorescent antibody tests

98. Protein A
    A. Reacts with all human immunoglobulins
    B. Is purified from *Staphylococcus aureus*
    C. Binds to antibody only after the antibody has reacted with antigen
    D. Cannot be used in immunoelectron microscopy
    E. Is actually a polysaccharide

99. Which of the following can be used as a quantitative serologic test?
    A. Nephelometry
    B. Western blotting
    C. Passive hemagglutination inhibition
    D. RIST
    E. All of the above

100. Which of the following is considered the most difficult to treat successfully?
    A. Chédiak-Higashi syndrome
    B. Hairy-cell leukemia
    C. Chronic mucocutaneous candidiasis
    D. Bruton's agammaglobulinemia
    E. Hereditary angioneurotic edema

Final Examination Key

1. B	26. E	51. A	76. B
2. C	27. C	52. C	77. A
3. A	28. B	53. E	78. C
4. D	29. B	54. B	79. D
5. D	30. D	55. B	80. A
6. A	31. D	56. D	81. D
7. E	32. A	57. E	82. E
8. B	33. C	58. A	83. A
9. A	34. E	59. B	84. E
10. D	35. B	60. D	85. C
11. E	36. E	61. E	86. B
12. E	37. C	62. D	87. D
13. C	38. D	63. B	88. A
14. B	39. A	64. C	89. C
15. A	40. A	65. A	90. E
16. E	41. E	66. B	91. C
17. D	42. E	67. C	92. C
18. A	43. B	68. C	93. C
19. B	44. D	69. B	94. A
20. E	45. C	70. D	95. B
21. E	46. A	71. D	96. E
22. B	47. C	72. E	97. C
23. B	48. E	73. E	98. B
24. C	49. E	74. C	99. E
25. D	50. A	75. E	100. A

Index

A "t" indicates a table; "f" indicates a figure.

◆